Ultrasound in Obstetrics and Gynecology

Series Editor

Valentina De Robertis, Fetal Medicine Unit, Di Venere Hospital Bari, Bari, Italy

This book series offers a comprehensive overview of the primary female reproductive organs and covers the care of women throughout every stage of their lives, including pregnancy. It is highly clinically relevant, with a specific emphasis on the diagnosis, management, and treatment of disorders and abnormalities. The content of the series is fully aligned with medical school curricula, ensuring its relevance and usefulness to doctors and operators in the field of ultrasound in obstetrics and gynecology.

This comprehensive collection serves as a resource for healthcare professionals, researchers, educators, and students seeking to deepen their understanding and expertise in the field of obstetrics and gynecology ultrasound.

The primary target audience for this book series includes medical professionals specializing in obstetrics and gynecology, such as obstetricians, gynecologists, sonographers, radiologists, and midwives. Furthermore, it serves as an essential reference for residents and students in the field, providing them with a comprehensive and up-to-date resource to support their learning journey.

Paolo Volpe • Tullio Ghi
Editors

Fetal Neurosonography

Springer

Editors
Paolo Volpe
Fetal Medicine Unit
Di Venere Hospital
Bari, Italy

Tullio Ghi
Department of Woman and Child Health
Catholic University of Sacred Heart
Fondazione Policlinico Gemelli IRCCS
Rome, Italy

ISSN 3004-8591 ISSN 3004-8605 (electronic)
Ultrasound in Obstetrics and Gynecology
ISBN 978-3-031-70191-7 ISBN 978-3-031-70192-4 (eBook)
https://doi.org/10.1007/978-3-031-70192-4

This Springer imprint is published by the registered company Springer Nature Switzerland AG
The registered company address is: Gewerbestrasse 11, 6330 Cham, Switzerland

Series Preface

Ultrasound technology has revolutionized the field of obstetrics and gynecology, providing invaluable insights into the development and health of both the mother and the fetus. The ability to visualize the internal structures of the body in real-time has not only enhanced diagnostic accuracy but also improved patient care and outcomes. This series of books *Ultrasound in Obstetrics and Gynecology* has been promoted by the Italian Society of Ultrasound in Obstetrics and Gynecology (SIEOG), a registered non-profit association with over 4 decades of experience in promoting the advancement of ultrasound science in Obstetrics and Gynecology, as well as education for the benefit of the public. Each volume of this series has been thought to delve into various aspects of ultrasound applications with the aim of bridging the gap between theory and practice by presenting detailed, evidence-based information on the latest technological innovations, procedural techniques, and clinical applications. From fundamental principles and basic techniques to advanced imaging and diagnostic challenges, this series is designed to enhance both the understanding and practical skills of practitioners at all levels of experience. The international credibility of the society has allowed to involve insights from pioneering experts who have shaped the practice over the years. We are deeply grateful to the contributing authors, who bring a wealth of experience and expertise to these volumes. Their dedication to advancing the field is evident in the depth and breadth of the content covered, ensuring that readers will find valuable information no matter if they are seasoned practitioners or new to the field.

As you embark on this journey through the world of ultrasound in obstetrics and gynecology, we hope this series will serve as a reference, inspire ongoing learning, and contribute to the continued improvement of patient care.

IRCCS Istituto Giannina Gaslini, Genova, Italy Federico Prefumo
Fetal Medicine Unit, Di Venere Hospital, Bari, Italy Valentina De Robertis

Preface

In recent years, significant advances have been made in fetal neurosonography. It is now possible to diagnose a wide range of cerebral pathologies that were previously misinterpreted, thanks to improved technological and cultural expertise and close collaboration among specialists in fetal medicine, pediatric neuroradiology, and genetics.

In this volume, we have sought to capture the collective experience of numerous national and international experts in the field. Their contributions have allowed us to present an updated and extensive collection of imaging. Moreover, given the crucial and complementary role of magnetic resonance imaging (MRI) in the study of the fetal brain, we have included numerous images from this modality, offering additional insights beyond those provided by ultrasound.

In the hope that we have done our best to meet the needs of the readers of this volume, we would like to extend our thanks to all the colleagues who have participated in this insightful journey toward a deeper understanding of fetal brain pathologies.

Bari, Italy — Paolo Volpe
Rome, Italy — Tullio Ghi

Preface

Contents

List of Videos

Destructive Lesions of the Brain: Intracranial Hemorrhage and Stroke

Video 1 ICH grade IV at 34 gestational weeks. Axial view demonstrating severe bilateral ventriculomegaly as well as dilatation of the third ventricle (secondary to aqueduct of Sylvius obstruction). Note the intraventricular clot with the hyperechoic margins and the hypoechoic core

Video 2 ICH grade IV at 34 gestational weeks. Parasagittal and coronal views demonstrating the parenchymal lesion and the intraventricular clot. Note the porencephalic cyst communicating with the ventricular lumen and the hyperechogenicity of ventricular lining

Video 3 ICH grade IV at 34 gestational weeks. Parasagittal and coronal views demonstrating the parenchymal lesion and the intraventricular clot. Note the porencephalic cyst communicating with the ventricular lumen and the hyperechogenicity of ventricular lining

Neural Tube Defects

Video 1 Sagittal view of a fetus with open spinal dysraphism (spina bifida) showing the spinal defect and the protrusion of an anechoic mass (meningocele)

Contributors

Emiliana Angilletta Obstetric Unit, IRCCS Azienda Ospedaliero-Universitaria di Bologna, Bologna, Italy

Giulia Biancotto Fetal Medicine and Surgery Unit, Istituto IRCCS G. Gaslini, Genoa, Italy

Simona Boito Prenatal Diagnosis and Fetal Surgery Unit, Fondazione IRCCS Fondazione Cà Granda, Ospedale Maggiore Policlinico, Milan, Italy

Mariachiara Bosco Unit of Obstetrics and Gynecology, Department of Surgery, Dentistry, Pediatrics and Gynecology, University of Verona, AOUI Verona, Verona, Italy

Andrea Dall'Asta Department of Medicine and Surgery, Obstetrics and Gynecology Unit, University of Parma, Parma, Italy

Alice D'Amico Center for Fetal Care and High-Risk Pregnancies, University of Chieti, Chieti, Italy

Francesco D'Antonio Department of Obstetrics and Gynecology, Centre for Fetal Care and High-Risk Pregnancy, University of Chieti, Chieti, Italy

Center for Fetal Care and High-Risk Pregnancies, University of Chieti, Chieti, Italy

Sara Doroldi Obstetric Unit, IRCCS Azienda Ospedaliero-Universitaria di Bologna, Bologna, Italy

Tiziana Fanelli Fetal Medicine Unit, Di Venere Hospital Bari, Bari, Italy

Ilaria Fantasia Fetal Medicine Unit, Di Venere Hospital Bari, Bari, Italy

Nevena Fileva Neuroradiology Unit, Istituto Giannina Gaslini, Genoa, Italy

Department of Diagnostic Imaging, Medical University Sofia, Sofia, Bulgaria

Tullio Ghi Department of Woman and Child Health, Catholic University of Sacred Heart, Fondazione Policlinico Gemelli IRCCS, Rome, Italy

Pierre Mace Image 2 Center, Marseille, France

Prenatal Screening and Diagnostic Unit, Beauregard Hospital, Marseille, France

Ilenia Mappa Department of Obstetrics and Gynecology, Fondazione Policlinico Tor Vergata, University of Rome Tor Vergata, Rome, Italy

Daniele Di Mascio Department of Maternal and Child Health and Urological Sciences, Umberto I University Hospital, Sapienza University of Rome, Rome, Italy

Elisa Montaguti Obstetric Unit, IRCCS Azienda Ospedaliero-Universitaria di Bologna, Bologna, Italy

Giovanni Morganelli Department of Medicine and Surgery, Obstetrics and Gynecology Unit, University of Parma, Parma, Italy

Claudiana Olivieri Fetal Medicine Unit, Di Venere Hospital Bari, Bari, Italy

Dario Paladini Fetal Medicine and Surgery Unit, Istituto IRCCS G. Gaslini, Genoa, Italy

Elvira Di Pasquo Department of Medicine and Surgery, Obstetrics and Gynecology Unit, University of Parma, Parma, Italy

Nicola Persico Prenatal Diagnosis and Fetal Surgery Unit, Fondazione IRCCS Fondazione Cà Granda, Ospedale Maggiore Policlinico, Milan, Italy

Gianluigi Pilu Obstetric Unit, IRCCS Azienda Ospedaliero-Universitaria di Bologna, Bologna, Italy

Ritsuko K. Pooh Fetal Brain Center, CRIFM Prenatal Medical Clinic, Osaka, Japan

Edwin Quarello Image 2 Center, Marseille, France

Department of Obstetrics—Gynecology and ART, St Joseph Hospital, Marseille, France

Andrea Righini Pediatric Radiology and Neuroradiology Department, Children's Hospital V. Buzzi, Milan, Italy

Giuseppe Rizzo Department of Maternal and Child Health and Urological Sciences, Umberto I University Hospital, Sapienza University of Rome, Rome, Italy

Valentina De Robertis Fetal Medicine Unit, Di Venere Hospital Bari, Bari, Italy

Andrea Rossi Neuroradiology Unit, Istituto Giannina Gaslini, Genoa, Italy

Department of Health Sciences (DISSAL), University of Genoa, Genoa, Italy

Margherita Scarrone Prenatal Diagnosis and Fetal Surgery Unit, Fondazione IRCCS Fondazione Cà Granda, Ospedale Maggiore Policlinico, Milan, Italy

Irina Stavarache Donna Medical Center, Bucharest, Romania

Grazia Volpe Prenatal Diagnosis and Fetal Surgery Unit, Fondazione IRCCS Fondazione Cà Granda, Ospedale Maggiore Policlinico, Milan, Italy

Nicola Volpe Department of Medicine and Surgery, Obstetrics and Gynecology Unit, University of Parma, Parma, Italy

Paolo Volpe Fetal Medicine Unit, Di Venere Hospital Bari, Bari, Italy

Ruben Ramirez Zegarra Department of Medicine and Surgery, Obstetrics and Gynecology Unit, University of Parma, Parma, Italy

Normal Anatomy of the Fetal Brain and Spine: Screening Planes and Fetal Neurosonography

Valentina De Robertis, Tiziana Fanelli, Mariachiara Bosco, and Paolo Volpe

Abstract

With advancements in imaging technology, prenatal care has undergone a transformative shift, enabling clinicians to evaluate the fetal brain with unprecedented detail. This chapter explores the fascinating realm of normal ultrasonographic anatomy of the fetal central nervous system (CNS), providing a comprehensive examination of the intricacies defining its critical developmental changes.

The chapter begins by elucidating the fundamental views for a basic examination of the fetal CNS in the first and second trimester of pregnancy. Special emphasis is placed on the dynamic nature of these structures throughout gestation, providing clinicians with valuable insights into the variations that may be encountered during routine imaging assessments. Subsequently, the narrative unfolds to reveal the ultrasonographic planes for targeted fetal neurosonography—an expert diagnostic procedure crucial for patients at an elevated risk of CNS malformations.

Incorporating illustrative figures depicting both normal and abnormal aspect of the ultrasonographic planes, readers are guided through the visual nuances of ultrasonographic images, enabling them to discern the subtleties defining normal fetal CNS anatomy.

"Normal Ultrasonographic Anatomy of the Fetal CNS" serves as an indispensable resource for practitioners in the field of maternal-fetal medicine, radiology, and obstetrics. It offers a thorough examination of the normal fetal CNS anatomy, equipping clinicians with the expertise needed for accurate prenatal assessments.

Keywords

Fetal central nervous system · Ultrasound · Neurosonography · Anomaly scan · First trimester

1 Introduction

Assessing the fetal brain through sonography has consistently posed a significant challenge in both screening and diagnostic contexts. This challenge arises from the complex nature of cerebral anatomy on the one hand, and the continuous changes in the appearance of the brain throughout gestation on the other. Notably, the fetal brain is unique

V. De Robertis (✉) · T. Fanelli · P. Volpe
Fetal Medicine Unit, Di Venere Hospital Bari, Bari, Italy
e-mail: derobertis_v@libero.it

M. Bosco
Unit of Obstetrics and Gynecology, Department of Surgery, Dentistry, Pediatrics and Gynecology, University of Verona, AOUI Verona, Verona, Italy
e-mail: mariachiara.bosco@univr.it

P. Volpe, T. Ghi (eds.), *Fetal Neurosonography*, Ultrasound in Obstetrics and Gynecology,
https://doi.org/10.1007/978-3-031-70192-4_1

among organs, undergoing substantial developmental changes from the embryonic phase through postnatal life. Although there are fetuses at high risk for central nervous system (CNS) anomalies due to specific risk factors, necessitating referral targeted neurosonography [1], the majority of CNS malformations typically occur in "low risk" pregnancies. Therefore, analogous to fetal echocardiography for congenital heart disease, routine US screening of the CNS is key in prenatal detection of CNS anomalies. According to national [2] and international guidelines [3–5], most efforts to diagnose CNS anomalies are focused around mid-gestation, at time of midtrimester anomaly scan; however, the increasingly widespread ultrasound screening for chromosomal anomalies in the first trimester [6, 7] coupled with the introduction of high-frequency transabdominal probes has made it evident that several CNS malformations can be diagnosed at earlier gestational stages. Indeed, a systematic review conducted by Karim et al. [8] has shown that the detection rate for fetal structural anomalies in the first trimester ranged from 32 to 61%, according to the type of anomalies and population characteristics, thus demonstrating that first-trimester US has potential to identify large proportion of fetuses with structural anomalies. Of note, results from a large retrospective study on more than 100,000 singleton pregnancy demonstrated that some major brain structural defects (i.e., acrania, alobar holoprosencephaly, encephalocele) can be identified virtually in all cases in the first trimester [6]. Consequently, the thorough assessment of the fetal head and brain to identify major CNS anomalies is considered among the minimum requirements for scan at 11 + 0 to 14 + 0-weeks' gestation [9, 10]. However, given that a significant proportion of fetal brain malformations is detectable mainly or only in the midtrimester (e.g., agenesis of the corpus callosum), the anomaly scan at 19–21 weeks' gestation remains the cornerstone in the screening for CNS abnormalities [2–5]. Lastly, although there is no unanimous agreement among scientific societies on the role of third-trimester US in the screening for fetal anomalies, several structural anomalies become evident only at this gestational age, including some CNS anomalies [6]. Indeed, neuronal development, especially the migration process, occurs later during gestation [11]. Additionally, a wide range of acquired conditions, such as brain hemorrhage/stroke, tumors, and arachnoid cysts are known to be more common in the third trimester [6]. Therefore, in cases where a third-trimester scan is performed for any indication, some assessment of the fetal CNS is warranted using the trans-thalamic and trans-ventricular axial planes.

2 Basic Examination of the Fetal Brain and Spine at the *First Trimester Scan*

2.1 Axial Plane of the Fetal Head and Brain

The axial view of the head and brain (Fig. 1a) is listed among the minimum requirements for scan at 11 + 0–14 + 0 weeks' gestation by the latest guidelines for the first-trimester examination [9, 10]. This view enables to visualize ossification of the skull and the symmetry of the developing brain structures. Cranial bone ossification should be visible by 11 completed gestational weeks [10]. In this section, the two lateral ventricles are visible, predominantly occupied by the hyperechoic choroid plexuses which create the "*butterfly sign*" [12]. The two hemispheres, similar in size, are separated by a straight, uninterrupted midline echo (interhemispheric fissure and falx). The cortex appears very thin and most clearly observed anteriorly, lining the large fluid-filled ventricles. In selected cases, the biparietal diameter (BPD) may be measured on the axial view, primarily for dating purposes [9].

2.2 Midsagittal Plane of the Face and Brain

It is the same plane obtained for the measurement of the nuchal translucency and assessment of nasal bone (Fig. 1b). This plane can also be

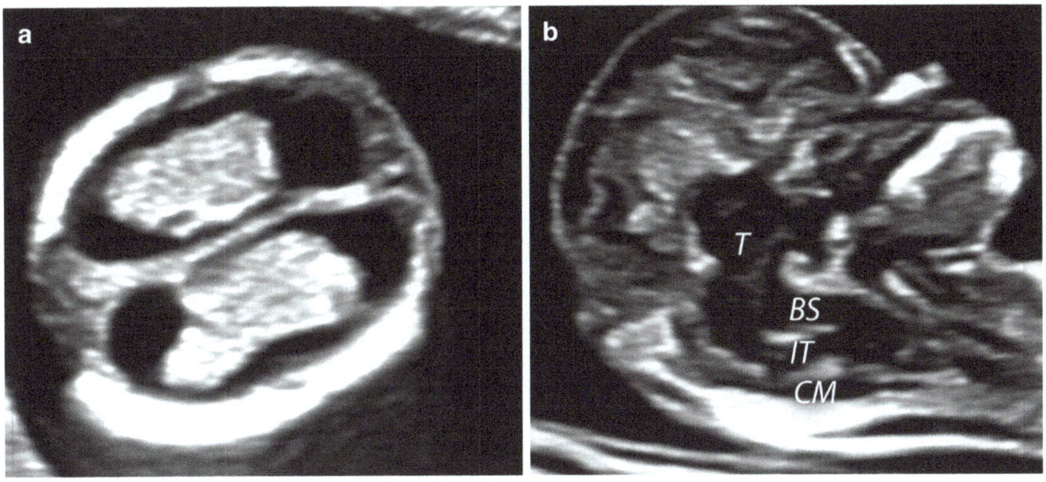

Fig. 1 Fetal head and brain at 12 weeks' gestation. (**a**) Axial view of the fetal head. (**b**) Midsagittal view of the fetal head: it is possible to visualize the cranial posterior fossa structures, including the brainstem (BS), the intracranial translucency (IT), and the cisterna magna (CM) appearing as three anechoic spaces, roughly similar in size. *T* thalami

Table 1 Major anomalies always, potentially, and never detectable in the first trimester

Always	Potentially	Never
Acrania/exencephaly/anencephaly	Spina bifida	Corpus callosum agenesis
Alobar holoprosencephaly	Cystic posterior fossa anomalies	Hemorrhage
Encephalocele		Microcephaly

used to assess the posterior fossa and visualize the intracranial translucency (IT, fourth ventricle), as well as the brainstem, serving as screening method for early diagnosis of open neural tube defects and cystic posterior fossa malformations [13–17]. In the midsagittal view, the diencephalon can be visualized as anechoic round-shaped structure in the middle of the fetal brain. More posteriorly, the structures of the posterior fossa structures, including the brainstem (BS), the fourth ventricle (4th V), and the cisterna magna (CM), appear as three anechoic spaces, roughly similar in size (Fig. 1b). According to the WAPM guidelines [9], the routine adoption of the midsagittal plane is recommended for assessing the posterior fossa and for evaluating the presence of the three parallel anechoic spaces of similar size. While the routine measurement of these spaces is not advised, it might be of use when abnormalities are suspected. Conversely, the ISUOG guidelines does not include the midsagittal plane as part of the basic examination for CNS anomaly screening at 11 + 0–14 + 0 weeks' gestation [10].

Table 1 shows major CNS malformations subdivided into three groups according to the chance of detection in the first trimester: always detectable, potentially detectable, and undetectable.

2.3 Sagittal View of the Fetal Spine

The assessment of fetal spine should be performed, when possible, in sagittal view. This view allows the evaluation of vertebral alignment and the integrity of the skin above the spine. Ossification of vertebral bodies is evident from 12 weeks' gestation. First trimester evaluation of fetal spine is of particular importance in presence of any intracranial sign suspicious for open spina bifida [9, 15].

3 Basic Examination of the Brain and Spine at *Midtrimester Anomaly Scan*

In the midtrimester, the basic ultrasound examination of the CNS is traditionally performed using a transabdominal probe and includes the evaluation of the fetal head and spine [3–5].

3.1 Head and Brain

Standard assessment of the fetal brain relies on the visualization of three axial planes (i.e., trans-thalamic, trans-ventricular, and trans-cerebellar). However, a notable disadvantage of these planes is the limited visualization the of the hemisphere proximal to the transducer and the difficult depiction of midline brain structures, particularly the corpus callosum and the cerebellar vermis, due to their anatomical location and orientation. To address this challenge, recent guidelines [4] recommended supplementing the traditional axial planes with the median/midsagittal view of the fetal brain. This plane allows for direct assessment of the normal anatomy of the corpus callosum and cerebellar vermis. Usually, adequate demonstration of fetal brain structures in the midtrimester can be achieved by standard transabdominal ultrasonography. However, in fetuses with cephalic fetal presentation, a transvaginal scan can provide higher resolution evaluation.

3.2 Spine

The basic examination of fetal spine includes a longitudinal view to assess the presence of open and closed spinal dysraphism.

Any suspicion of CNS or spinal malformations at routine midtrimester screening ultrasound or at nuchal translucency scan is an indication for "targeted fetal neurosonography" referral as diagnostic examination. This examination requires a high level of expertise in both transabdominal and transvaginal approaches as well as the use of high-resolution transducers.

Recently, a consensus has been published regarding the description and interpretation of the US abnormal findings in each trimester suggestive of the most common CNS anomalies [18]. This effort to standardize the reporting of suspected findings may not only influence the management of referrals, but also impact on the obstetrician training. Ultimately, adopting a standardized approach could contribute to reduce the prevalence of false-positive cases at routine examination.

4 Targeted Fetal Neurosonography

Targeted fetal neurosonography is a dedicated, multiplanar, diagnostic examination indicated for fetuses at high risk or with suspicion of CNS or spinal malformation [1]. Common indications for referral are listed in Table 2. Targeted fetal neurosonography is recognized having a much greater diagnostic potential than does the basic screening examination and is particularly helpful in the evaluation of complex malformations [1, 4]. Nonetheless, proficiency in this technique requires a high level of expertise, encompassing not only dexterity in conducting the scan, but also a comprehensive understanding of cerebral developmental and acquired lesions as well as genetics.

Table 2 Common indications for targeted fetal neurosonography

Suspicion of CNS or spinal malformation at routine screening ultrasound examinations
Family history of inheritable CNS or spinal malformations
Previous pregnancy complicated by fetal brain or spinal malformation
Fetus with congenital heart disease
Monochorionic twins
Suspected congenital intrauterine infection
Exposure to teratogens known to affect neurogenesis
Chromosomal microarray findings of unknown significance

CNS central nervous system
Modified from Malinger G, et al. [5]

Since CNS anomalies can be detected at various gestational ages depending on the specific anomaly, fetal neurosonography must be tailored to the gestational age period during which the anomaly is observed.

The primary characteristics distinguishing fetal neurosonography from the screening examination are as follows:

- The transvaginal approach should be always attempted as it is the preferred method to perform an adequate high-resolution targeted neurosonographic examination. When this is not technically feasible (e.g., breech presentation, twin pregnancy), the use of high-resolution microconvex transducers is encouraged, as they provide higher resolution than convex probes [1].
- The basis of the neurosonographic examination of the fetal brain and spine is the multiplanar approach with a combination of axial, coronal, and sagittal planes.
- The use of the three-dimensional (3D) multiplanar image correlation is highly recommended when performing fetal neurosonography.

5 Cerebral Anomalies by Scanning View

Here we provide a comprehensive description of the planes visualized during targeted fetal neurosonography, detailing the structures that can be imaged in each of these planes and the possible associated malformations. The description specifically focuses on structures that can be visualized from the midtrimester onwards.

5.1 Axial Planes

5.1.1 Axial Trans-ventricular Plane and Related Malformations

This is the most cephalad axial plane of the fetal head demonstrating the lateral ventricles (Fig. 2a), with the anterior (or frontal) horns and the continuum between the atria and the occipital horns, posteriorly. The frontal horns appear as two comma-shaped, fluid-filled structure with well-defined lateral wall, and they are separated centrally by the cavum septi pellucidi (CSP). The CSP is a box-like fluid-filled cavity between two thin membranes. The formation of CSP begins as early as 12 weeks' gestation, it is usually fully formed by 15–16 weeks' gestation, and it starts to close at approximately 6 months gestational age. Therefore, it should always be demonstrable between 18 and 37 weeks while failure to detect the CSP prior to 15–16 weeks or later than 37 weeks is a normal finding [19]. The frontal horns of the lateral ventricles and the CSP are main components of the "anterior complex" (Fig. 2b) [20], a key anatomical structure observed in the routine trans-ventricular plane. The importance of visualizing this complex is because its abnormal appearance is associated with midline cerebral anomalies. In the anterior complex, a cross-section of the genu of the corpus callosum is also visible (Fig. 2b). From 16 weeks of gestation, choroid plexuses begin to shrink, and the atria with the occipital horns become more evident. Each atrium is characterized by the presence of the glomus of the choroid plexus, which is highly echogenic, while the occipital horn is filled with cerebrospinal fluid. Especially during the second trimester of gestation, both medial and lateral walls of each ventricle run parallel to the midline, making them clearly visible on this plane as two regular echogenic lines (Fig. 3a). Under normal circumstances, the glomus of the choroid plexus fills the cavity of the ventricle at the level of the atrium, closely contacting both the medial and lateral walls. However, in some normal cases, a small fluid rim may exist between the medial wall and the choroid plexus [21]. To exclude the presence of ventriculomegaly (VM), the width of the atrium distal to the transducer is measured at the level of the glomus of the choroid plexus. The measurement is performed perpendicular to the ventricular axis by positioning the calipers on the inner sides of the echogenic ventricular walls (inner to inner borders) [4, 5] (Fig. 3b). The width should be less than 10 mm, irrespective of gestational age [22]. The measurement site at the level

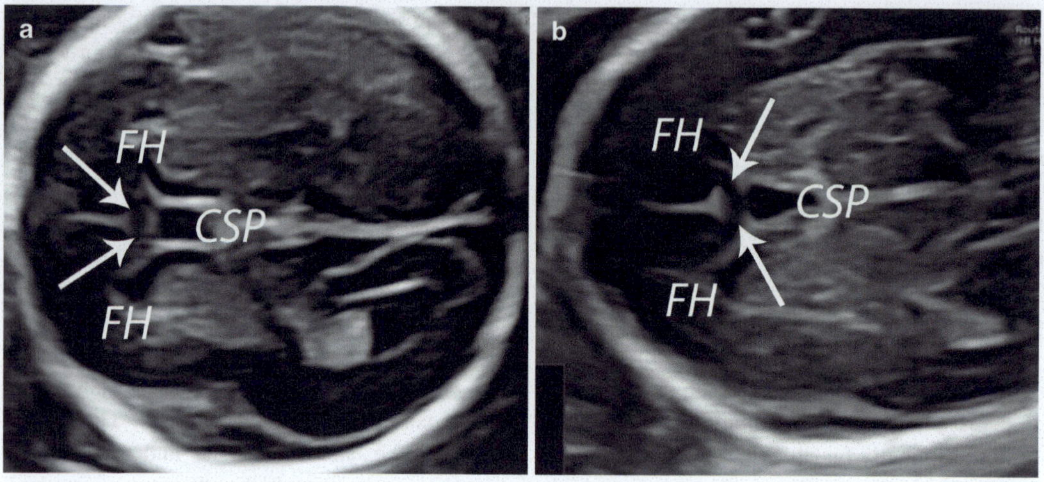

Fig. 2 The trans-ventricular plane. (**a**) In this plane, the cavum septi pellucidi (CSP), the two frontal horns (FH), and the genu of the corpus callosum (arrows) are visible. (**b**) The anterior complex is constituted of (from anterior to posterior): the interhemispheric fissure, the genu of the corpus callosum (arrows), the CSP and, laterally, the anterior horns of the lateral ventricles (FH)

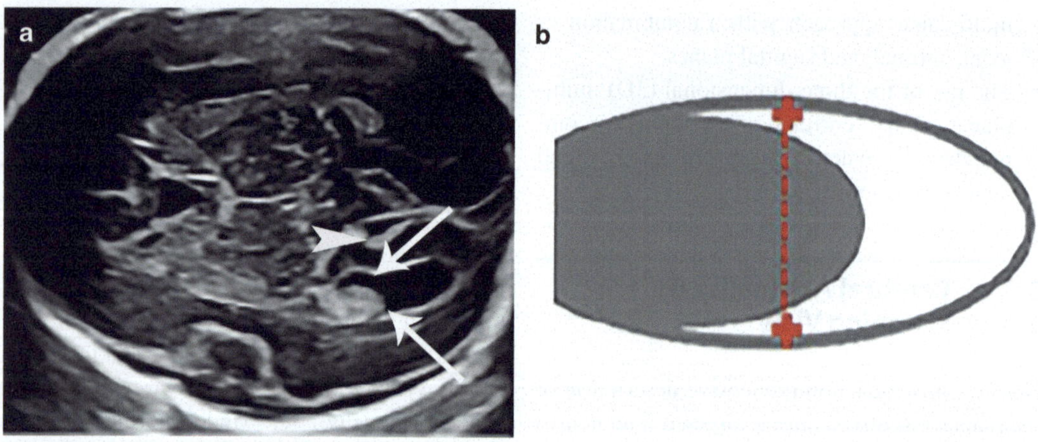

Fig. 3 Measurement of the atrium of the lateral ventricle distal to the transducer. (**a**) The measurement of the atrium (arrows) is performed at the level of parieto-occipital fissure (arrowhead). (**b**) The drawing shows the correct placement of the calipers, at the level of the glomus of the choroid plexus, inside the echoes generated by the ventricular walls. The calipers are aligned perpendicular to the long axis of the ventricle

of the glomus is chosen because regardless the etiology, dilatation of the lateral ventricle typically begins at the caudal portion (atrium and posterior horn). The trans-ventricular plane serves as starting point for both basic and advanced assessment of the fetal brain. This plane allows for the examination of the normal shape, ossification, and mineralization of the fetal skull. Additionally, it is used to assess the symmetry and proper separation of the cerebral hemispheres. Under normal conditions, the cerebral hemispheres are completely separated by a hyperechoic straight line representing the interhemispheric fissure and the falx. The only interruption of this line is where the CSP lies [16]. It is important to note that, due to artifacts in the near field of the image caused by shadowing from the proximal parietal bone, the standard trans-ventricular plane typically allows clear visualization only of the hemisphere and the lateral ventricle distal to the transducer (Fig. 2a). The limited visualization of the lateral ventricle proximal to the transducer might restrict the detection rate of unilateral VM. Detecting unilateral VM affecting the proximal ventricle often depends on its qualitative assessment, as the measurement is generally suboptimal. In cases where a subjective impression suggests a proximal ventricle significantly larger than the distal one, it is advisable to refer the patient for fetal neurosonography [23]. For the same reason, on this plane, the evaluation of the symmetry of the hemispheres might be challenging. However, in the absence of major distortion of the falx, symmetry of the brain can be assumed, at least in the context of screening examinations. On the trans-ventricular view, Sylvian fissure (SF) opercularization can be easily assessed prenatally by ultrasound [24]. Although always visible, the appearance of the SF changes during gestation. At 20 weeks' gestation, the SF is smooth without any angularity (Fig. 4a), and SF opercularization typically becomes more evident after 24 weeks' gestation (Fig. 4b). The above-mentioned anatomic structures—CSP, lateral ventricles and midline—should be carefully assessed on the trans-ventricular view. In fact, a large group of mild and severe malformations can be suspected on this key plane of the fetal head (Fig. 5).

5.1.2 Axial Trans-cerebellar Plane and Related Malformations

This plane is slightly caudal to the trans-ventricular one, and it is obtained tilting the transducer slightly toward the posterior fossa, from the trans-thalamic axial plane. The trans-cerebellar plane is used to visualize the posterior fossa: the cerebellar hemispheres, the cerebellar vermis, and the cisterna magna (CM). On this plane, the cerebellum appears as a butterfly-shaped (or dumb-bell shaped) structure formed by the round cerebellar hemispheres joined in the middle by the slightly more echogenic cerebellar vermis (Fig. 6a). The cerebellar hemispheres should be homogeneous and symmetrically round shaped, with smooth borders. The trans-cerebellar diameter should be measured in this section, as the distance between its lateral edges (cerebellar diameter) in millimeters correspond to the gestational age in weeks (Fig. 6a). If the probe is moved slightly downwards, the fourth ventricle is also visible as a tiny anechoic space between the vermis and the brain stem (Fig. 6b). While the normal appearance of the cerebellar hemispheres and fourth ventricle is expected to be seen by this axial scan, a thorough evaluation of the vermis requires serial axial plans to demonstrate the different portions of the cerebellar vermis [4]. The cisterna magna is a fluid-filled space posterior to the cerebellum. It normally contains thin septations, which are thought to represent the remnants of the Blake's pouch that

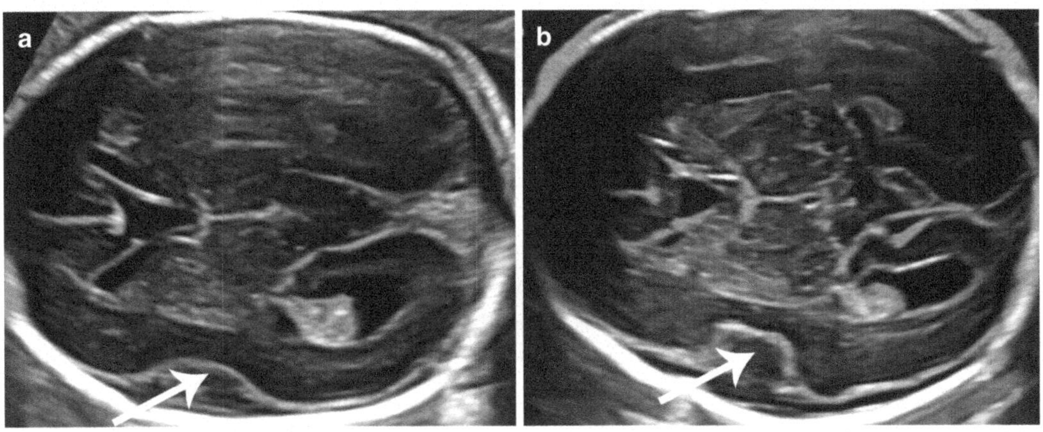

Fig. 4 The Sylvian fissure. (**a**) In a fetus at 20 weeks' gestation: the Sylvian fissure (arrow) is smooth without any angularity. (**b**) In a fetus at 24 weeks' gestation: opercularization (arrow) becomes more evident

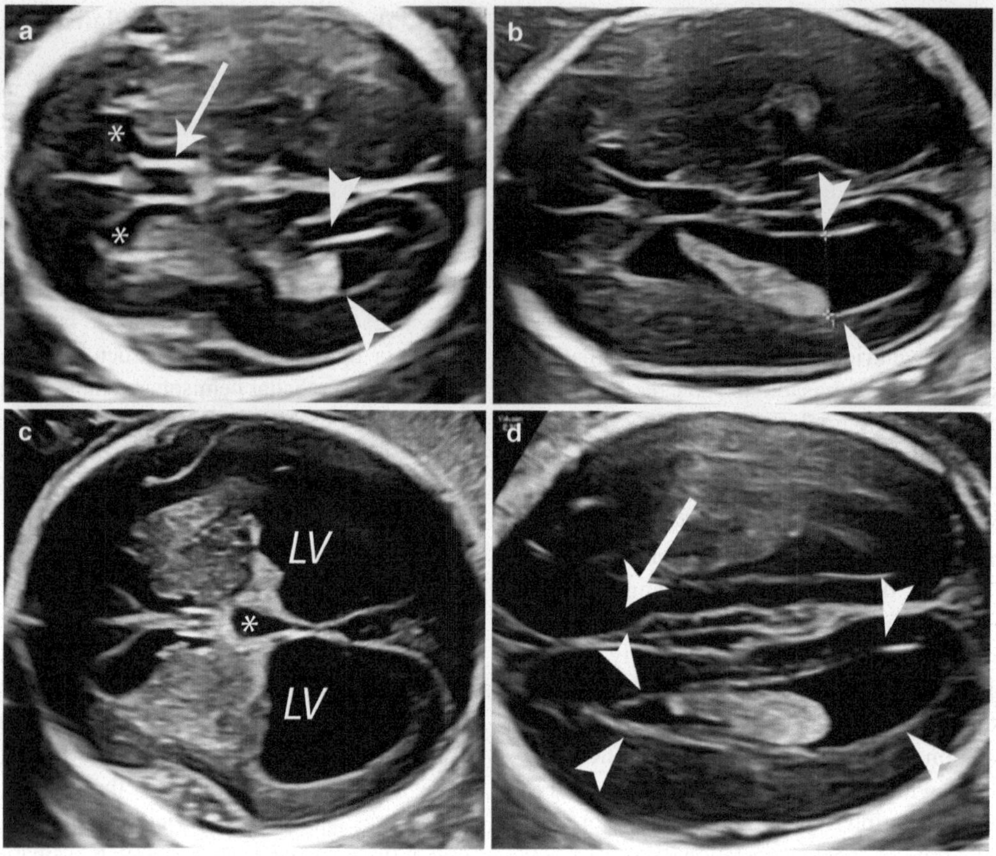

Fig. 5 The trans-ventricular plane. (**a**) Normal aspect of the trans-ventricular plane showing the frontal horns (*), the cavum septi pellucidi (arrow), and the atrium of the lateral ventricle distal to the transducer (arrowheads). (**b**) Mild ventriculomegaly: the atrium of the lateral ventricle distal to the transducer (arrowheads) is >10 mm. (**c**) Severe ventriculomegaly (aqueductal stenosis). Note the severe dilatation of both lateral ventricles (LV) and of the third ventricle (*). (**d**) Complete agenesis of the corpus callosum. The CSP is not visible (arrow), and the atrium is rounded and tear drop-shaped (colpocephaly) (arrowheads)

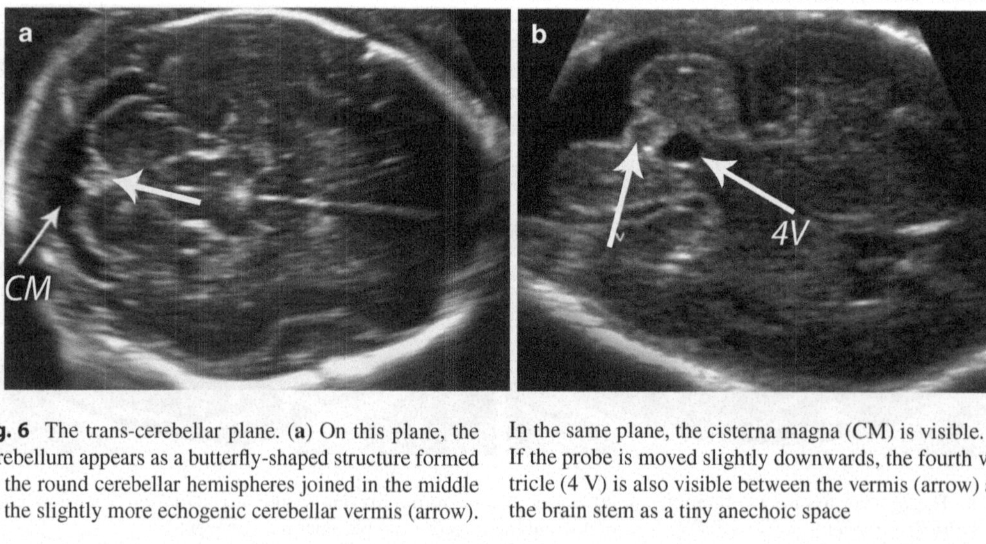

Fig. 6 The trans-cerebellar plane. (**a**) On this plane, the cerebellum appears as a butterfly-shaped structure formed by the round cerebellar hemispheres joined in the middle by the slightly more echogenic cerebellar vermis (arrow). In the same plane, the cisterna magna (CM) is visible. (**b**) If the probe is moved slightly downwards, the fourth ventricle (4 V) is also visible between the vermis (arrow) and the brain stem as a tiny anechoic space

physiologically ruptures at about 13 gestational weeks, to form the Magendie foramen (see chapter "First Trimester Neurosonography") [25]. The antero-posterior diameter of the CM may be measured in this section as the distance between the vermis and the inner border of the occipital bone, and it should not exceed 10 mm (Fig. 6a). While assessing the posterior fossa, particularly before 19 weeks' of gestation, it should be taken into account that the rotation of the vermis may be still incomplete; in this case, the fourth ventricle may be visible in between the two cerebellar hemispheres, creating a misleading impression of a vermian defect. As a rule of thumb, by 19 gestational weeks, there should be no midline fluid-filled space between the two cerebellar hemispheres. Care should be taken to avoid "overtilting" of the probe, since this increases the likelihood of false-positive diagnosis of a vermian anomaly. Several anomalies of the cerebellum and the posterior fossa can be suspected or diagnosed through the trans-cerebellar view (Fig. 7). However, only certain diagnoses can be confirmed on this plane, such as the Chiari II

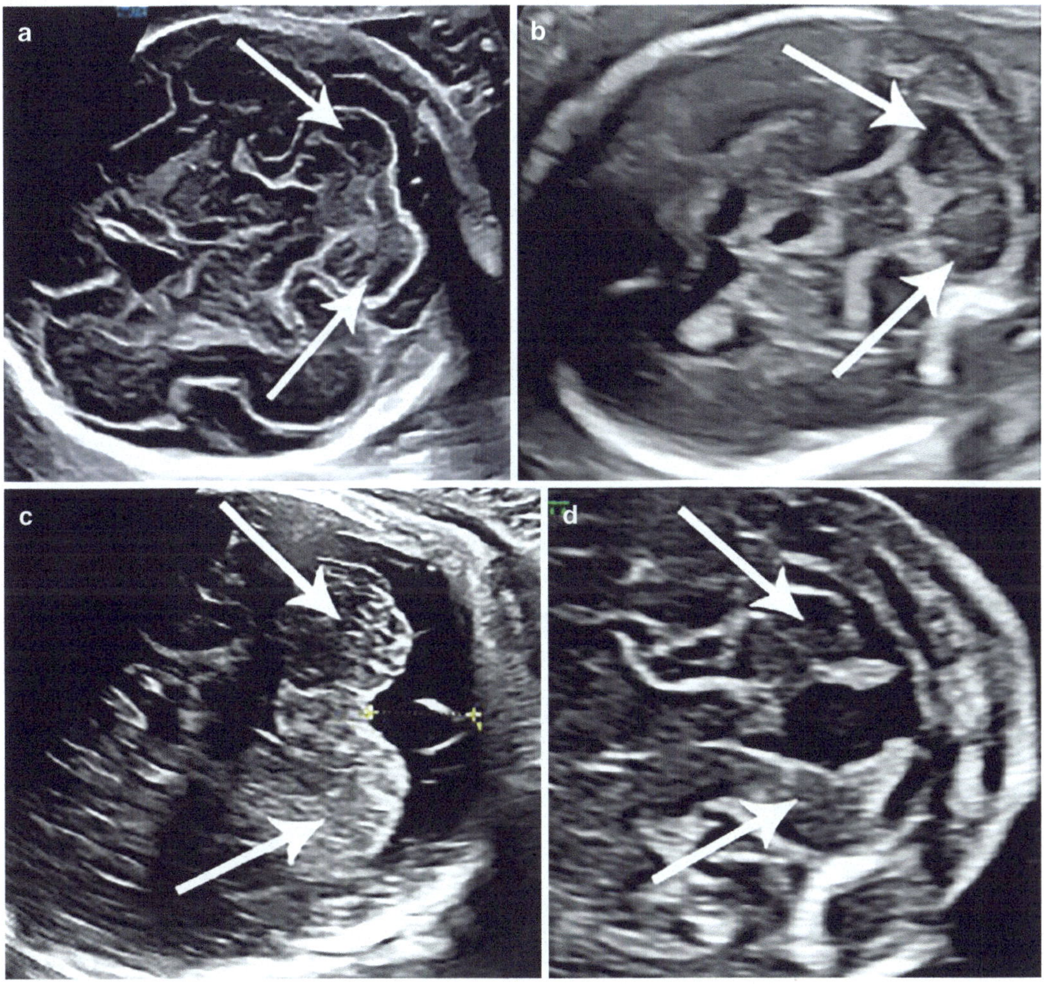

Fig. 7 The trans-cerebellar plane. (**a**) Normal aspect of the plane: round cerebellar hemispheres (arrows) are homogeneous and symmetrically round shaped, with smooth borders. (**b**) Chiari II malformation in open spina bifida. The cisterna magna is collapsed, and the cerebellum is dysmorphic (arrows; banana sign) and displaced downwardly, toward the foramen magnum. (**c**) Mega cisterna magna. The antero-posterior diameter of the cisterna magna is increased. (**d**) Keyhole sign in a fetus with Blake's pouch cyst. The cerebellar hemispheres (arrows) are mildly splayed and, in between, the fourth ventricle's continuity with the cisterna magna is seen

malformation, associated with open spinal dysraphisms (Fig. 7b), and the megacisterna magna (Fig. 7c). Conversely, when the cerebellar hemispheres are splayed and the vermis is not visible (Fig. 7d), a cystic abnormality of the posterior fossa is suspected. However, in this scenario, only the midsagittal view can effectively distinguish among various cystic posterior fossa anomalies, including Dandy–Walker malformation (DWM), Blake's pouch cyst (BPC), and vermian hypoplasia.

5.1.3 Axial Trans-thalamic Plane and Related Malformations

This plane is obtained parallel but caudal to the trans-ventricular plane. The anatomic landmarks include, from anterior to posterior, the frontal horns of the lateral ventricles, the CSP, the thalami, and the hippocampal gyri (Fig. 8a). It is commonly referred to as the biparietal diameter (BPD) plane as this plane is used for measuring the BPD to assess fetal size. This because the insonation of this plane has been shown to be eas-

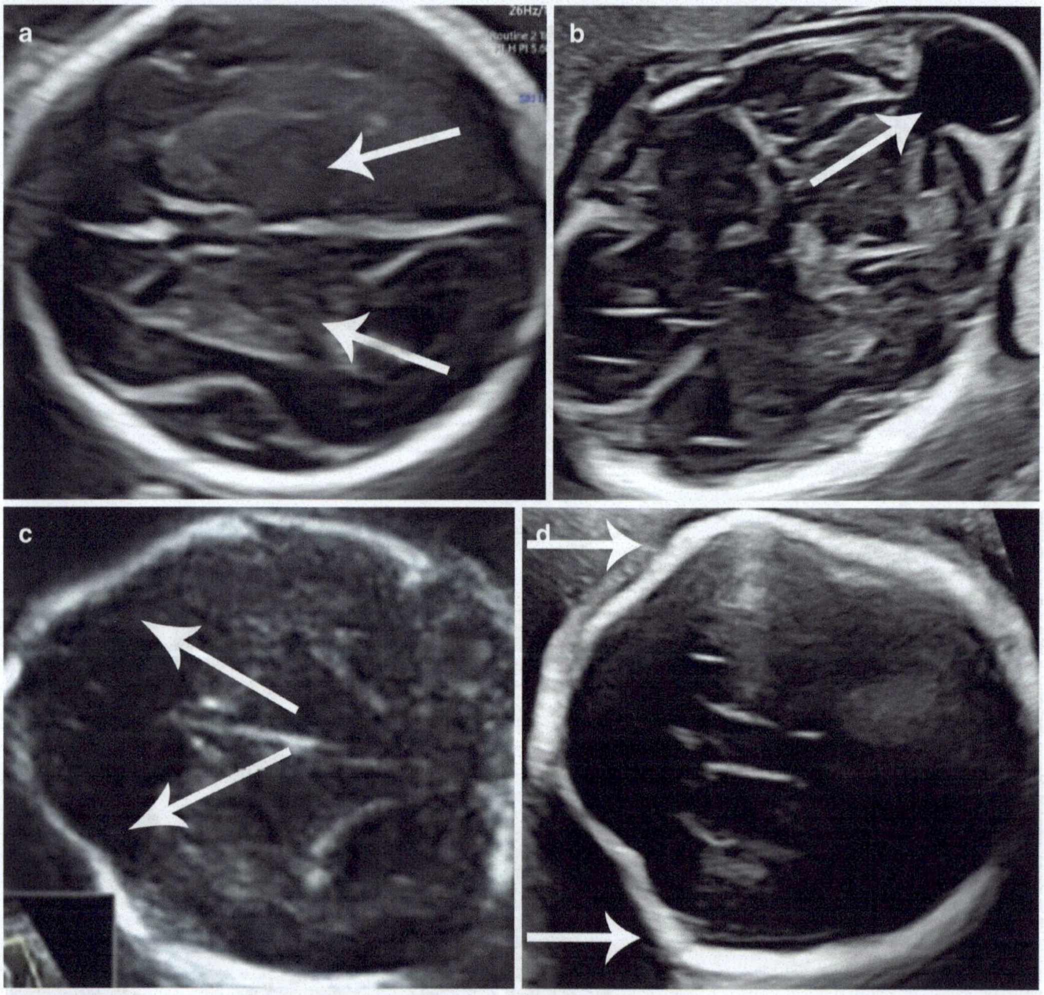

Fig. 8 The trans-thalamic plane. (**a**) Normal trans-thalamic plane: The two thalami (arrows) are depicted on either side of the midline. (**b**) Occipital cephalocele (arrow). Note the bony defect of the occipital bone through which the cephalocele herniates. (**c**) Chiari II malformation in open spina bifida. The fetal head has an abnormal shape (arrows; lemon sign). (**d**) Coronal synostosis in Apert syndrome. Note the indentations at the level of the prematurely sealed fronto-parietal sutures (arrows)

ily obtained in late gestation and therefore it allows a more reproducible measurements throughout pregnancy than other planes [26]. Apart from this use in the setting of the fetal biometry, the trans-thalamic view allows the detection of several malformations of the skull and brain (Fig. 8b–d).

5.2 Sagittal Planes

5.2.1 Midsagittal (or Median) Plane

This plane should be acquired through the anterior and posterior fontanelle (Fig. 9). The selection of the fontanelle depends on the specific area of interest or pathology. If the examination focuses on the posterior part of the brain (i.e., posterior fossa), then imaging plane should be acquired through the posterior fontanelle. Conversely, for a comprehensive assessment of the midline anatomic structures, the midsagittal plane should be obtained through the anterior fontanelle or through the unossified sagittal suture (Fig. 9a). This median view is the reference plane for assessing all major midline organs such as the corpus callosum (CC) and its components (rostrum, genu, body, and splenium), and its close relationship with the CSP and cavum vergae, when present. Below the CSP, the third ventricle can be identified as a hypoechoic structure, while its cranial portion appears hyperechoic due to the presence of the tela choroidea (choroid plexus of the third ventricle). As illustrated in Fig. 9a, the anterior approach also allows access to the infratentorial area. However, if the focus is on this specific area, a posterior approach through the posterior fontanelle is also recommended (Fig. 9b). In the latter scenario, care should be taken to avoid shadowing from the occipital bone, as this artifact can significantly limit the anatomical assessment of the hindbrain. The posterior midsagittal view enables a thorough assessment of all midline anatomical structures of the posterior fossa, such as the vermis (with the primary fissure and, later in gestation, the secondary fissure), the choroid plexus of the fourth ventricle (4th V-CP), the fourth ventricle, the tentorium, the cisterna magna, and the brain stem. After 18–19 weeks' gestation, the vermis is formed and it closes the fourth ventricle; there-

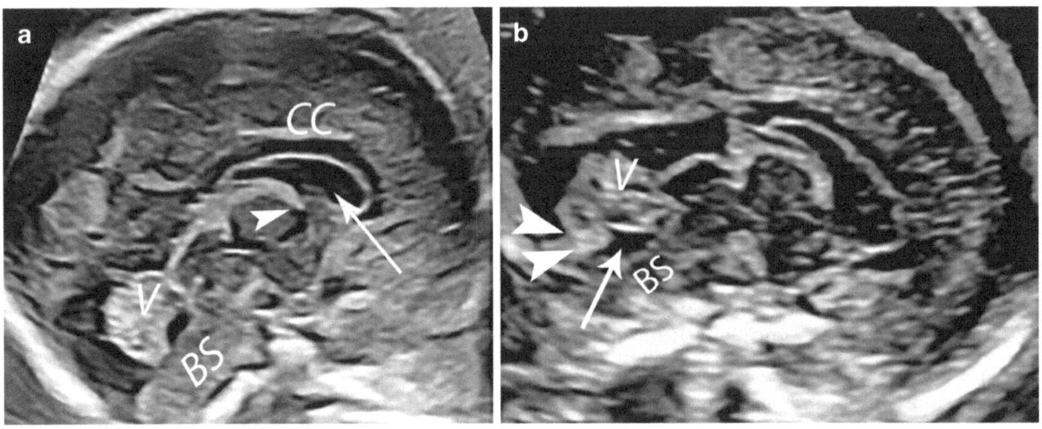

Fig. 9 The midsagittal plane of the fetal brain. This plane can be obtained through the anterior or the posterior fontanelle depending on the elements of interest (supratentorial or infratentorial anatomy, respectively). (**a**) Midsagittal (median) plane at 21 gestational weeks obtained through the unossified sagittal suture. In particular, the corpus callosum (CC) with the CSP (arrow) is visible in the central part of the brain. The hyperechoic tela choroidea (small arrow) represents the roof of the third ventricle. Finally, the midline structures of the posterior fossa [cerebellar vermis (V); brain stem (BS)] are also visible. (**b**) Midsagittal (median) plane at 21 gestational weeks obtained through the posterior fontanelle. It allows an optimal visualization of the posterior fossa. In this plane, the following anatomic structures will be depicted: the vermis (V), the fourth ventricle (arrow) and the brain stem (BS). The medial portion of choroid plexus of fourth ventricle can be seen (arrowheads) between the vermis (V) and the brainstem (BS) as a separate structure attached to the inferior part of the cerebellar vermis

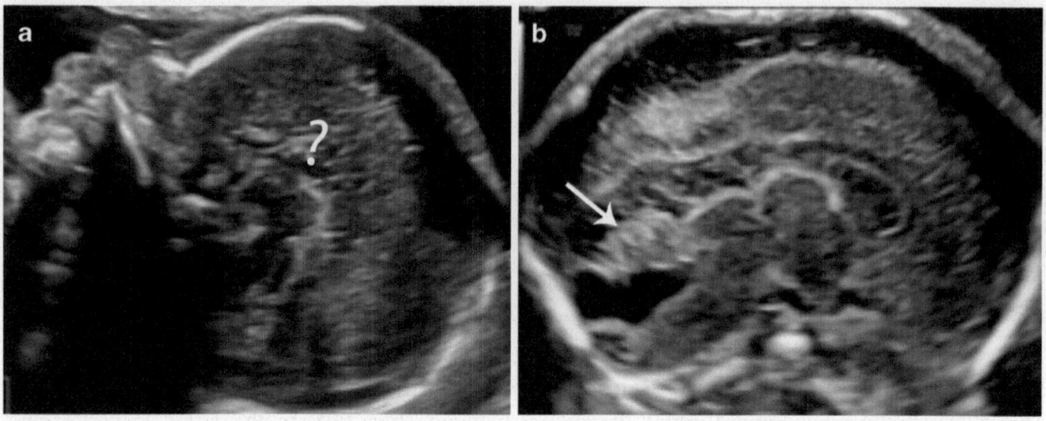

Fig. 10 Abnormal midsagittal (median) plane. (**a**) Complete agenesis of the corpus callosum. In the median plane, the corpus callosum is absent (?). (**b**) Blake's pouch cyst. In the median plane, through the posterior fontanelle, an upward displacement of a normal vermis (arrow) and an open fourth ventricle, communicating with the cisterna magna, is seen

fore, the demonstration of an opening may be indicative of a cystic posterior fossa anomaly. Recently, it has been demonstrated that the 4th V-CP has been misinterpreted as the lower portion of the vermis and that the closure of the fourth ventricle is determined from the 4th V-CP and not only from the vermis (see chapter "Cystic Posterior Fossa Anomalies") [25]. The medial portion of the 4th V-CP can be seen as a separate structure attached to the inferior part of the cerebellar vermis using high-frequency transabdominal (TA) and high- or standard-frequency transvaginal (TV) transducers (Fig. 9b). Additionally, the position of the 4th V-CP could inform on the differential diagnosis of fetal cystic posterior fossa abnormalities, characterized by an open fourth ventricle, such as the DWM and the BPC, which have a significant different prognosis [25, 27–29]. Adequate diagnosis of several forebrain and hindbrain anomalies requires the median plane (Fig. 10).

5.2.2 Parasagittal Plane

Parasagittal Plane (Left and Right). These planes are obtained by slowly tilting the transducer laterally from the midsagittal plane. On these planes, the following anatomic structures can be visualized: the lateral ventricles with the choroid plexuses, the periventricular brain parenchyma and, mainly in the third trimester, the gyri of the cortex, on the convex surface of the brain, as well as a variable portion of the insulae/Sylvian fissures (Fig. 11a). If the transducer is tilted more laterally, the temporal horns of the ventricles and the insulae will become visible (Fig. 11b). Abnormalities of the cortex can be detected in this view (Fig. 11c).

5.3 Coronal Planes

5.3.1 Coronal Transfrontal Plane (Fig. 12a)

This represents the most anterior coronal plane included in the neurosonographic examination, acquired via the anterior fontanelle. It displays the interhemispheric fissure and the frontal lobes of the brain. The skull base, with the sphenoid bone, and, occasionally the orbits, are visible. This plane constitutes the key plane for excluding fusion of the frontal lobes, especially when suspecting lobar holoprosencephaly (see chapter "Holoprosencephaly and Its Variants").

5.3.2 Coronal Transcaudate Plane (Fig. 12b)

This plane is also acquired through the anterior fontanelle, slightly tilting posteriorly the trans-

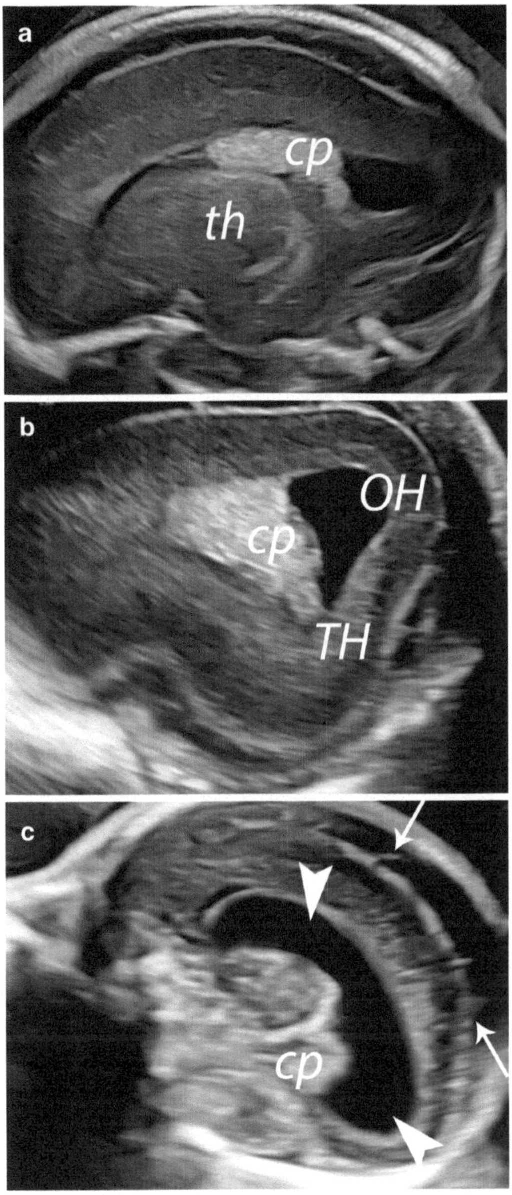

Fig. 11 The parasagittal planes. (**a**) A normal parasagittal plane at 19 gestational weeks. This plane is mostly employed to assess the cortex, the temporal lobe, and the thalamus (th). Most of the lateral ventricle is also displayed, with the temporal and occipital horns. The choroid plexus (cp) is also visible. (**b**) When the transducer is tilted further laterally, the temporal horns (TH) of the ventricles are seen. Most of the lateral ventricle is also depicted, with the occipital horns (OH). The choroid plexus (cp) is visible. (**c**) This figure shows a severe ventriculomegaly (arrowheads) with an associated shrinking of the choroid plexus (cp). The cerebral cortex has the typical aspect of lissencephaly in a fetus at 27 gestational weeks

ducer from the transfrontal plane. It likely represents one of the most important neurosonographic plane, alongside the midsagittal ones. On this plane, the following anatomic structures can be demonstrated: the frontal horns of the lateral ventricles, the CSP (a triangular/ trapezoid structure below the CC and between the two frontal horns), the cross-section of the anterior part of the body of the CC (appearing as a mildly hypoechoic band on top of the CSP and between the frontal horns), the cerebral falx, the ganglionic eminence, and the caudate nuclei. This view allows the identification of several CNS malformations (Fig. 12c, d).

5.3.3 Coronal Trans-thalamic Plane (Fig. 13a)

This plane is positioned just posterior to the transcaudate one. To achieve the optimal view, the transducer should be tilted slightly more posteriorly or, alternatively, slid along the yet unossified sagittal suture. The midline marker of this plane is the slit-like third ventricle with the two Monro foramina. Close to the skull base, the basal cistern contains the blood vessels of the circle of Willis and the optic chiasm. Of note, the Sylvian fissure is best displayed on this view. However, to visualize this structure effectively, the tip of the transducer should firmly indent the fontanelle; otherwise, the parietal bone will cast a shadow that hinders the visualization of the insulae and the Sylvian fissures.

5.3.4 Coronal Trans-cerebellar Plane (Fig. 13b)

This represents the only coronal plane that needs be obtained through the posterior fontanelle. In this plane, the posterior sections of the hemispheres, as well as the infratentorial structures, are visualized. Specifically, the following anatomic landmarks are identifiable: the occipital horns of the lateral ventricles, the interhemispheric fissure, the calcarine, and, at a deeper level, the parieto-occipital fissures. Beneath the tentorium, the cerebellar hemispheres and relatively hyperechoic vermis are seen in cross-section.

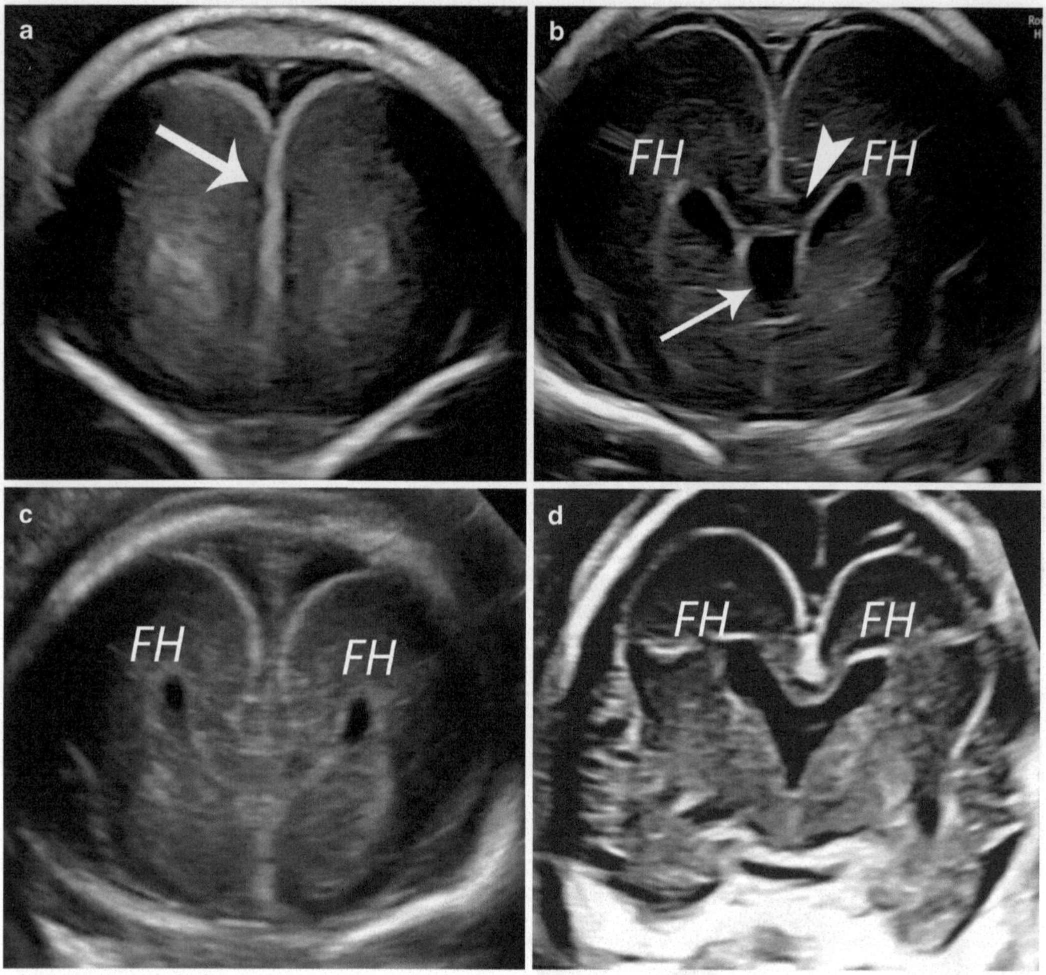

Fig. 12 The coronal planes of the fetal brain. (**a**) The transfrontal plane. This is the most anterior of the coronal planes and shows the frontal lobes with the interhemispheric fissure (arrow). (**b**) The transcaudate plane. On this plane, the following anatomic structures are depicted: the frontal horns of the lateral ventricles (FH), the CSP (arrow), the cross-section of the anterior part of the body of the CC (arrowhead), appearing as a mildly hypoechoic band on top of the CSP and between the frontal horns. (**c**) Abnormal transcaudate plane in a fetus with corpus callosum agenesis: the two frontal horns (FH) are typically distorted and dislodged laterally (*bullhorn*-like). (**d**) Abnormal transcaudate plane in a fetus with agenesis of the cavum septi pellucidi: the cavum is absent, and the frontal horns (FH) are fused

6 Fetal Spine

Under normal circumstances, the spine appears as an S-shaped line without any abnormal curvatures, and the skin above the spine appears uninterrupted [4]. To assess the integrity of the spine, three scanning planes can be employed, depending on the fetal position [5]. During the anomaly scan, it is essential to obtain a longitudinal section of the spine to screen for open and closed spinal dysraphism [4, 5]. Although efforts should be made to demonstrate the intactness of the skin overlying the spine, it is acknowledged that this examination requires expertise, and the results

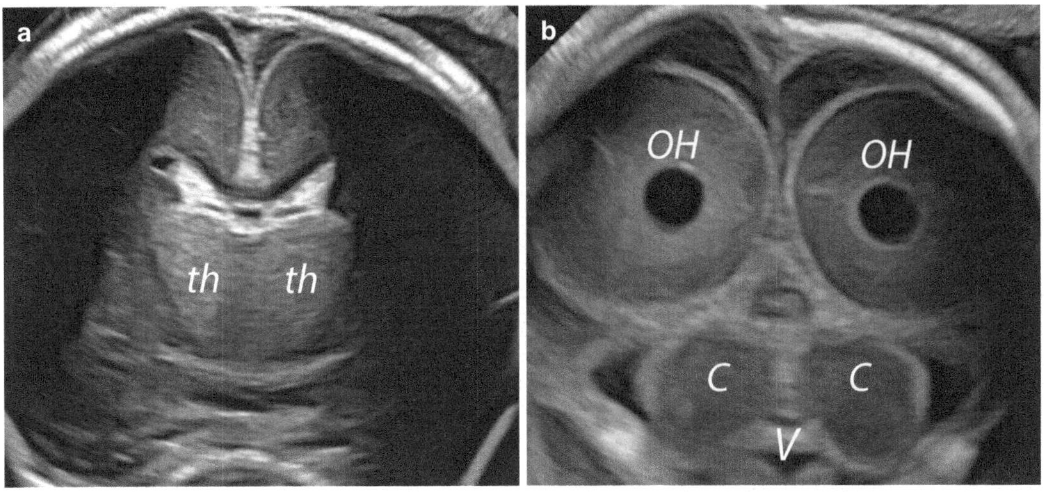

Fig. 13 (**a**) The coronal trans-thalamic plane. This plane, which lies just posterior to the transcaudate one, allows visualization of the thalami (th). (**b**) The coronal trans-cerebellar plane of the fetal brain showing the occipital horns of the lateral ventricles (OH). Below the tentorium, the cerebellar hemispheres (**c**) and the relatively hyperechoic vermis (V) are also visible in cross-section

are significantly influenced by the fetal position. In cases where suspicions of spinal malformations arise during routine screening US, a targeted fetal neurosonography is indicated, involving a multiplanar evaluation of the spine with a combination of sagittal, coronal, and axial planes.

6.1 Sagittal Plane (Fig. 14a)

When the fetus is in a prone position, obtaining a true sagittal section is possible by directing the ultrasound beam across the non-ossified spinous process. This allows imaging of the spinal canal and the contained spinal cord (Fig. 14a). In the late second and third trimesters, the conus medullaris is usually observed at the level of the second/third lumbar vertebrae (L2–L3) [30–32]. The integrity of the neural canal can be deduced from the regular arrangement of the ossification centers of the spine and from the presence of soft tissue covering it. If a true sagittal section is obtained, the visualization of the conus medullaris in its normal location provides additional confirmation of normality [5]. The use of high-frequency transabdominal transducers improves the assessment of the spinal cord and conus medullaris in the midsagittal view of the spine. The ability to visualize the conus medullaris lying on the ventral border of the spinal canal, close to the vertebral bodies, serves as valuable indicator for determining the normality of the lumbosacral spine.

6.2 Paramedian Sagittal Plane

In this plane, the normal spine appears as two parallel lines formed by the vertebral bodies anteriorly and the ossification centers of the lateral processes posteriorly converging in the sacrum.

6.3 Transverse or Axial Planes

In transverse or axial planes (Fig. 14b), the examination of the spine is a dynamic process, performed by sweeping the transducer along the entire length of the spine [1]. The vertebrae have different anatomic configurations at different levels: fetal thoracic and lumbar vertebrae have a triangular shape; the cervical vertebrae are quadrangular in shape; and sacral vertebrae are flat.

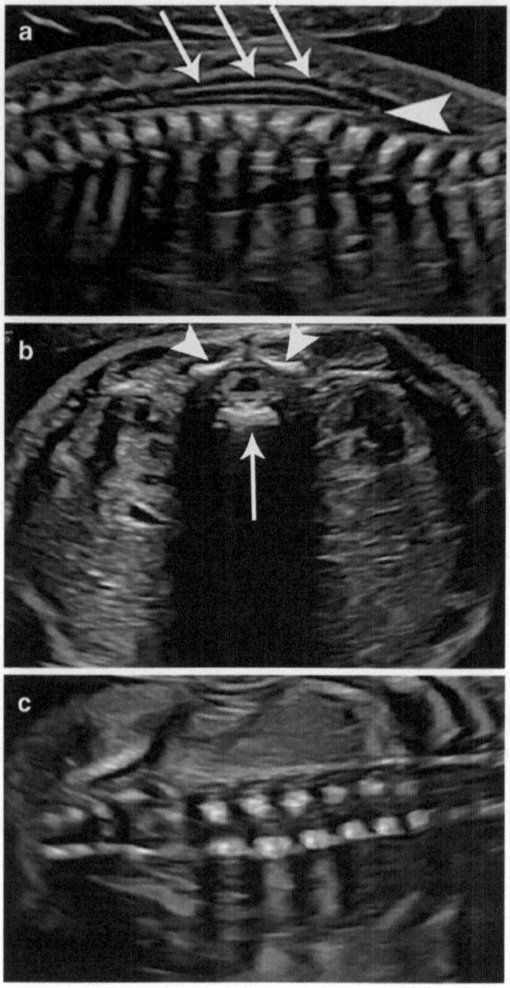

Fig. 14 The normal fetal spine. (**a**) A sagittal view showing the spinal canal and the spinal cord within it (arrows). After 20 weeks, the conus medullaris (arrowhead) is normally positioned at level of second/third lumbar (L2–L3) vertebrae. (**b**) An axial view of the spine at lumbar level shows three ossification centers of the lumbar vertebrae (arrows). (**c**) The coronal view of the spine showing the vertebral bodies and posterior arches

6.4 Coronal Planes

In coronal planes of the spine (Fig. 14c), one, two, or three parallel lines are seen, depending upon the orientation of the ultrasound beam. These correspond to cutting planes across, from ventral to dorsal, the vertebral bodies (one line), the vertebral bodies and posterior arches (three lines), or the posterior arches (two lines) [1]. The visualization of these planes is more effectively demonstrated through 3D imaging, as discussed below.

7 Three-dimensional (3D) Ultrasound of the CNS Anatomy

The use of a 3D ultrasound approach is recommended in targeted neurosonography [1]. Firstly, the utilization of multiplanar image correlation enables the acquisition of precisely aligned views on the three orthogonal planes (Fig. 15). Secondly, the possibility of displaying thicker "slices" of the brain enhances the signal-to-background noise ratio on all three planes, significantly improving image quality. These advantages support our recommendation to use a 3D approach in neurosonography. Moreover, the assessment of the fetal spine sees advantages with a 3D approach. Usually, only two scanning planes are possible in any given case, but 3D ultrasound can be used to obtain the third plane when necessary. Additionally, the assessment of the fetal spine benefits from 3D rendering and reconstruction of the coronal planes at the level of the vertebral bodies and/or posterior arches in normal (Fig. 16a) and abnormal cases (Fig. 16b).

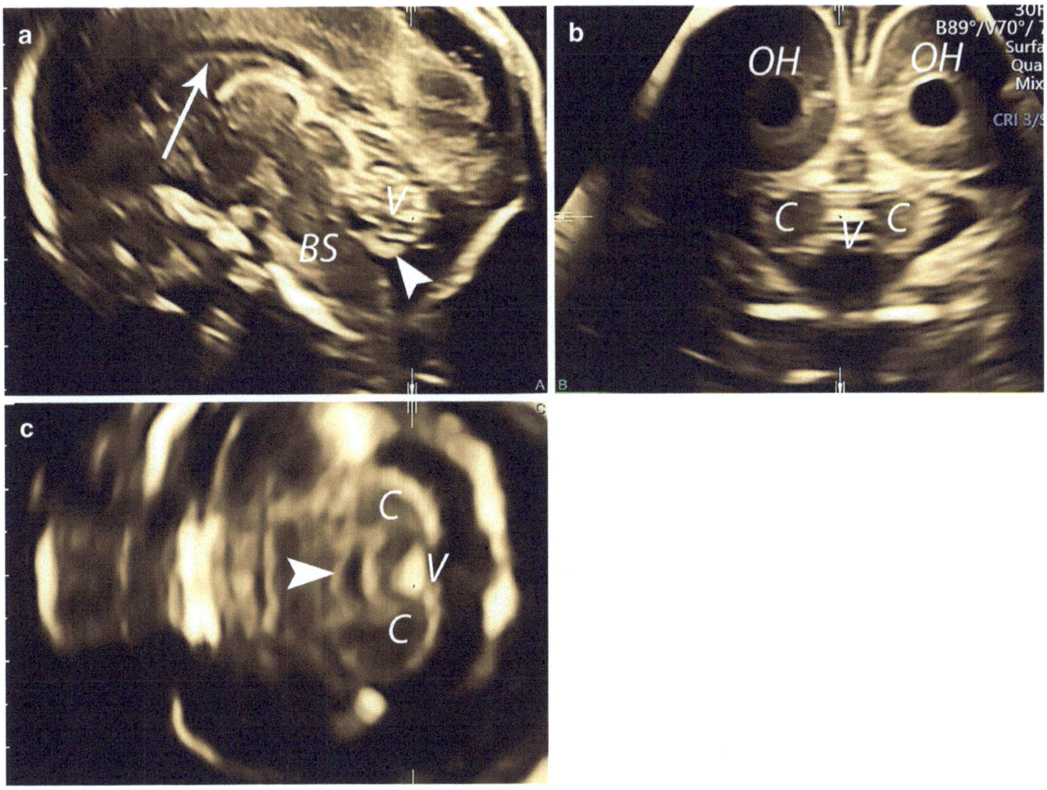

Fig. 15 Three-dimensional ultrasound of fetal brain. (**a**) Three-dimensional multiplanar image correlation of a normal fetal brain allowing visualization of all major cerebral structures in three planes: in midsagittal plane (**plane a**) corpus callosum (arrow) together with vermis (V) and the brainstem (BS) are visible. Between the cerebellar vermis and the brainstem, the choroid plexus of the fourth ventricle (arrowhead) is detectable. (**b**) The coronal trans-cerebellar plane (**plane b**) shows the occipital horns of the lateral ventricles (OH), the cerebellar hemispheres (C), and the relatively hyperechoic vermis (V). (**c**) The **Plane C** shows the axial trans-cerebellar plane: the cerebellar hemispheres (C) with the vermis (V) and the fourth ventricle (arrowhead) are visible

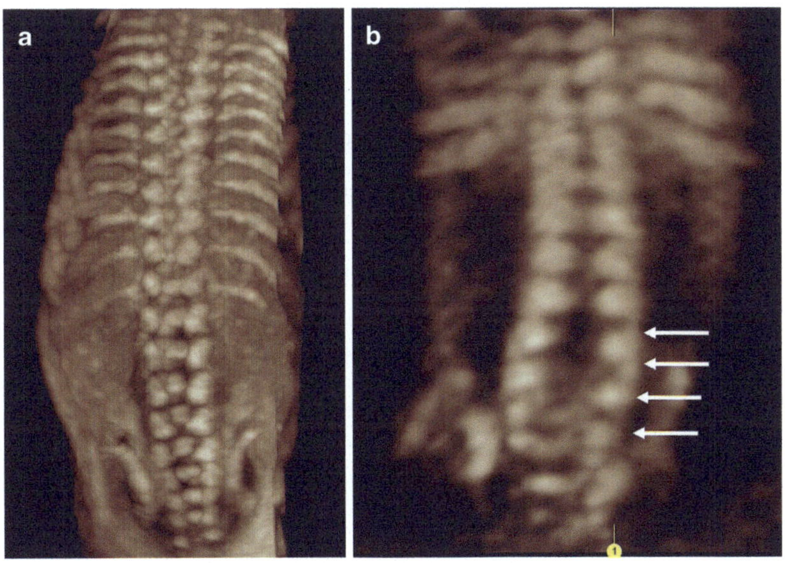

Fig. 16 Maximum-mode rendering of the spine and thorax on a coronal plane at the level of the vertebral bodies and/or posterior arches. (**a**) Normal fetus. (**b**) Fetus with open spina bifida: it is possible to identify the spinal defects (arrows)

References

1. Paladini D, Malinger G, Birnbaum R, Monteagudo A, Pilu G, Salomon LJ, et al. ISUOG practice guidelines (updated): sonographic examination of the fetal central nervous system. Part 2: performance of targeted neurosonography. Ultrasound Obstet Gynecol. 2021;57(4):661–71. https://doi.org/10.1002/uog.23616.
2. The Italian Society for Ultrasound in Obstetrics and Gynecology Sieog. The Italian guidelines on ultrasound in obstetrics and gynecology: executive summary of recommendations for practice. Eur J Obstet Gynecol. 2022;279:176–82.
3. Salomon LJ, Alfirevic Z, Berghella V, Bilardo CM, Chalouhi GE, Da Silva CF, et al. ISUOG practice guidelines (updated): performance of the routine mid-trimester fetal ultrasound scan. Ultrasound Obstet Gynecol. 2022;59(6):840–56. https://doi.org/10.1002/uog.24888.
4. De Robertis V, Sen C, Timor-Tritsch I, Chaoui R, Volpe P, Galindo A, et al. WAPM-world association of perinatal medicine practice guidelines: fetal central nervous system examination. J Perinat Med. 2021;49(9):1033–41. https://doi.org/10.1515/jpm-2021-0183.
5. Malinger G, Paladini D, Haratz KK, Monteagudo A, Pilu GL, Timor-Tritsch IE. ISUOG practice guidelines (updated): sonographic examination of the fetal central nervous system. Part 1: performance of screening examination and indications for targeted neurosonography. Ultrasound Obstet Gynecol. 2020;56(3):476–84. https://doi.org/10.1002/uog.22145.
6. Syngelaki A, Hammami A, Bower S, Zidere V, Akolekar R, Nicolaides KH. Diagnosis of fetal non-chromosomal abnormalities on routine ultrasound examination at 11-13 weeks' gestation. Ultrasound Obstet Gynecol. 2019;54(4):468–76. https://doi.org/10.1002/uog.20844.
7. Syngelaki A, Chelemen T, Dagklis T, Allan L, Nicolaides KH. Challenges in the diagnosis of fetal non-chromosomal abnormalities at 11-13 weeks. Prenat Diagn. 2011;31(1):90–102. https://doi.org/10.1002/pd.2642.
8. Karim JN, Roberts NW, Salomon LJ, Papageorghiou AT. Systematic review of first-trimester ultrasound screening for detection of fetal structural anomalies and factors that affect screening performance. Ultrasound Obstet Gynecol. 2017;50(4):429–41. https://doi.org/10.1002/uog.17246.
9. Volpe N, Sen C, Turan S, Sepulveda W, Khalil A, Rolnik DL, et al. First trimester examination of fetal anatomy: clinical practice guideline by the world association of perinatal medicine (WAPM) and the perinatal medicine foundation (PMF). J Perinat Med. 2022;50(7):863–77. https://doi.org/10.1515/jpm-2022-0125.
10. International Society of Ultrasound in Obstetrics and Gynecology, Bilardo CM, Chaoui R, Hyett JA, Kagan KO, Karim JN, et al. ISUOG practice guidelines (updated): performance of 11-14-week ultrasound scan. Ultrasound Obstet Gynecol. 2023;61(1):127–43. https://doi.org/10.1002/uog.26106.
11. Cohen-Sacher B, Lerman-Sagie T, Lev D, Malinger G. Sonographic developmental milestones of the fetal cerebral cortex: a longitudinal study. Ultrasound Obstet Gynecol. 2006;27(5):494–502. https://doi.org/10.1002/uog.2757.
12. Sepulveda W, Wong AE. First trimester screening for holoprosencephaly with choroid plexus morphology ("butterfly" sign) and biparietal diameter. Prenat Diagn. 2013;33(13):1233–7. https://doi.org/10.1002/pd.4235.
13. Chaoui R, Nicolaides KH. Detecting open spina bifida at the 11-13-week scan by assessing intracranial translucency and the posterior brain region: mid-sagittal or axial plane? Ultrasound Obstet Gynecol. 2011;38(6):609–12. https://doi.org/10.1002/uog.10128.
14. Lachmann R, Chaoui R, Moratalla J, Picciarelli G, Nicolaides KH. Posterior brain in fetuses with open spina bifida at 11 to 13 weeks. Prenat Diagn. 2011;31(1):103–6. https://doi.org/10.1002/pd.2632.
15. Chaoui R, Benoit B, Mitkowska-Wozniak H, Heling KS, Nicolaides KH. Assessment of intracranial translucency (IT) in the detection of spina bifida at the 11-13-week scan. Ultrasound Obstet Gynecol. 2009;34(3):249–52. https://doi.org/10.1002/uog.7329.
16. Volpe P, Persico N, Fanelli T, De Robertis V, D'Alessandro J, Boito S, et al. Prospective detection and differential diagnosis of cystic posterior fossa anomalies by assessing posterior brain at 11-14 weeks. Am J Obstet Gynecol MFM. 2019;1(2):173–81. https://doi.org/10.1016/j.ajogmf.2019.06.004.
17. Volpe P, Contro E, Fanelli T, Muto B, Pilu G, Gentile M. Appearance of fetal posterior fossa at 11-14 weeks in fetuses with Dandy-Walker malformation or chromosomal anomalies. Ultrasound Obstet Gynecol. 2016;47(6):720–5. https://doi.org/10.1002/uog.14883.
18. De Robertis V, Sen C, Timor-Tritsch I, Volpe P, Galindo A, Khalil A, Volpe N, Gil MM, Birnbaum R, Villalain C, Malinger G. Clinical Practice Guidelines and Recommendations by The World Association of Perinatal Medicine and Perinatal Medicine Foundation—Reporting Suspected Findings from Fetal Central Nervous System Examination. Fetal Diagn Ther. 2024;51(3):203–15. https://doi.org/10.1159/000535917.
19. Falco P, Gabrielli S, Visentin A, Perolo A, Pilu G, Bovicelli L. Transabdominal sonography of the cavum septum pellucidum in normal fetuses in the second and third trimesters of pregnancy. Ultrasound Obstet Gynecol. 2000;16(6):549–53. https://doi.org/10.1046/j.1469-0705.2000.00244.x.

20. Viñals F, Correa F, Gonçalves-Pereira PM. Anterior and posterior complexes: a step towards improving neurosonographic screening of midline and cortical anomalies. Ultrasound Obstet Gynecol. 2015;46(5):585–94. https://doi.org/10.1002/uog.14735.
21. Pilu G, Reece EA, Goldstein I, Hobbins JC, Bovicelli L. Sonographic evaluation of the normal developmental anatomy of the fetal cerebral ventricles: II. The atria. Obstet Gynecol. 1989;73(2):250–6.
22. Cardoza JD, Goldstein RB, Filly RA. Exclusion of fetal ventriculomegaly with a single measurement: the width of the lateral ventricular atrium. Radiology. 1988;169(3):711–4. https://doi.org/10.1148/radiology.169.3.3055034.
23. Guibaud L. Fetal cerebral ventricular measurement and ventriculomegaly: time for procedure standardization. Ultrasound Obstet Gynecol. 2009;34(2):127–30. https://doi.org/10.1002/uog.6456.
24. Quarello E, Stirnemann J, Ville Y, Guibaud L. Assessment of fetal Sylvian fissure operculization between 22 and 32 weeks: a subjective approach. Ultrasound Obstet Gynecol. 2008;32(1):44–9. https://doi.org/10.1002/uog.5353.
25. Volpe P, De Robertis V, Volpe G, Boito S, Fanelli T, Olivieri C, et al. Position of the choroid plexus of the fourth ventricle in first- and second-trimester fetuses: a novel approach to early diagnosis of cystic posterior fossa anomalies. Ultrasound Obstet Gynecol. 2021;58(4):568–75. https://doi.org/10.1002/uog.23651.
26. Snijders RJ, Nicolaides KH. Fetal biometry at 14–40 weeks' gestation. Ultrasound Obstet Gynecol. 1994;4(1):34–48. https://doi.org/10.1046/j.1469-0705.1994.04010034.x.
27. Volpe P, De Robertis V, Volpe G, Olivieri C, Fanelli T, Boito S, et al. Evaluation of cerebellar vermis at 12–22 weeks of gestation: why is traditional assessment incorrect? Ultrasound Obstet Gynecol. 2023;61(3):415–6. https://doi.org/10.1002/uog.26059.
28. Paladini D, Donarini G, Parodi S, Volpe G, Sglavo G, Fulcheri E. Hindbrain morphometry and choroid plexus position in differential diagnosis of posterior fossa cystic malformations. Ultrasound Obstet Gynecol. 2019;54(2):207–14. https://doi.org/10.1002/uog.20120.
29. Volpe P, De Robertis V, Fanelli T, Volpe G, Olivieri C, Boito S, et al. Impact of choroid plexus size in prenatal diagnosis of normal and abnormal closure of fourth ventricle. Ultrasound Obstet Gynecol. 2023;62(6):875–81. https://doi.org/10.1002/uog.26278.
30. Perlitz Y, Izhaki I, Ben-Ami M. Sonographic evaluation of the fetal conus medullaris at 20 to 24 weeks' gestation. Prenat Diagn. 2010;30(9):862–4. https://doi.org/10.1002/pd.2572.
31. Mottet N, Saada J, Jani J, Martin A, Riethmuller D, Zerah M, et al. Sonographic evaluation of fetal conus medullaris and filum terminale. Fetal Diagn Ther. 2016;40(3):224–30. https://doi.org/10.1159/000443731.
32. Rodríguez MA, Prats P, Rodríguez I, Comas C. Prenatal evaluation of the fetal conus medullaris on a routine scan. Fetal Diagn Ther. 2016;39(2):113–6. https://doi.org/10.1159/000441295.

Cerebral Ventriculomegaly. Hydrocephalus

Daniele Di Mascio, Ilenia Mappa, Francesco D'Antonio, and Giuseppe Rizzo

Abstract

Fetal cerebral "ventriculomegaly" and congenital "hydrocephalus" are two terms that have been commonly used indistinctly in the literature. Nonetheless, "ventriculomegaly" usually refers to the overall enlargement of the ventricles of the brain, regardless of etiopathogenesis, natural history, or outcome; conversely, "hydrocephalus" is used to define the pathological dilation of cerebral ventricles caused by an increased cerebrospinal fluid (CSF) pressure, often related to an imbalanced CSF production and/or absorption.

The main causes of ventriculomegaly are structural, genetic, or infective conditions.

Ventriculomegaly is diagnosed at screening ultrasound by placing the calipers at the level of the parieto-occipital sulcus, with a ventricular dilation of more than 10 mm. Fetal MRI plays an important role in detecting additional anomalies which may be overlooked also at expert brain ultrasound (so-called neurosonography), particularly when the severity of the dilation increases.

The presence of associated anomalies detected either at antenatal or postnatal imaging, the severity of the condition, and the persistence and/or progression of ventricular dilation are the main determinants of postnatal outcome in fetuses initially presenting with mild to moderate ventriculomegaly.

In utero ventriculo-amniotic shunting for severe fetal ventriculomegaly did not demonstrate to yield a clear improvement in outcome over expectant management. There is no proven evidence on different timing or mode of delivery to improve perinatal and neonatal outcomes in mild or moderate ventriculomegaly, and therefore timing and type of delivery should follow standard obstetric indications. For fetuses with severe ventriculomegaly or hydrocephalus and macrocephaly, elective cesarean delivery could be a reasonable option

Supplementary Information The online version contains supplementary material available at https://doi.org/10.1007/978-3-031-70192-4_2.

D. Di Mascio (✉) · G. Rizzo
Department of Maternal and Child Health and Urological Sciences, Umberto I University Hospital, Sapienza University of Rome, Rome, Italy
e-mail: daniele.dimascio@uniroma1.it; giuseppe.rizzo@uniroma2.it

I. Mappa
Department of Obstetrics and Gynecology, Fondazione Policlinico Tor Vergata, University of Rome Tor Vergata, Rome, Italy

F. D'Antonio
Department of Obstetrics and Gynecology, Centre for Fetal Care and High-Risk Pregnancy, University of Chieti, Chieti, Italy
e-mail: francesco.dantonio@unich.it

P. Volpe, T. Ghi (eds.), *Fetal Neurosonography*, Ultrasound in Obstetrics and Gynecology,
https://doi.org/10.1007/978-3-031-70192-4_2

to avoid obstructed labor due to cephalopelvic disproportion although there is no univocal cut-off for head circumference to guide the decision about mode of delivery.

Keywords
Ventriculomegaly · Hydrocephalus
Neurosonography · Fetal brain · Fetal MRI

1 Definition

Fetal cerebral "ventriculomegaly" and congenital "hydrocephalus" are two terms that have been commonly used indistinctly in the literature. Nonetheless, "ventriculomegaly" usually refers to the overall enlargement of the ventricles of the brain, regardless of etiopathogenesis, natural history, or outcome; conversely, "hydrocephalus" is used to define the pathological dilation of cerebral ventricles caused by an increased cerebrospinal fluid (CSF) pressure, often related to an imbalanced CSF production and/or absorption. Thus, the term "ventriculomegaly" does not refer to a single, specific disorder, but rather to a sonographic sign which represents the endpoint of different conditions with different prognosis. In this context, congenital hydrocephalus is virtually always associated with fetal ventriculomegaly, but fetal ventriculomegaly is not always related to congenital hydrocephalus. However, these two definitions are occasionally used interchangeably also because cerebral ventricular pressure cannot be assessed during fetal life [1].

With this premise, fetal ventriculomegaly is normally defined as the dilatation (≥10 mm) of the posterior part of the lateral ventricles measured at the level of the parieto-occipital sulcus, with or without dilatation of the third or fourth ventricles. Ventriculomegaly has been classified according to the severity of ventricular dilatation into either mild (10–14.9 mm) and severe (≥15 mm) or mild (10–12.9 mm), moderate (13–14.9 mm), and severe (≥15 mm) [2]. This further stratification into three classes of severity is generally preferred due to a stronger association with the postnatal outcome, as the short- and long-term prognosis worsens as the dilation increases [2].

Ventriculomegaly can also be further differentiate into "isolated" ventriculomegaly, when no other additional central nervous system (CNS) or extra-CNS anomalies are present, or into "unilateral" vs "bilateral" ventriculomegaly, when the dilation, respectively, involves only one or both lateral cerebral ventricles. Finally, other criteria for classification regard the evolution of the lesion (whether it is transient, stable over time, or progressive) and the symmetry (whether there is or not a relatively significant discrepancy between the dilation of the two ventricles).

Congenital hydrocephalus is defined as the dilatation of fetal cerebral ventricles (usually presenting as a severe ventriculomegaly), potentially involving also third and fourth ventricles, due to an excessive production and/or a reduced reabsorption of CSF [1].

2 Epidemiology

Ventriculomegaly is the most common CNS abnormal sonographic finding detected antenatally, although establishing the prevalence of this condition might be challenging to define since it varies in accordance with a list of factors, such as the severity of the dilation, the gestational age at diagnosis, the type of sonographic assessment (i.e., screening vs expert examination), and the evaluation of one or both fetal cerebral hemispheres [1].

The reported prevalence for mild and moderate ventriculomegaly (i.e., <15 mm) ranges from 1:50 to 1:1000 fetuses, while the incidence of severe VM is about 1:1000 [1–3].

About 50%–60% of ventriculomegaly are unilateral, although the diagnosis of bilateral ventriculomegaly might be more difficult to be established, as the ventricle which is closer to the ultrasound beam (within the proximal hemisphere) cannot be properly measured on the axial plane, due to the shadow cast from the parietal bone [3–5].

Isolated ventriculomegaly might be found in 0.39–0.87 per 1000 births, while the prevalence of non-isolated ventriculomegaly is greatly influenced from the severity of the dilation (less than 10% in case of mild ventriculomegaly and up to 60% in case of severe ventriculomegaly) [1].

The risk of progression from mild to severe ventriculomegaly has been reported to be approximately 15% and progression also poses a significant risk of subsequent neurodevelopmental delay, compared with persistence or resolution of ventriculomegaly. Conversely, 43–75% tend of cases to stabilize and 14–62% normalize their ventricular size [1].

Ventriculomegaly is more often diagnosed in male compared with female fetuses, with a male-to-female ratio of 7:1 [2, 3], and in those with other larger fetal biometric measurements, such as head circumference, biparietal diameter, femur length, and estimated fetal weight [6].

3 Etiology/Pathogenesis

As already mentioned, ventriculomegaly is the epiphenomenon of different disorders with different outcomes, but might also represent a normal variant, mostly when isolated in fetuses with normal karyotype and negative infectious screening (Table 1).

The etiopathological mechanism causing most of the cases of isolated mild and moderate fetal ventriculomegaly is still unknown. An anecdotic cause for these mild cases has been associated with a delayed fenestration of the Blake's pouch, in particular in the presence of a communication between fourth ventricle and the cisterna magna [1].

The association with genetic abnormalities will be more extensively discussed in the dedicated section of this chapter (see "Genetic Background"), but genetic etiology should always be taken into account, especially when dealing with severe forms of ventriculomegaly and/or those associated with other CNS/extra-CNS structural anomalies.

Another potential cause of ventriculomegaly is congenital infection, mostly toxoplasmosis or cytomegalovirus infection. Rare cases of ventriculomegaly have also been reported to be associated with other infective agents (i.e., mumps virus, enterovirus, parainfluenza virus type 3, parvovirus B19, and lymphocytic choriomeningitis virus) [2, 3, 7]. Ventriculomegaly due to an infectious cause rarely appears as an isolated condition, but it is rather associated with typical signs of brain infection/inflammation such as microcephaly, hyperechogenic ventricular walls, hyperechogenic periventricular calcifications (toxoplasmosis), intraventricular synechiae, periventricular cysts, or halo (CMV) [8, 9]. Moreover, additional extra-CNS anomalies are usually present in these cases, including fetal growth restriction, hepatosplenomegaly, placentomegaly and, in the most severe cases, fetal hydrops [10].

A prognostically important but uncommon etiology of severe ventriculomegaly is also intracranial hemorrhage. This condition is frequently associated with severe ventriculomegaly, presence of blood clots, irregular ventricular walls due to fibrin deposition, and common involvement of brain parenchyma [11].

Table 1 Main potential causes of ventriculomegaly

Structural	Genetic	Infectious
Delayed fenestration of the Blake's pouch	Chromosomal anomalies	Toxoplasmosis
Stenosis of the aqueduct of Sylvius and the fourth ventricular foramina	X-linked aqueductal stenosis (MASA syndrome, CRASH syndrome)	Cytomegalovirus
Obstruction of fourth ventricular CSF egress through the foramina of Magendi and/or Luschka	Ciliopathies (i.e., Meckel-Gruber syndrome, Joubert syndrome), dystroglycanopathies (Walker-Warburg syndrome), and tubulinopathies (TUBA1A)	More rare infections (mump virus, enterovirus, parainfluenza virus type 3, parvovirus B19, and lymphocytic choriomeningitis virus)
Intraventricular hemorrhage		

According to its pathogenesis fetal hydrocephalus could be further differentiated into "obstructive" or "noncommunicating" hydrocephalus, when the enlargement of fetal ventricles is caused by an obstruction of CSF flow upstream or at the fourth ventricular foramina, or "communicating" hydrocephalus, that is conversely caused by an impaired absorption of the CSF flow distal to the fourth ventricular foramina (e.g., in the subarachnoid spaces or arachnoid granulations) [1].

In obstructive hydrocephalus, the obstruction is generally located at the level of the aqueduct of Sylvius and the fourth ventricular foramina, thus resulting into an enlargement of the lateral and third ventricles, with a normal size of the fourth ventricle. Conversely, in case of obstruction of fourth ventricular CSF egress through the foramina of Magendie and/or Luschka, the hydrocephalus is tetraventricular (i.e., involving all the four ventricular spaces) [1].

The main structural defects causing congenital hydrocephalus are the above-mentioned aqueductal stenosis and posterior fossa anomalies, such as myelomeningocele with the Chiari type II malformation and the Dandy–Walker complex that might obstruct the CSF flow at aqueduct, foramina, and subarachnoid levels [1].

4 Genetic Background

The prevalence of genetic anomalies in the context of fetal ventriculomegaly mostly depends on the severity of the lesion and the presence of associated anomalies.

With this perspective, in case of apparently isolated mild and moderate ventriculomegaly, the rate of chromosomal anomalies (mostly represented by trisomy 21) ranges from 3% to 5% [2, 3, 12]. Beside abnormal karyotype, pathogenic copy number variants are found at chromosomal microarray (CMA) in up to 10–15% [2]. The laterality and the severity of the lesion, and the presence of additional structural anomalies are among the main predictors of chromosomal aberrations at CMA [13, 14].

In case of severe ventriculomegaly, chromosomal anomalies have been reported in around 5% of fetuses on standard karyotyping and 23% on CMA. Therefore, despite good diagnostic yield obtained with CMA, the majority of fetuses with severe ventriculomegaly still remain without a genetic diagnosis. In this scenario, exome sequencing (ES) has been recently investigated to ascertain whether it could be associated with a higher diagnostic yield, compared with standard karyotyping and CMA. A diagnostic yield of 54% was obtained for severe ventriculomegaly associated with extracranial anomalies, followed by a diagnostic yield of 38% and 35% in case of severe ventriculomegaly associated or not with other intracranial anomalies, respectively, highlighting a potential role for ES even in cases of isolated severe ventriculomegaly [15].

Ventriculomegaly has also been described to be associated with single gene disorders, such as the mutation of L1 cell adhesion molecule (L1CAM) [16], which is a neuronal cell adhesion molecule with important functions in the development of the CNS. The gene encoding L1 is located near the telomere of the long arm of the X chromosome in Xq28 and this mutation may result in an X-linked form of aqueductal stenosis causing hydrocephalus. The syndrome represents a spectrum of disorders including X-linked hydrocephalus with stenosis of the aqueduct of Sylvius (HSAS); mental retardation, ataxia, shuffling gait and adducted thumbs (MASA) syndrome; corpus callosum hypoplasia, retardation, adducted thumbs, spastic paraplegia, and hydrocephalus (CRASH) syndrome [17].

Although less common, other genetic conditions aside from X-linked aqueductal stenosis have been associated with ventriculomegaly (usually associated with other CNS anomalies), such as ciliopathies (i.e., Meckel-Gruber syndrome, Joubert syndrome), dystroglycanopathies (i.e., Walker-Warburg syndrome), and tubulinopathies (i.e., TUBA1A) [18].

5 Sonographic Findings

The evaluation of fetal lateral ventricles is recommended by the main guidelines on the screening examination of the fetal CNS during the second trimester anatomy scan and is to be accomplished through the examination of the axial transventricular plane that shows the anterior and the posterior portions of the lateral ventricle in the distal brain hemisphere (Fig. 1) [19, 20]. The anterior horns look like two comma-shaped, fluid-filled structures, divided medially by the cavum septi pellucidi (CSP). The posterior part of the lateral ventricles (also called "occipital horns") is defined as a complex made by the atrium that continues posteriorly into the occipital horn. The atrium is recognized by the presence of the glomus of the choroid plexus (highly echogenic), while the occipital horn is usually filled with cerebrospinal fluid (anechoic) (Fig. 2) [19].

The assessment of fetal ventricles includes both a qualitative and a quantitative evaluation of the atrial width as this is recognized as the most effective method to confirm the normal appearance and size of the ventricular system [19].

Although initially the measurement of the atrium was performed at the level of the glomus of the choroid plexus [19], a standardized method is to place the calipers on the inner edge of ventricular wall at the level of the parieto-occipital sulcus and aligned perpendicular to long axis of ventricle. This may be particularly useful in the third trimester when the lateral ventricles have a more complex architecture [18].

At mid-trimester, the posterior ventricle has a mean diameter of 6–8 mm and is defined as "normal" when is less than 10 mm, as this is the 95th centile, based on the available charts (Fig. 3) [19]. The term "borderline ventriculomegaly" (either used when the ventricular measurement is close to the standard threshold of 10 mm or between 10 and 15 mm) is no longer used and should indeed be avoided, as it has unclear significance in terms of clinical relevance [21].

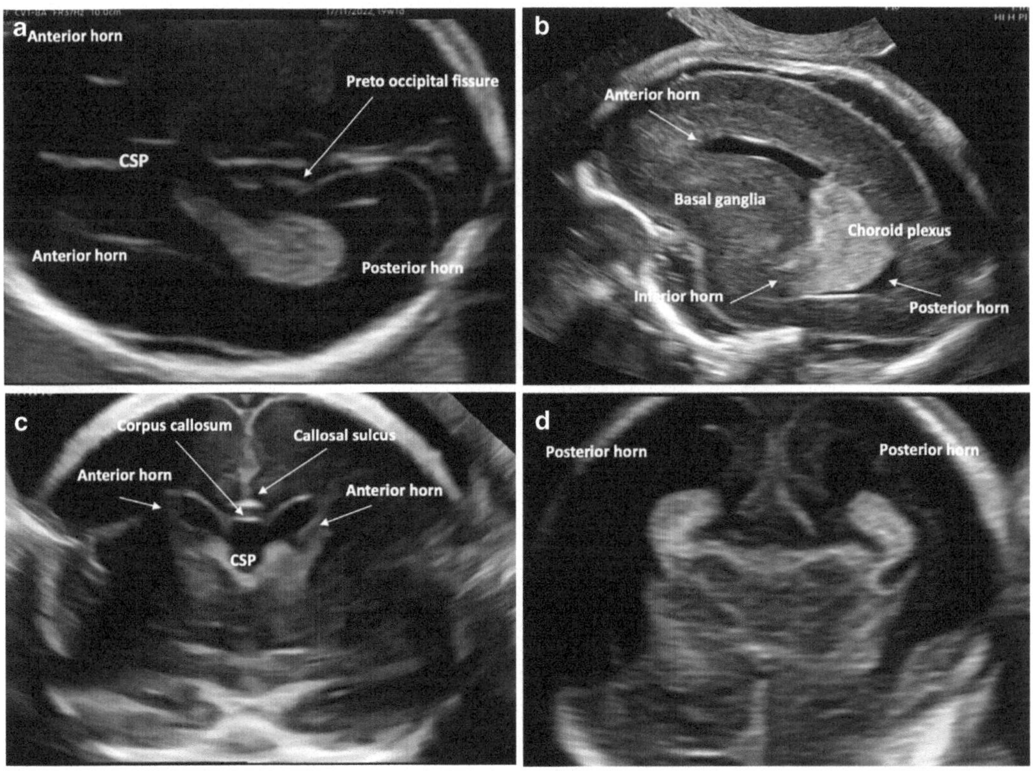

Fig. 1 Anatomy of the ventricular system on a multiplanar assessment

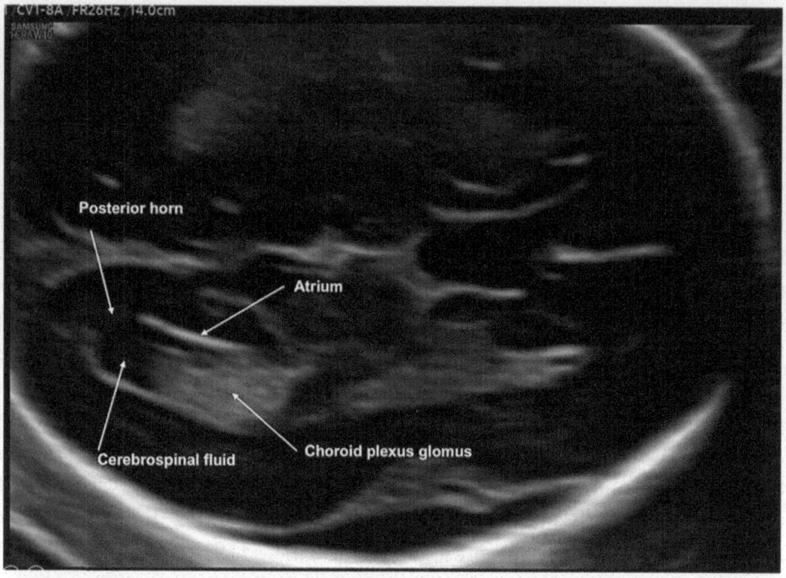

Fig. 2 Anatomy of the posterior part of the lateral ventricles (also called "occipital horns")

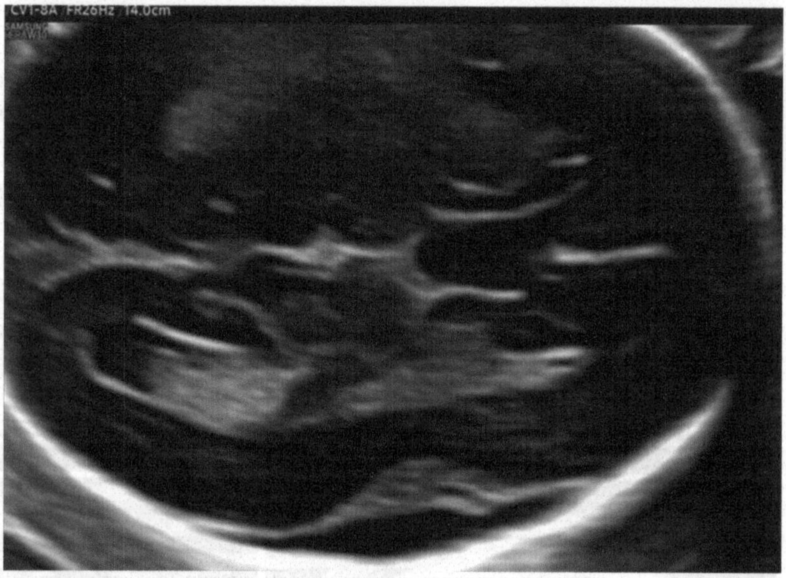

Fig. 3 Normal diameter of the posterior ventricle

When ventriculomegaly is found at routine ultrasound (Fig. 4), a targeted fetal neurosonography should be performed [19, 22] in a referral center, as this examination performed by experienced specialists has a much higher diagnostic potential to rule out or detect additional CNS anomalies (Fig. 5; Videos 1, 2, and 3) [22, 23].

Regarding ventriculomegaly, a systematic etiological approach to assess fetuses with ventriculomegaly has been proposed almost 10 years ago by Guibaud, based on a set of etiological diagnostic features which consist in [24]:

1. Investigation of an "obstructive pattern" causing ventriculomegaly, regardless of the cause of the obstruction (i.e., malformative, tumoral, vascular origin), assessing fetal head size, shape of the CSP, evaluation of the third ventricle size, pericerebral spaces, and suprapineal recess.

2. Investigation of "vascular/clastic pattern," particularly when dealing with asymmetrical or unilateral ventriculomegaly, suggesting the presence of ischemic or hemorrhagic lesion. It involves the assessment of the echogenicity of the ventricular wall, the presence of echogenic deposits within the ventricular cavity potentially extending to the periventricular zone and brain parenchyma, suggesting intracranial hemorrhage.

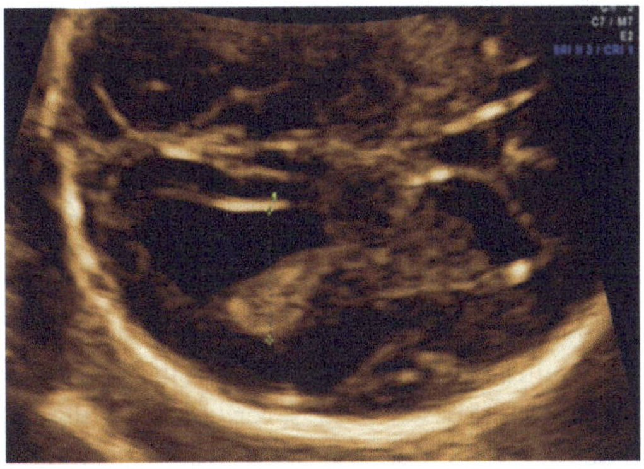

Fig. 4 Severe ventriculomegaly on axial view

3. Assessment of CSF flow from the diencephalon to the posterior fossa, which includes a detailed evaluation of the entire ventricular system from the supratentorial structures to the infra-cerebellar cisterna, in order to rule out impaired circulation of the CSF.
4. Assessment of brain gyration and myelinization, mainly obtained by the evaluation of the Sylvian fissure as the main landmark of gyration, in order to rule out neuronal migration disorders.
5. Assessment of the fetal ventricular wall, ventricular lumen, and periventricular area, to exclude congenital and acquired conditions including infections, hemorrhage, and heterotopia (Fig. 6 and 7).
6. Systematic analysis of the pericerebral spaces, to rule out micro- or macrocephaly.

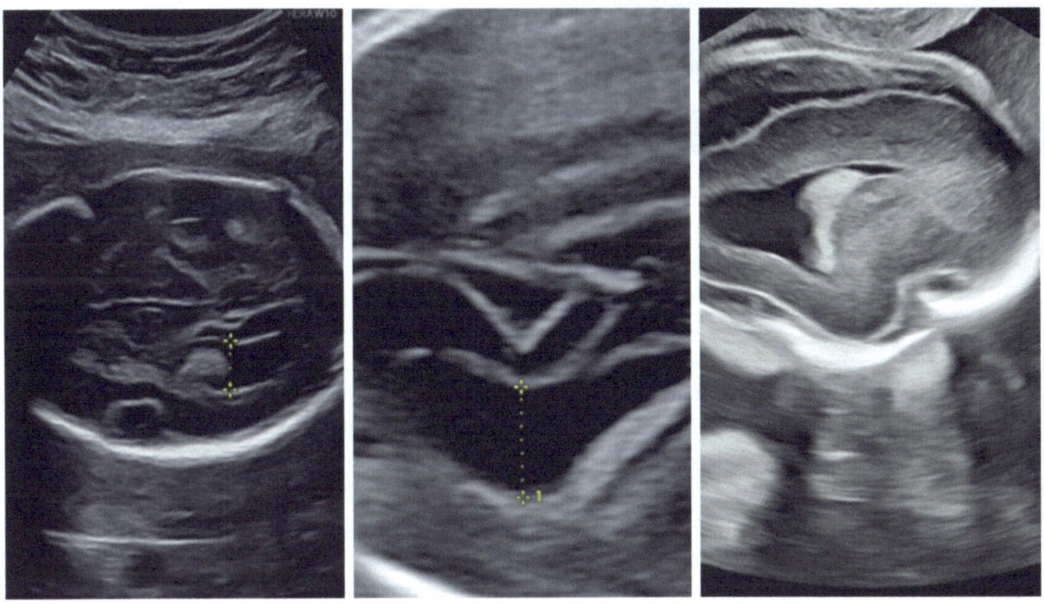

Fig. 5 Severe ventriculomegaly on multiplanar assessment

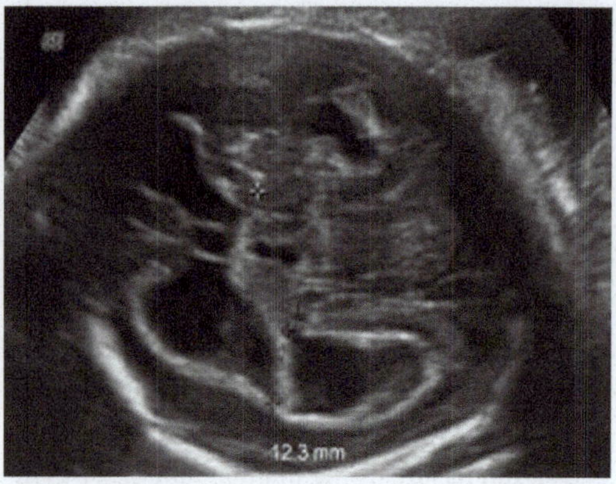

Fig. 6 Intraventricular synechia in a fetus affected by congenital CMV infection

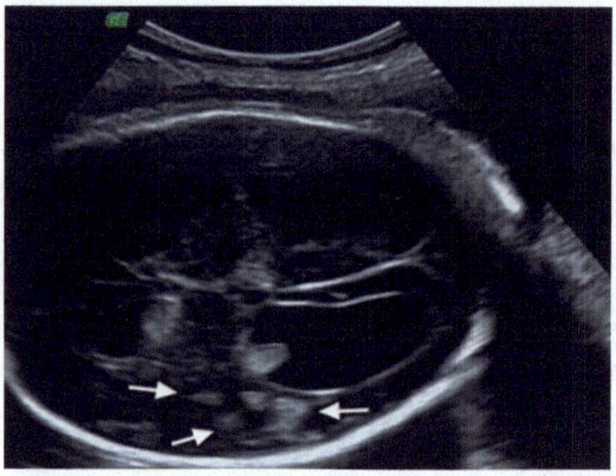

Fig. 7 Severe ventriculomegaly associated with periventricular nodular heterotopia

6 Differential Diagnosis

While the antenatal diagnosis of ventriculomegaly is usually accomplished by non-expert sonographers on the axial plane, a skilled operator performing a mutiplanar assessment of the fetal brain is required for the differential diagnosis of those conditions which may mimic ventriculomegaly, such as hydranencephaly, holoprosencephaly, or enlarged CSP or cavum velum interpositum. Whether neurosonography is not conclusive, fetal brain MRI is indicated to clarify the diagnosis [1].

In more severe cases, ventriculomegaly should be properly differentiated from more complex anomalies such as intracranial hemorrhage (ICH), cortical malformations, or X-linked hydrocephalus spectrum. Also for these peculiar situations, antenatal MRI may help in distinguishing the anomaly [25].

7 MRI

Fetal magnetic resonance imaging (MRI) is an important diagnostic adjunct to ultrasonography, especially for evaluation of the fetal brain [26].

In case of fetal ventriculomegaly, antenatal MRI plays an important role in detecting or excluding additional anomalies even when diagnostic ultrasound is performed in referral centers and particularly when the severity of the dilation increases, as demonstrated by two recent multinational studies (Fig. 8) [5, 27–29].

In case of mild to moderate isolated ventriculomegaly diagnosed with neurosonography, the rate of additional anomalies detected exclusively by fetal MRI was 5.4%, with the most common types of anomalies which were missed at ultrasound involving supratentorial intracranial hemorrhage and malformations of cortical development (i.e., lissencephaly, heterotopia). Factors independently associated with a higher incidence of additional findings detected only at fetal MRI were gestational age at MRI at or after 24 weeks, moderate ventricular dilation and higher maternal body mass index (BMI). Finally, there was also a small rate (3.8%) of associated anomalies diagnosed exclusively after birth and missed at prenatal imaging (both neurosonography and MRI) [5].

When focusing on isolated severe ventriculomegaly, the rate of additional anomalies only found at fetal MRI was 18.1%. Most anomalies detected exclusively on prenatal MRI were malformations of cortical development (i.e., lissencephaly, heterotopia, or polymicrogyria) and midline anomalies (i.e., hypoplasia or dysgenesis of the corpus callosum), the latter probably underdiagnosed because of the

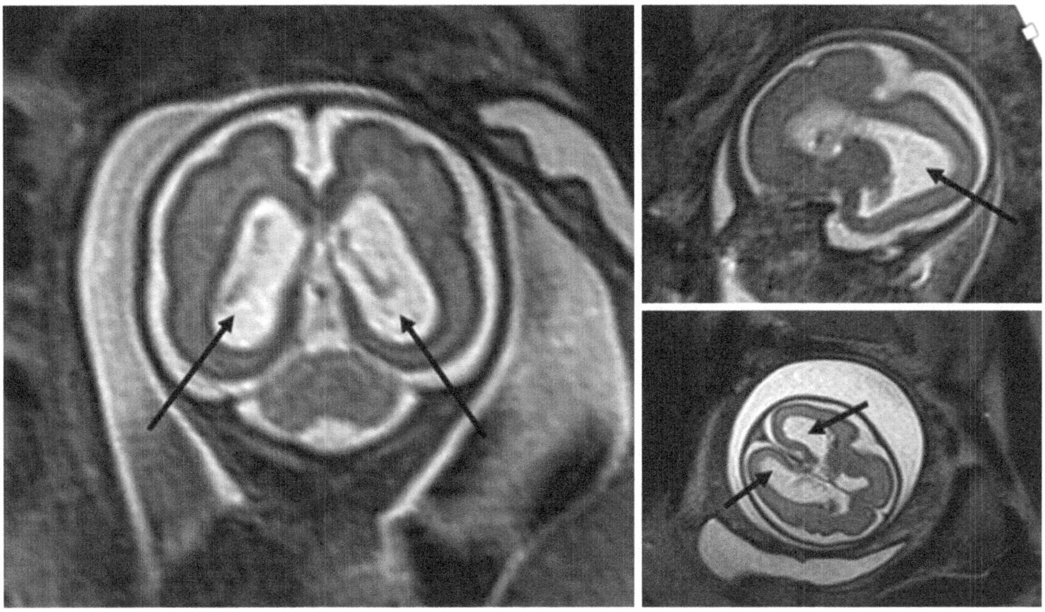

Fig. 8 Isolated ventriculomegaly at MRI (courtesy of Dr. Lucia Manganaro). Lateral ventricles are indicated by black arrows

increased size of lateral ventricles that may hamper a clear assessment of the midline structures. The bilaterality of the lesion was independently associated with a higher chance of detecting anomalies at MRI. Finally, the rate of associated anomalies detected exclusively after birth and missed at prenatal imaging was 13.6% [29].

8 Prognosis

Ventriculomegaly, particularly when mild and isolated, is generally associated with excellent survival, while mortality rate in case of congenital hydrocephalus or in the setting of a more complex syndrome might be tangible but it is to be assessed on an individual basis. The survival rate in apparently isolated mild and moderate ventriculomegaly has been estimated to be around 97%–98%, while the survival rate in case of severe ventriculomegaly is about 88% [18].

In terms of neurological short- and long-term morbidity, the presence of associated anomalies detected either at antenatal or postnatal imaging, the severity of the condition (i.e., size of the posterior ventricle) and the persistence and/or progression of ventricular dilation are the main determinants of postnatal outcome in fetuses initially presenting with mild to moderate ventriculomegaly.

In a meta-analysis including 652 cases of mild and moderate isolated ventriculomegaly with postnatal neurological assessment at a mean age of 27.7 months, a diagnosis of neurodevelopmental impairment was made in 7.9% of cases [12], that is similar to what found also by another meta-analysis evaluating only unilateral cases of mild and moderate ventriculomegaly, where the prevalence of abnormal neurodevelopmental outcome was 5.9% in apparently isolated cases and 7.0% in truly isolated unilateral cases [30].

Furthermore, no significant difference in the rate of abnormal scores between either mild/moderate and symmetric/asymmetric ventriculomegaly was also confirmed by a recent prospective study on 133 cases of isolated ventriculomegaly assessed at both ultrasound and fetal MRI [31].

Finally, a recent Danish nationwide registry-based study on all fetuses diagnosed prenatally with isolated mild and moderate ventriculomegaly and followed up until the age of 2–7 years reported an incidence of neurodevelopmental delay of 5.6%, including disorders such as autism spectrum disorder, epilepsy, and abnormal psychomotor development, with no case of severe intellectual disability or cerebral palsy [32].

Progression of ventricular dilatation, particularly when beyond 15 mm, is associated with a higher risk of impaired neurodevelopment, which has been reported to be around 50% in older series [33, 34].

Regarding severe ventriculomegaly, the vast majority of cases present with multiple associated anomalies which account for a high rate of termination of pregnancy and long-term neurological sequelae. However, a 2018 meta-analysis of eleven studies investigating the neurological outcome of a total of 110 fetuses with apparently isolated severe ventriculomegaly reported no disability in 42.2% of cases, mild/moderate disability in 18.6%, and severe disability in 39.6% of cases [35].

However, it should be clearly acknowledged that the definition of "isolated" at antenatal imaging is only presumptive, even when neurosonography and fetal MRI are performed, as there is still a small portion of abnormalities that might be missed prenatally and only detected after birth [5, 26]. This is an important issue that should be always taken into account by maternal fetal specialists, in particular when counselling the prospective parents about short- and long-term prognosis of such a condition.

Finally, as mentioned earlier in this chapter, the postnatal outcome is also negatively impacted by the presence of additional CNS anomalies or by an underlying specific syndrome.

9 Options of Treatment

In utero ventriculo-amniotic shunting for severe fetal ventriculomegaly has been performed in the years eighties of the past century. The results from the first procedures did not demonstrate a clear improvement in outcome over expectant management, with a procedure-related death rate of 10.3% and a rate of serious and less severe neurologic handicaps of 52.9% and 11.8%, respectively [36].

The clinical usefulness of antenatal ventriculo-amniotic shunting for drainage of severe fetal cerebral ventriculomegaly has been recently reassessed on the data from a tertiary fetal therapy center. In this series, shunt insertion was successfully carried out at a median gestational age of 25 weeks with a good outcome in terms of survival rate (38 out of 41 live births at a median gestational age of 37 weeks). However, neurodevelopment at 2 years of age using the Bayley scale was moderately or severely impaired in 29.6% of cases with isolated ventriculomegaly and in 81.8 of cases with non-isolated ventriculomegaly [37].

The need for and timing of postnatal neurosurgical intervention in children with ventriculomegaly/hydrocephalus mainly depends on the severity of symptoms (i.e., headache, neurovegetative symptoms, neurologic deficits, papilledema) and/or neuroimaging findings (i.e., progression of ventriculomegaly or overt obstruction of the CSF). However, neurosurgical management and prognosis of obstructive and communicating hydrocephalus in children are beyond the scope of this chapter.

10 Obstetric Management

There is no proven evidence that different timing or mode of delivery would improve perinatal outcome in cases with antenatal diagnosis of mild to moderate ventriculomegaly, and therefore timing and type of delivery should follow standard obstetric indications.

For fetuses with severe ventriculomegaly or hydrocephalus and macrocephaly, elective cesarean delivery could be a reasonable option to avoid obstructed labor due to cephalopelvic disproportion although there is no univocal cut-off for head circumference to guide the decision about the mode of delivery. A recent study on fetuses with severe fetal ventriculomegaly reported an overall rate of cesarean delivery of 65.3%, with those with macrocrania (head circumference larger than 95th centile) having the highest rate of cesarean delivery (86.1%), thus suggesting an individualized delivery plan to improve to a certain extent neonatal outcomes and minimize harm to the mother [38].

References

1. du Plessis AJ, Robinson S, Volpe JJ. Congenital hydrocephalus. In: Neurology of the Newborn, Elsevier. 6th ed. Philadelphia, PA; 2018.
2. Society for Maternal-Fetal Medicine (SMFM), Fox NS, Monteagudo A, Kuller JA, Craigo S, Norton ME. Mild fetal ventriculomegaly: diagnosis, evaluation, and management. Am J Obstet Gynecol. 2018;219:B2–9.
3. Melchiorre K, Bhide A, Gika AD, Pilu G, Papageorghiou AT. Counseling in isolated mild fetal ventriculomegaly. Ultrasound Obstet Gynecol. 2009;34:212–24.
4. Falip C, Blanc N, Maes E, Zaccaria I, Oury JF, Sebag G, Garel C. Postnatal clinical and imaging follow-up of infants with prenatal isolated mild ventriculomegaly: a series of 101 cases. Pediatr Radiol. 2007;37:981.
5. ENSO Working Group. Role of prenatal magnetic resonance imaging in fetuses with isolated mild or moderate ventriculomegaly in the era of neurosonography: international multicenter study. Ultrasound Obstet Gynecol. 2020;56:340–7.
6. Fishel-Bartal M, Shai D, Shina A, Achiron R, Katorza E. Correlation between fetal mild ventriculomegaly and biometric parameters. J Matern Fetal Neonatal Med. 2019;32:243–7.
7. Bascietto F, Liberati M, Murgano D, Buca D, Iacovelli A, Flacco ME, Manzoli L, Familiari A, Scambia G, D'Antonio F. Outcome of fetuses with congenital parvovirus B19 infection: systematic review and meta-analysis. Ultrasound Obstet Gynecol. 2018;52:569–76.
8. Hawkins-Villarreal A, Castillo K, Nadal A, Planas S, Moreno-Espinosa AL, Alarcón A, Rebollo-Polo M, Figueras F, Gratacós E, Eixarch E, Goncé A. Halo sign in fetal cytomegalovirus infection: cerebral imaging abnormalities and postmortem histopathology in 35 infected fetuses. Ultrasound Obstet Gynecol. 2023;61:749–57.
9. Simonazzi G, Guerra B, Bonasoni P, Pilu G, Lazzarotto T, Santini D, Rizzo N. Fetal cerebral periventricular halo at midgestation: an ultrasound finding suggestive of fetal cytomegalovirus infection. Am J Obstet Gynecol. 2010;202(599):e1–5.
10. Khalil A, Sotiriadis A, Chaoui R, da Silva CF, D'Antonio F, Heath PT, Jones C, Malinger G, Odibo A, Prefumo F, Salomon LJ, Wood S, Ville Y. ISUOG practice guidelines: role of ultrasound in congenital infection. Ultrasound Obstet Gynecol. 2020;56:128–51.
11. Sileo FG, Zöllner J, D'Antonio F, Islam S, Papageorghiou AT, Khalil A. Perinatal and long-term outcome of fetal intracranial hemorrhage: systematic review and meta-analysis. Ultrasound Obstet Gynecol. 2022;59:585–95.
12. Pagani G, Thilaganathan B, Prefumo F. Neurodevelopmental outcome in isolated mild fetal ventriculomegaly: systematic review and meta-analysis. Ultrasound Obstet Gynecol. 2014;44:254–60.
13. Chang Q, Yang Y, Peng Y, Liu S, Li L, Deng X, Yang M, Lan Y. Prenatal detection of chromosomal abnormalities and copy number variants in fetuses with ventriculomegaly. Eur J Paediatr Neurol. 2020;25:106–12.
14. Wang J, Zhang Z, Li Q, Zhu H, Lai Y, Luo W, Liu S, Wang H, Hu T. Prenatal diagnosis of chromosomal aberrations by chromosomal microarray analysis in foetuses with ventriculomegaly. Sci Rep. 2020;10:20765.
15. Mustafa HJ, Sambatur EV, Barbera JP, Pagani G, Yaron Y, Baptiste CD, Wapner RJ, Khalil A. Diagnostic yield with exome sequencing in prenatal severe bilateral ventriculomegaly: a systematic review and meta-analysis. Am J Obstet Gynecol MFM. 2023;5:101048.
16. Finckh U, Schröder J, Ressler B, Veske A, Gal A. Spectrum and detection rate of L1CAM mutations in isolated and familial cases with clinically suspected L1-disease. Am J Med Genet. 2000;92:40–6.
17. Fransen E, Lemmon V, Van Camp G, Vits L, Coucke P, Willems PJ. CRASH syndrome: clinical spectrum of corpus callosum hypoplasia, retardation, adducted thumbs, spastic paraparesis and hydrocephalus due to mutations in one single gene, L1. Eur J Hum Genet. 1995;3:273–84. Erratum in: Eur J Hum Genet 1996; 4:126
18. Giorgione V, Haratz KK, Constantini S, Birnbaum R, Malinger G. Fetal cerebral ventriculomegaly: what do we tell the prospective parents? Prenat Diagn. 2022;42:1674–81.
19. Malinger G, Paladini D, Haratz KK, Monteagudo A, Pilu GL, Timor-Tritsch IE. ISUOG Practice Guidelines (updated): sonographic examination of the fetal central nervous system. Part 1: performance of screening examination and indications for targeted neurosonography. Ultrasound Obstet Gynecol. 2020;56:476–84. Erratum in: Ultrasound Obstet Gynecol. 2022; 60:591
20. De Robertis V, Sen C, Timor-Tritsch I, Chaoui R, Volpe P, Galindo A, Achiron R, Pooh R, Khalil A, Volpe N, D'Antonio F, Birnbaum R. WAPM-world association of perinatal medicine practice guidelines: fetal central nervous system examination. J Perinat Med. 2021;49:1033–41.
21. Guibaud L. Fetal cerebral ventricular measurement and ventriculomegaly: time for procedure standardization. Ultrasound Obstet Gynecol. 2009;34:127–30.

22. Paladini D, Malinger G, Birnbaum R, Monteagudo A, Pilu G, Salomon LJ, Timor-Tritsch IE. ISUOG Practice Guidelines (updated): sonographic examination of the fetal central nervous system. Part 2: performance of targeted neurosonography. Ultrasound Obstet Gynecol. 2021;57:661–71. Erratum in: Ultrasound Obstet Gynecol. 2022; 60:591
23. D'Antonio F, Di Mascio D, Rizzo G. Should we expand indications for targeted fetal neurosonography? Ultrasound Obstet Gynecol. 2022 Feb;59(2):274–6. https://doi.org/10.1002/uog.24840.
24. Guibaud L, Lacalm A. Etiological diagnostic tools to elucidate 'isolated' ventriculomegaly. Ultrasound Obstet Gynecol. 2015;46:1–11.
25. Pilu G, Malinger G. A severe fetal cerebral ventriculomegaly. Visual Encyclopedia of Ultrasound in Obstetrics and Gynecology. www.isuog.org. 24 June 2013.
26. Prayer D, Malinger G, De Catte L, De Keersmaecker B, Gonçalves LF, Kasprian G, Laifer-Narin S, Lee W, Millischer AE, Platt L, Prayer F, Pugash D, Salomon LJ, Sanz Cortes M, Stuhr F, Timor-Tritsch IE, Tutschek B, Twickler D, Raine-Fenning N, ISUOG Clinical Standards Committee. ISUOG practice guidelines (updated): performance of fetal magnetic resonance imaging. Ultrasound Obstet Gynecol. 2023;61:278–87.
27. Di Mascio D, Sileo FG, Khalil A, Rizzo G, Persico N, Brunelli R, Giancotti A, Panici PB, Acharya G, D'Antonio F. Role of magnetic resonance imaging in fetuses with mild or moderate ventriculomegaly in the era of fetal neurosonography: systematic review and meta-analysis. Ultrasound Obstet Gynecol. 2019;54:164–71.
28. Di Mascio D, Khalil A, Rizzo G, Kasprian G, Caulo M, Manganaro L, Odibo AO, Flacco ME, Giancotti A, Buca D, Liberati M, Timor-Tritsch IE, D'Antonio F. Reference ranges for fetal brain structures using magnetic resonance imaging: systematic review. Ultrasound Obstet Gynecol. 2022 Mar;59(3):296–303. https://doi.org/10.1002/uog.23762.
29. Di Mascio D, Khalil A, Pilu G, Rizzo G, Caulo M, Liberati M, Giancotti A, Lees C, Volpe P, Buca D, Oronzi L, D'Amico A, Tinari S, Stampalija T, Fantasia I, Pasquini L, Masini G, Brunelli R, D'Ambrosio V, Muzii L, Manganaro L, Antonelli A, Ercolani G, Ciulla S, Saccone G, Maruotti GM, Carbone L, Zullo F, Olivieri C, Ghi T, Frusca T, Dall'Asta A, Visentin S, Cosmi E, Forlani F, Galindo A, Villalain C, Herraiz I, Sileo FG, Mendez Quintero O, Salsi G, Bracalente G, Morales-Roselló J, Loscalzo G, Pellegrino M, De Santis M, Lanzone A, Parazzini C, Lanna M, Ormitti F, Toni F, Murru F, Di Maurizio M, Trincia E, Garcia R, Bennike Bjørn Petersen O, Neerup L, Sandager P, Prefumo F, Pinelli L, Mappa I, Acuti Martellucci C, Flacco ME, Manzoli L, Giangiordano I, Nappi L, Scambia G, Berghella V, D'Antonio F. Role of prenatal magnetic resonance imaging in fetuses with isolated severe ventriculomegaly at neurosonography: a multicenter study. Eur J Obstet Gynecol Reprod Biol. 2021;267:105–10.
30. Scala C, Familiari A, Pinas A, Papageorghiou AT, Bhide A, Thilaganathan B, Khalil A. Perinatal and long-term outcomes in fetuses diagnosed with isolated unilateral ventriculomegaly: systematic review and meta-analysis. Ultrasound Obstet Gynecol. 2017;49:450–9.
31. Bar-Yosef O, Barzilay E, Dorembus S, Achiron R, Katorza E. Neurodevelopmental outcome of isolated ventriculomegaly: a prospective cohort study. Prenat Diagn. 2017;37:764–8.
32. Thorup E, Jensen LN, Bak GS, Ekelund CK, Greisen G, Jørgensen DS, Hellmuth SG, Wulff C, Petersen OB, Pedersen LH, Tabor A. Neurodevelopmental disorder in children believed to have isolated mild ventriculomegaly prenatally. Ultrasound Obstet Gynecol. 2019;54:182–9.
33. Li QM, Liao HZ, Wang WB, Zeng SY, Qiu XS, Ke S, Xiao J, Li QH, Xia XW, Li Y. Prognostic analysis and risk factors associated with fetal ventriculomegaly. Pediatr Neurosurg. 2021;56:407–15.
34. Baffero GM, Crovetto F, Fabietti I, Boito S, Fogliani R, Fumagalli M, Triulzi F, Mosca F, Fedele L, Persico N. Prenatal ultrasound predictors of postnatal major cerebral abnormalities in fetuses with apparently isolated mild ventriculomegaly. Prenat Diagn. 2015;35:783–8.
35. Carta S, Kaelin Agten A, Belcaro C, Bhide A. Outcome of fetuses with prenatal diagnosis of isolated severe bilateral ventriculomegaly: systematic review and meta-analysis. Ultrasound Obstet Gynecol. 2018;52:165–73. Erratum in: Ultrasound Obstet Gynecol. 2018; 52:684
36. Manning FA, Harrison MR, Rodeck C. Catheter shunts for fetal hydronephrosis and hydrocephalus. Report of the international fetal surgery registry. N Engl J Med. 1986;315:336–40.
37. Litwinska M, Litwinska E, Czaj M, Polis B, Polis L, Szaflik K. Ventriculo-amniotic shunting for severe fetal ventriculomegaly. Acta Obstet Gynecol Scand. 2019;98:1172–7.
38. Start AO, Ryan GA, Cathcart B, Hughes H, Higgins S, Corcoran S, Walsh J, Carroll S, Mahony R, Crimmins D, Caird J, Colleran G, McParland P, McAuliffe FM. Severe fetal ventriculomegaly: fetal morbidity and mortality, caesarean delivery rates and obstetrical challenges in a large prospective cohort. Prenat Diagn. 2022;42:109–17.

Holoprosencephaly

Elisa Montaguti and Gianluigi Pilu

Abstract

Holoprosencephaly derives from failed or incomplete cleavage of the prosencephalon; it is featured by varying degrees of fusion of the cerebral hemispheres and has a very severe prognosis in most cases. The alobar form shows a great distortion of normal brain anatomy with a single cerebral ventricle. Its prenatal sonographic diagnosis is straightforward since early gestation, and it is frequently associated with other anomalies or genetic conditions. Lesser degrees of anatomic alteration are associated with more subtle ultrasound findings and may be difficult to recognize or categorize unless a careful evaluation of both cavum septi pellucidi and frontal horns as well is conducted. In semilobar and lobar forms, the septum pellucidum is typically absent in axial planes, with fused hypoplastic frontal horns, while posterior fossa is usually normal. A recently described entity is the interhemispheric variant, in which a separation of the lateral ventricles anteriorly and posteriorly is seen, with various degree of fusion in their middle part. At multiplanar neurosonogram, anomalies involving corpus callosum and cortex development can be detected.

Keywords

Holoprosencephaly · Forebrain · Ultrasound · Neurosonography · Cavum septi pellucidi

1 Definition

Holoprosencephaly is a heterogeneous disorder involving the development of the prosencephalon and midface, with the failure of forebrain division into two separate lobes. This disorder leads to various degrees of incomplete cleavage of hemispheres.

2 Epidemiology

This brain disorder has an incidence of approximately 1–1.7 per 10,000 viable and unviable births and terminations [1–3], but the real incidence is probably higher, because the most severe forms of holoprosencephaly may result in early

Supplementary Information The online version contains supplementary material available at https://doi.org/10.1007/978-3-031-70192-4_3.

E. Montaguti (✉) · G. Pilu
Obstetric Unit, IRCCS Azienda Ospedaliero-Universitaria di Bologna, Bologna, Italy
e-mail: gianluigi.pilu@aosp.bo.it

P. Volpe, T. Ghi (eds.), *Fetal Neurosonography*, Ultrasound in Obstetrics and Gynecology,
https://doi.org/10.1007/978-3-031-70192-4_3

pregnancy loss [4], while minor forms may will not be recognized before birth because of the subtle ultrasound findings, thus escaping epidemiologic surveys.

3 Etiology and Pathogenesis

The term "holoprosencephaly" refers to a group of complex brain malformation and is commonly regarded as the result of a failure of cleavage of the prosencephalon [5, 6]. The prosencephalon is the most rostral of the three primitive cerebral vesicles and gives rise to the cerebral hemispheres and diencephalic structures (including neurohypophysis, thalami, and third ventricle). This differentiation process is thought to be induced by the prechordal mesenchyma, which is probably also responsible for the differentiation of the median facial structures (forehead, nose, interorbital structures, premaxilla, and upper lip).

An interference with the activity of the prechordal mesenchyma would lead to defects in both areas, brain and midface. The cerebral anomalies are due to varying degrees of failure of cleavage of the derivatives of the prosencephalon, with incomplete division of the cerebral hemispheres and underlying structures. The facial anomalies encompass a broad range of defects that are due to aplasia or varying degrees of hypoplasia of the median structures. Holoprosencephaly indeed fits the definition of a malformative sequence, featuring both cerebral and facial anomalies.

Holoprosencephaly etiology is quite heterogeneous; most cases are of unknown cause, others are derived from chromosomal or monogenic disorders. There are no environmental teratogens known to cause this malformation in humans, but in animals the condition can be induced by veratrum alkaloids and radiation. Ingestion of salicylates, retinoic acid, and ethyl alcohol in pregnancy has also been reported in relation to holoprosencephaly.

Some metabolic factors, such as pregestational diabetes, have also been suggested to play a causal role in this disorder; nevertheless, most cases remain of unknown origin.

4 Genetic Background

The risk of chromosomal anomalies is high (from 25% to 50% of cases) [7–10], in particular is well known the association with trisomy 13 and triploidy [11–13]. The risk of non-chromosomal syndromes is high as well, and is related to at least 12 loci on 11 chromosomes. The known holoprosencephaly-associated genes include Sonic hedgehog (SHH) on 7q36(MIM 600725), ZIC2 on 13q32 (MIM 603073), SIX3 on 2p21 (MIM 603714), and TG-interacting factor (TGIF) on 18p11.3 (MIM 602630). Hereditary holoprosencephaly has been reported with autosomal dominant (MIM 142945), autosomal recessive (MIM 236100), and X linked recessive (MIM 306990) inheritance.

These genes are related to the Sonic hedgehog (SHH) pathway, a protein involved in the regulation of ventral neural tube development. Aberrancies in the cells expression of SHH may result in abnormalities of forebrain cleavage.

Syndromes that include holoprosencephaly among their manifestations are numerous: Grote, Steinfeld, Di George, Meckel-Gruber, Kallmann's, campomelic dysplasia, Hall-Pallister, and Vasadi among others.

5 Sonographic Findings

Holoprosencephaly is a continuum of malformations with progressive severity of degrees. A widely accepted classification recognizes four major varieties (Fig. 1): the alobar, semilobar, and lobar type [14]. A fourth variant, defined as middle interhemispheric, has also more recently been described [15–17].

- **Alobar**. In the alobar variety, the most severe one, the interhemispheric fissure and the falx cerebrii are totally absent and there is a single primitive ventricle (Figs. 2 and 3); this ventricle balloons out superiorly through the incompletely enfolded cortex and forms a large cyst, commonly referred to as the "dorsal sac" (Fig. 4). The thalami are fused on the midline, and there is absence of all the midline struc-

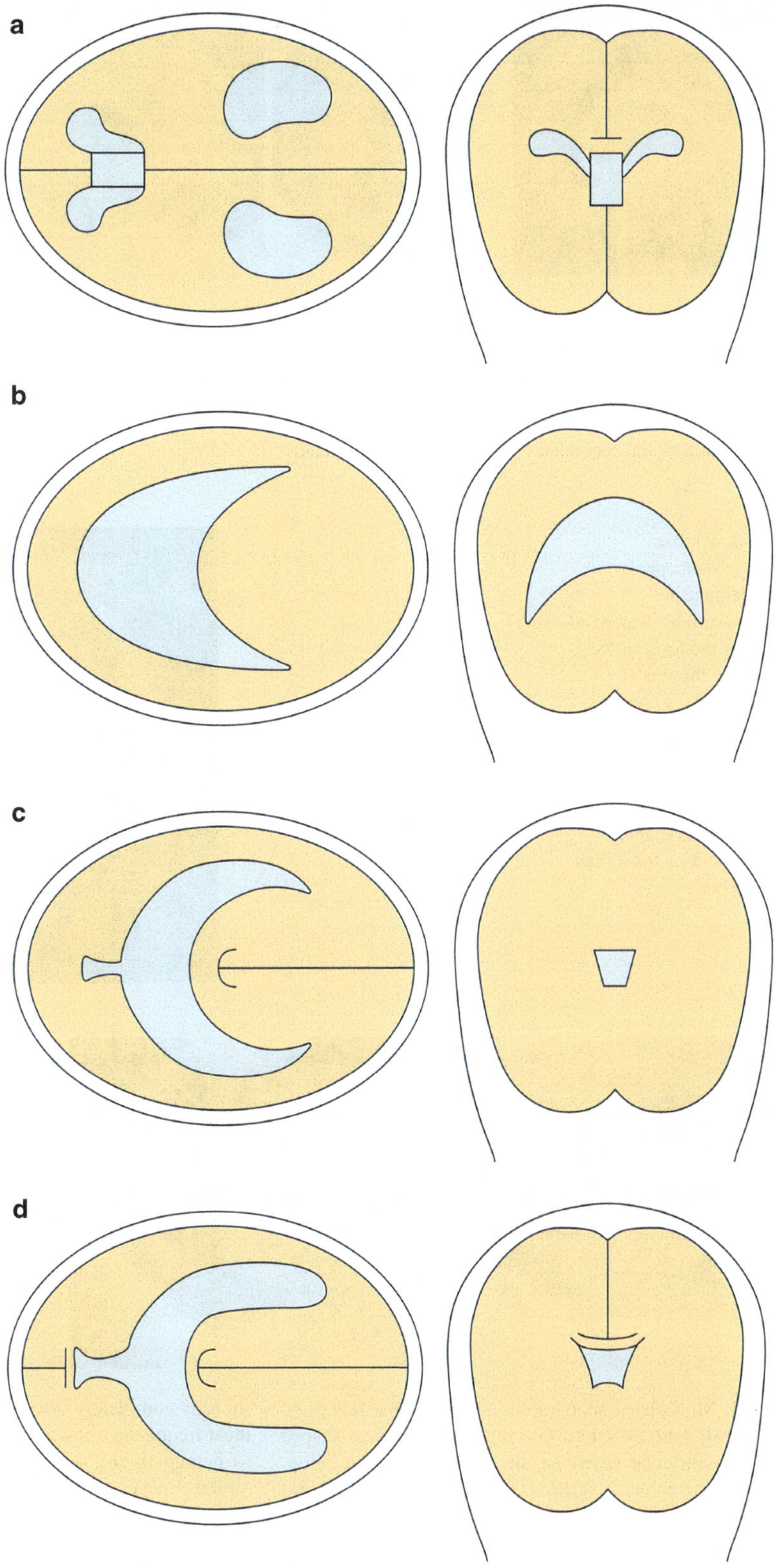

Fig. 1 Schematic representation of a normal brain compared with different varieties of holoprosencephaly. Normal brain (**a**): well-developed posterior ventricles, cavum septi pellucidi clearly separated from frontal horns. Alobar HPE (**b**): no interhemispheric fissure, single rudimentary ventricle, fused thalami, associated facial anomalies. Semilobar HPE (**c**): no midline structures in the anterior part of the brain. Lobar HPE (**d**): midline well developed but absence of the septum pellucidum and wide communication between frontal horns (modified from Montaguti E, Cariello L, Brunelli E, Youssef A, Livi A, Salsi G, Pilu G. Sonography of fetal holoprosencephaly: a guide to recognize the lesser varieties. J Matern Fetal Neonatal Med. 2022 Dec;35 (25):9717–9723)

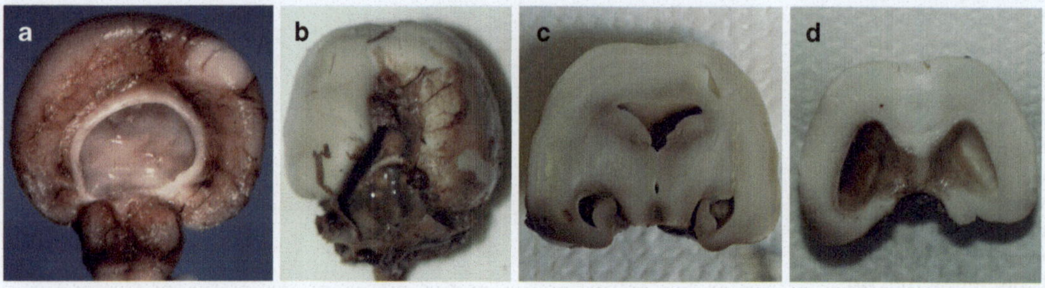

Fig. 2 Autoptic specimens of holoprosencephaly: (**a**) Alobar type: the brain mass is undivided and unfolded over the single rudimentary ventricular cavity; this appears in communication with a superior cystic cavity, the dorsal sac, whose thin wall was disrupted during the preparation of the specimen (courtesy of Philippe Jeanty, MD); (**b, c, d**) Semilobar type: the brain mass is divided only posteriorly; there is no anterior midline and a single ventricular cavity is present that however gives origin to separate posterior horns (courtesy of Paola Bonasoni, MD)

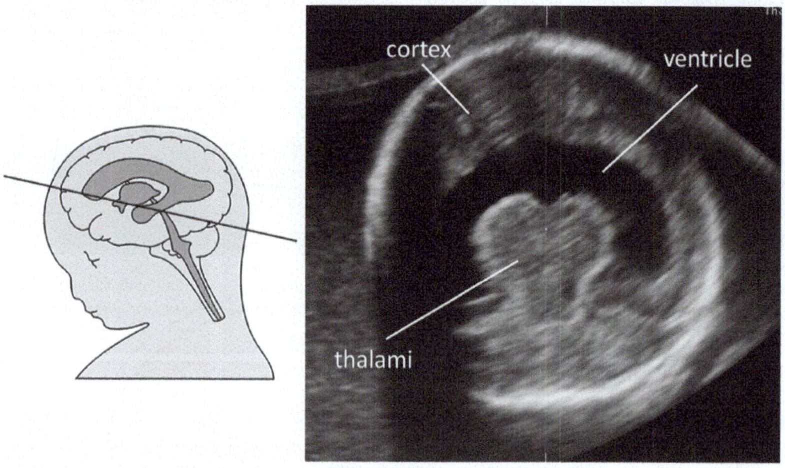

Fig. 3 Alobar holoprosencephaly appearance at midgestation: in an axial scan at the level of the thalami, there is no midline and a crescent-shaped ventricular cavity is seen between the anterior frontal cortex and the posterior bulb-shaped thalami. The posterior fossa may be normal

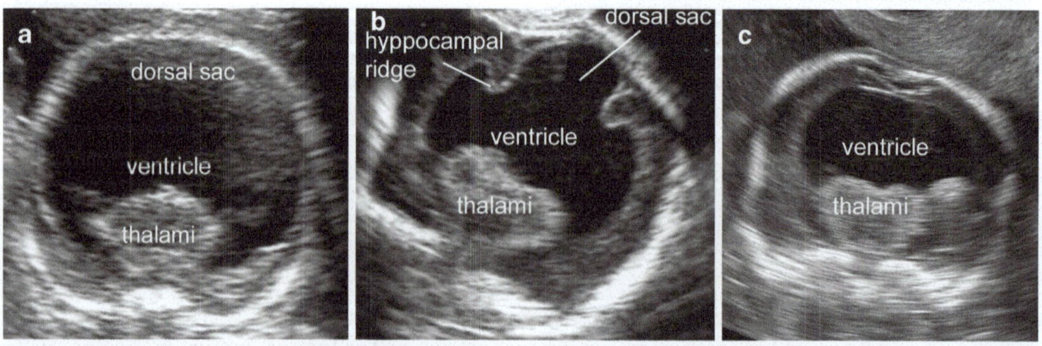

Fig. 4 Multiplanar sonography of fetal alobar holoprosencephaly with dorsal sacs on top of the crescent-shaped single ventricular cavity (**a, b**). The degree of development of the cortex is variable; (**a**) in some cases, it forms a thin rim at the base of the ventricles (pancake); (**b**) in some cases, it is more developed and is partially enfolded on top the ventricular cavity: (**c**) in some cases, the ventricle is completely covered and there is no dorsal sac; most frequently, these cases are pathologically diagnosed to belong to the semilobar variety. Modified from the Visual Encyclopedia of Ultrasound in Obstetrics and Gynecology, Pilu G, Malinger G, Chaoui R Holoprosenephaly. VISUOG, www.isuog.org, (January 2013)

tures, such as the interhemispheric fissure, the septum pellucidum, the corpus callosum, the third ventricle, neurohypophysis, olfactory bulbs, and tracts. The term arhinencephaly is indeed frequently used as a synonym of alobar holoprosencephaly. The alobar variant is also characterized by frequent associated anomalies, involving different fetal districts (i.e., face, heart, gastrointestinal, skeleton, and also kidneys). The sonographic findings of alobar holoprosencephaly are usually prominent and characterized by a major distortion of cerebral anatomy so that diagnosis is usually possible starting at around 9–10 weeks' gestation (Figs. 5 and 6) [18]. There is no midline echo, one central ventricular cavity and a typical bulb-like appearance of the thalami [14, 19–25]. The failure in the identification of the so-called butterfly sign during the first trimester ultrasound is an extremely sensitive and specific sign [23, 26, 27].

Demonstration of facial anomalies such as cyclopia, hypotelorism, and median cleft lip strengthens the diagnosis of holoprosencephaly based upon central nervous system findings (Figs. 7, 8, and 9). Conversely, should any of the mentioned facial features be serendipitously encountered, a careful examination of the intracranial contents is recommended [28].

- **Semilobar**. In the semilobar variety, the two cerebral hemispheres are partially separated posteriorly but there is still a single crescent-shaped ventricular cavity (Figs. 2 and 10). The single ventricular cavity divides posteriorly giving rise to posterior horns (Fig. 11); on the

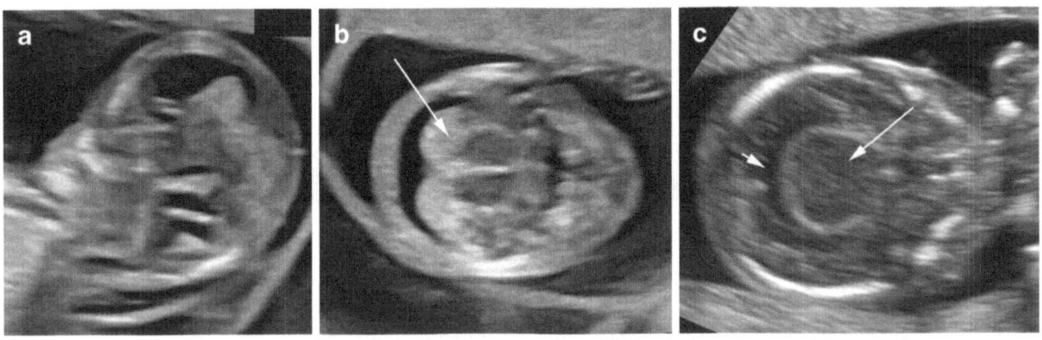

Fig. 5 Alobar holoprosencephaly in a 11 weeks' fetus: (**a**) Transabdominal scan demonstrating a flat face with no evidence of the nose; (**b**) in transabdominal axial scan of the fetal head, the midline echo is not seen and the choroid plexuses form a single undivided mass (arrow); (**c**) transvaginal coronal scan demonstrating a single crescent-shaped ventricular cavity (arrowhead) surrounding bulb-shaped undivided thalami (arrow)

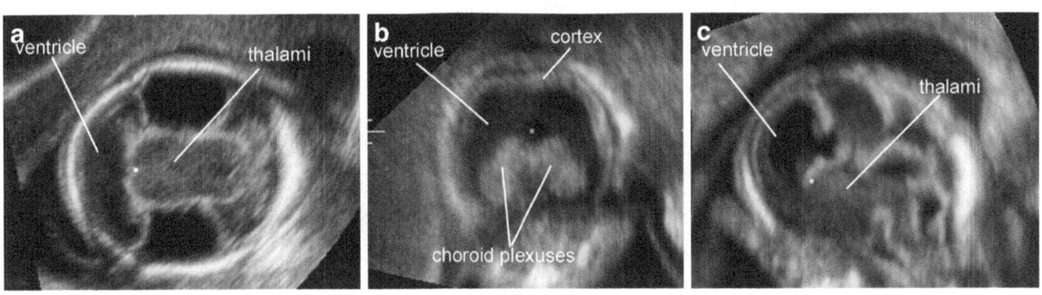

Fig. 6 High resolution transvaginal sonography of alobar holoprosencephaly in a 13 weeks fetus; the absence of the midline echo and the presence of a single rudimentary ventricular cavity are well demonstrated. (Modified from from: Tutschek B, Pilu G: Virtual reality ultrasound imaging of the normal and abnormal fetal central nervous system. Ultrasound Obstet Gynecol 2009 Sep;34(3):259–67)

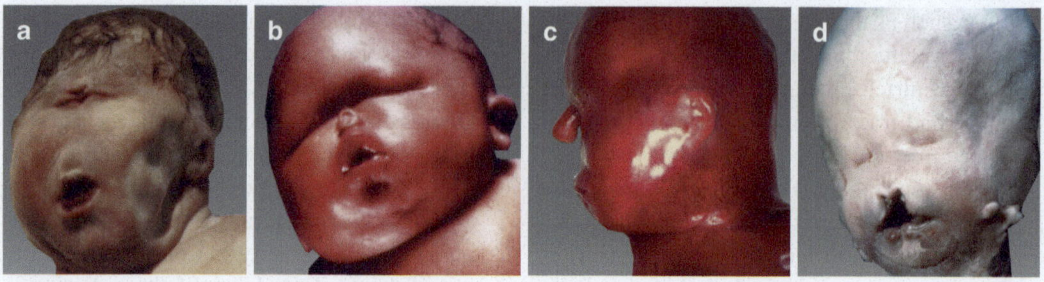

Fig. 7 Facial anomalies associated with alobar holoprosencephaly. (**a**) Cyclopia; (**b**) ethmocephaly; (**c**) cyclopia with proboscis; (**d**) median cleft lip with hypotelorism

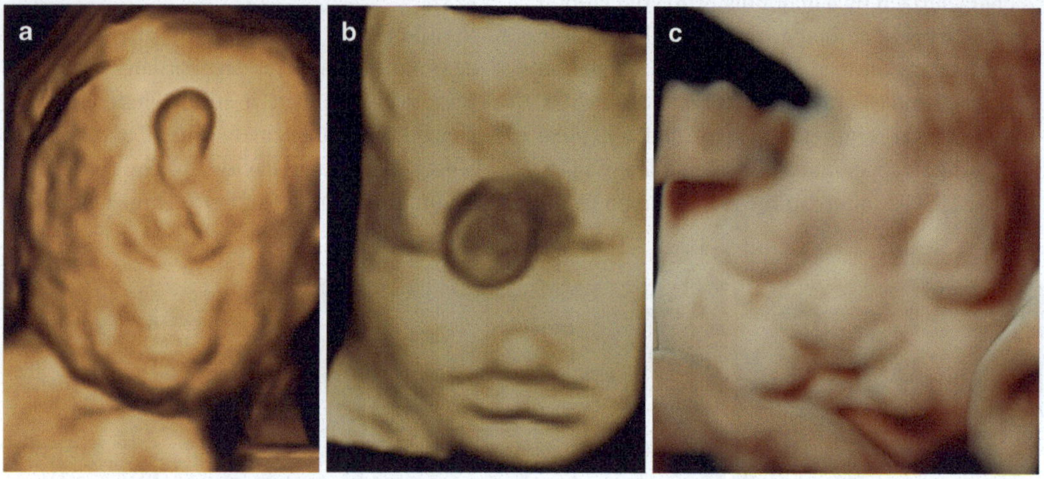

Fig. 8 Three-dimensional sonography of facial anomalies associated with alobar holoprosencephaly. (**a**) Cyclopia; (**b**) ethmocephaly; (**c**) median cleft lip and hypotelorism

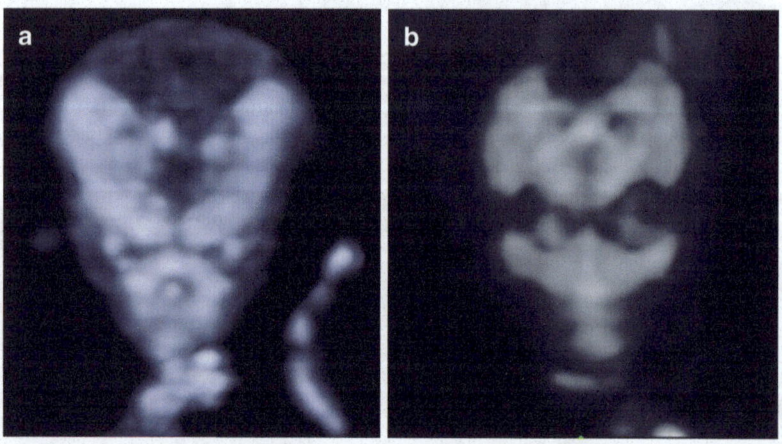

Fig. 9 Three-dimensional sonograms of the cranio-facial skeleton in a normal fetus (**a**) and in a case of alobar holoprosencephaly (**b**) at 12 weeks' gestation. In the normal fetus, the bregmatic fontanel and metopic sutures are large; in the holoprosencephalic fetus the bregmatic fontanel is restricted, the metopic suture is fused, and the orbits are close

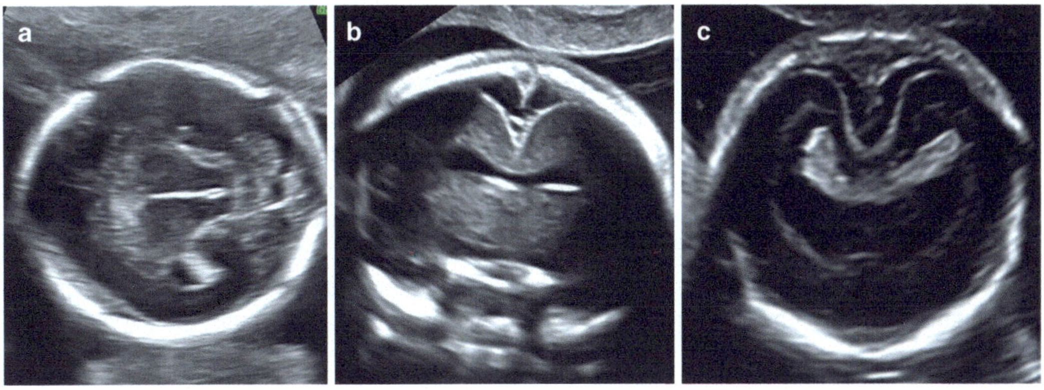

Fig. 10 Semilobar holoprosencephaly. (**a**) In the axial views, the most prominent finding is the complete absence of the cavum septi pellucidi and frontal horns. (**b**, **c**): a definitive diagnosis is made by demonstrating with multiplanar sonography that there is one single boomerang-shaped ventricular cavity

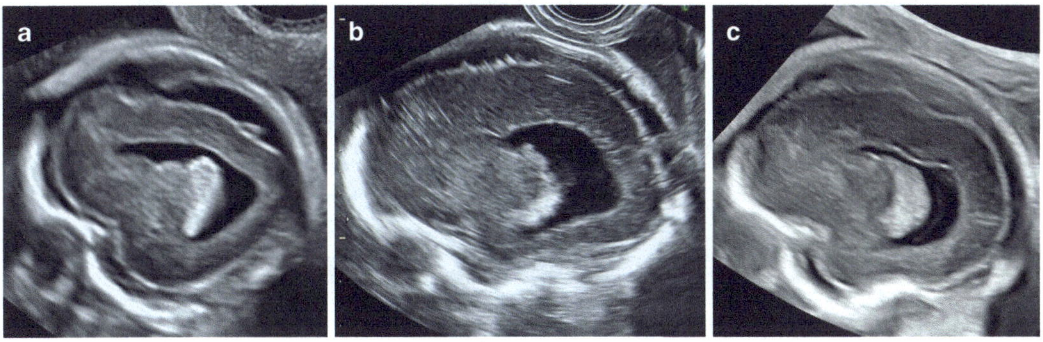

Fig. 11 Sagittal views demonstrating the posterior horns in midtrimester fetuses with semilobar (**a**) and lobar holoprosencephaly (**b**, **c**). The aspect is similar, and the images demonstrate ventricles with a rudimentary configuration lacking a well-developed occipital horn

contrary, anterior horns are absent. The interhemispheric fissure and the falx cerebri are present posteriorly, but there is no evidence of the midline in the anterior brain instead [29]. The thalami are partially fused, and there is a partial agenesis of corpus callosum. In axial views, commonly employed for screening the most remarkable finding is either the complete absence or no visualization of the anterior complex (frontal horns and cavum septi pellucidi).

The other types of classical holoprosencephaly are associated with similar, but less severe, sonographic findings that overlap, and differentiation with antenatal sonography is often difficult.

- **Lobar**. With lobar holoprosencephaly, the anatomical derangement is more subtle, as pathologic studies demonstrate that the brain is almost completely divided into two distinct hemispheres (Fig. 12), with the only exception of a variable degree of fusion at the level of the cingulate gyrus and frontal horns of lateral ventricles. The septum pellucidum is always absent, even if a squared cavity may be demonstrated. The olfactory bulbs and tracts and the corpus callosum may be present but not completely developed in particular in their anterior portion [29–32]. Differential diagnosis between lobar holoprosencephaly, agenesis of the septum pellucidum, and other conditions associated with absence of the septum pellucidum may not be immediate. A box-like structure interrupting the anterior midline resembling the cavum septi pellucidi could be seen in the axial views, but the frontal horns are not identified (Figs. 13, 14, and 15, Video 1).

Multiplanar sonography demonstrates the typical findings of lobar holoprosencephaly: incomplete separation of frontal lobes, with anterior midline present albeit incomplete, diminutive frontal horns without evidence of the septum pellucidum, fusion of the midbodies of the lateral ventricles that communicate amply with the inferior third ventricle, an irregular corpus callosum-like structure, and anterior displacement of the loop formed by the anterior cerebral arteries.

The most consistent finding is however the presence of a large communication between the bodies of the lateral ventricles and a parenchymal bridge connecting the parietal lobes,

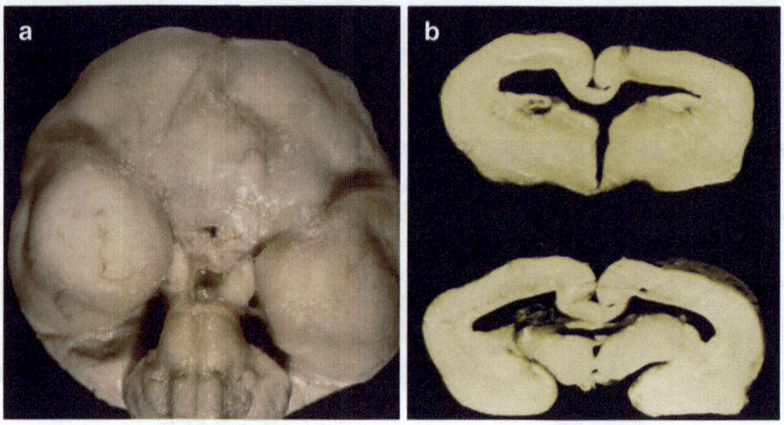

Fig. 12 Autoptic specimen of lobar holoprosencephaly. (**a**) The frontal lobes are fused inferiorly; note the absence of the olfactory tracts; (**b**) coronal sections demonstrating a single ventricular cavity. (Modified from: Pilu G, Sandri F, Perolo A, Giangaspero F, Cocchi G, Salvioli GP, Bovicelli L. Prenatal diagnosis of lobar holoprosencephaly. Ultrasound Obstet Gynecol. 1992 Mar 1;2 [2]:88–94)

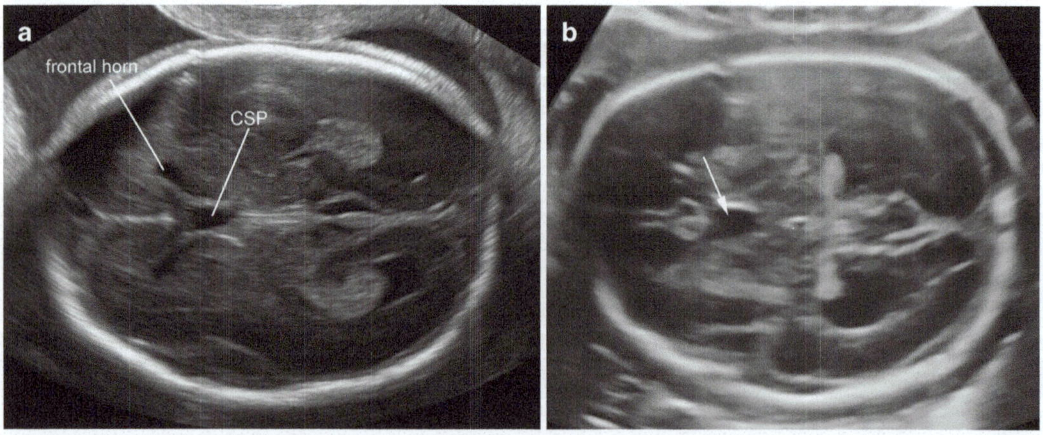

Fig. 13 In a basic sonographic examination, the findings of lobar holoprosencephaly are subtle and may be easily overlooked. Compared to normal (**a**), the most important clue is probably the absence of the complex formed by frontal horns and cavum septi pellucidi (CSP). In its place, only a square shaped fluid filled area is seen (**b**, arrow) resembling the cavity of the septum pellucidum but representing the most anterior part of the single ventricular cavity. Frontal horns are either diminutive or not seen

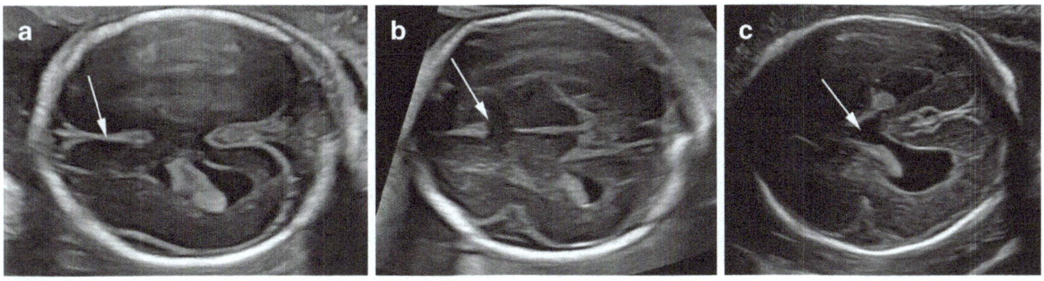

Fig. 14 Lobar holoprosencephaly in the axial planes. (**a**) The midline echo is present anteriorly; (**b**) the complex formed by frontal horns and interposed cavum septi pellucidi is not present and only a square shaped quadrangular area representing the most anterior part of the ventricular cavity is seen; (**c**) posterior horns are present but they converge anteriorly into a single anterior cavity (arrow)

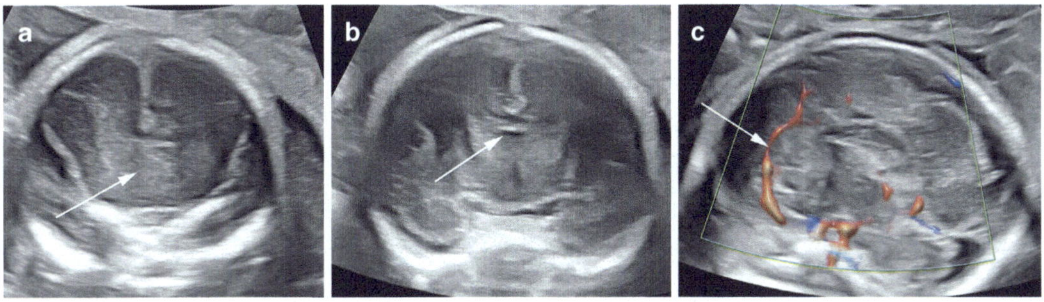

Fig. 15 A case of lobar holoprosencephaly in coronal and sagittal planes at midgestation ultrasound examination. (**a**) The midline is present but incomplete with inferior fusion of the frontal lobes (arrow); (**b**) the complex formed by frontal horns and cavum septi pellucidi is not seen and a only a small quadrangular fluid filled area is seen on the midline, representing the most anterior part of the ventricular cavity; (**c**) the anterior cerebral artery runs on the surface of the brain

which can be easily demonstrated in an axial view slightly superior to the standard transventricular plane (Fig. 16). In general, the axial and coronal scan are most helpful. Median planes demonstrate the absence of the complex formed by corpus callosum, cavum septi pellucidi, and third ventricle but these findings usually are not specific (Fig. 17).

Additional findings that are consistently present and may corroborate the diagnosis include: color Doppler demonstration that the anterior cerebral artery is displaced under the skull, running more anteriorly than normal, along the surface of the undivided frontal lobes rather than the within the interhemispheric fissure ("serpent crawling under the skull" sign, Fig. 15) [33].

- The middle interhemispheric variant of holoprosencephaly is intermediate between the lobar and alobar variety (Fig. 18). When compared to the alobar variety, the frontal lobes are more differentiated than usual with recognizable frontal horns but the cavum septi pellucidi is typically absent. The basal forebrain, anterior frontal, and occipital lobes are normally separated, while the posterior parts of the frontal lobe and the parietal lobe are partially fused. Posteriorly, however, there is one single ventricular cavity with a hypoplastic diencephalon [15]. Similarly lateral ventricles are divided anteriorly and posteriorly, with various degree of fusion in the middle part.

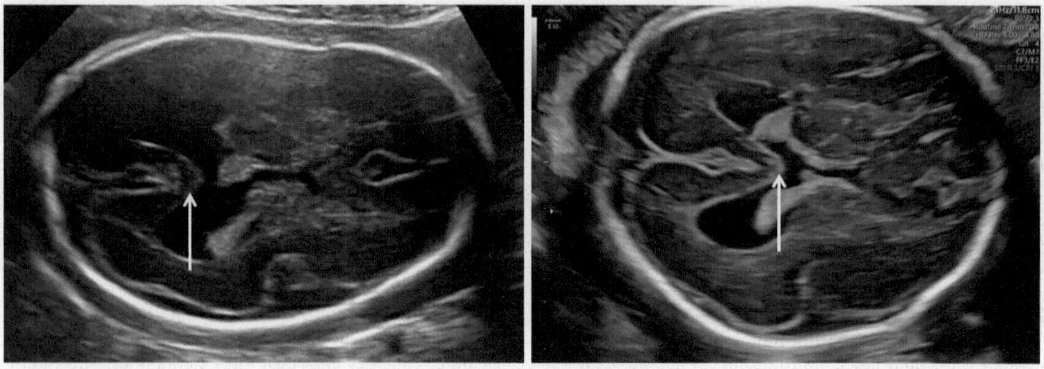

Fig. 16 Third trimester ultrasound of two cases of lobar holoprosencephaly. A large communication between the bodies of the lateral ventricles and a characteristic parenchymal bridge between the parietal lobes (arrows) can be demonstrated in an axial view slightly superior to the standard transventricular plane

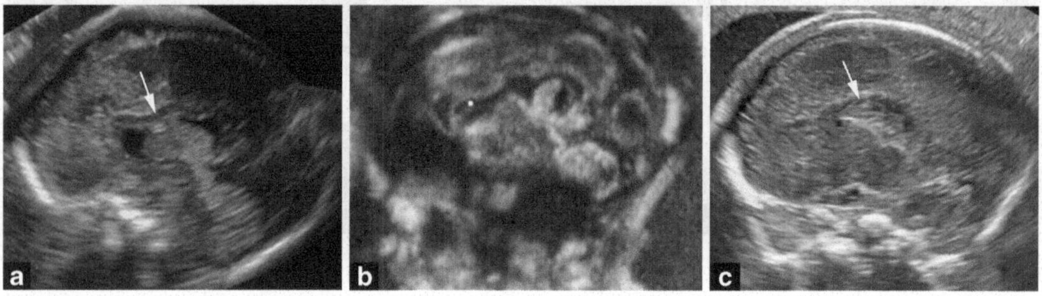

Fig. 17 Lobar holoprosencephaly. The median scans demonstrate abnormal anatomy but are not specific. The corpus callosum is not clearly seen (**b**) and in Figures **a** and **c** an irregular ridge of tissue is seen bridging the hemispheres posteriorly (arrow)

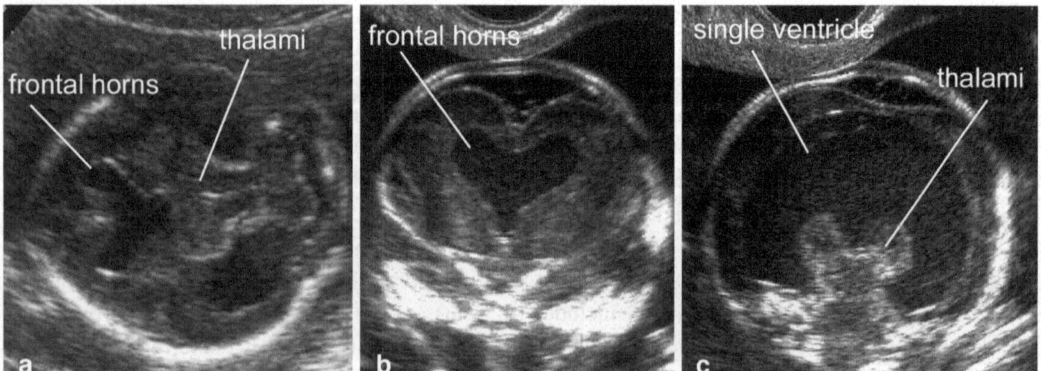

Fig. 18 Middle interhemispheric variant of holoprosencephaly in the axial (**a**), anterior coronal (**b**), and midcoronal plane (**c**). The frontal horns are well developed, and there is a partial formation of the interhemispheric fissure. However, the midcoronal plane reveals a common ventricular cavity with hypoplastic undivided thalami

6 Associated Anomalies

Holoprosencephaly reflects a very early derangement of embryogenesis and is very frequently associated with other malformations [7, 14]. Apart from facial anomalies, that are considered a part of the malformative sequence, and other telencephalic anomalies such as interhemispheric cysts and lipomas, holoprosencephaly has a striking association with two other conditions: chromosomal aberrations and Dandy–Walker malformation. The list of chromosomal aberrations found in patients with holoprosencephaly includes more than 35 conditions, but among them only seven are frequently described: Trisomy 13, del(13q), del(18p), Trisomy 18, Tripoidy, dup(3p), and del (pter+q32) [7]. It has been estimated that over 60% of infants with trisomy 13 have holoprosencephaly; conversely, holoprosencephaly is associated with trisomy 13 in about 20% of cases [12]. Holoprosencephaly is often associated with microcephaly, less frequently with macrocephaly, which is invariably due to internal obstructive hydrocephalus.

Extracranial malformation may also be present and include renal dysplasia or cysts, omphalocele, congenital heart disease, clubfoot, myelomeningocele, and intestinal abnormalities.

Pleomorphic facial anomalies are a part of the holoprosencephaly sequence (Figs. 7, 8, 9, and 19) [28]. In particular are described: cyclopia (single eye or single orbit, arrhinia with proboscis), ethmocephaly (extreme hypotelorism and arrhinia with proboscis), cebocephaly (orbital hypotelorism, proboscis like nose, no cleft), median cleft with flat nose, and hypotelorism, agnathia-astomia (hypoplasia or absence of the mandible, small or absent mouth, abnormal position of the ears).

Facial anomalies are usually encountered with the alobar and semilobar types, rarely with lobar holoprosencephaly, in which facial findings may be more subtle or even normal. Flat profile with hypotelorism is described, but the presence of a single median incisor tooth is the most remarkable in our own experience and a single maxillary incisor may be detected even in prenatal life (Figs. 19 and 20) [14, 29, 30].

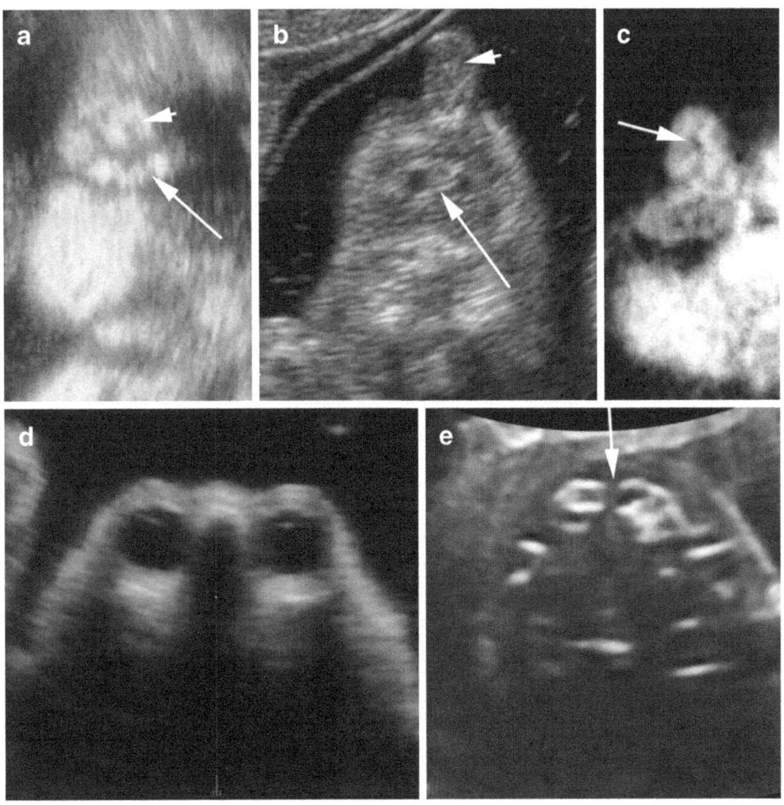

Fig. 19 Two-dimensional sonography of facial anomalies associated with alobar holoprosencephaly. (**a**, **b**) Cyclopia: proboscis (arrowhead) and single orbit (arrow); (**c**) proboscis with single central cavity (arrow); (**d**) hypotelorism; (**e**) median cleft lip and palate (arrow)

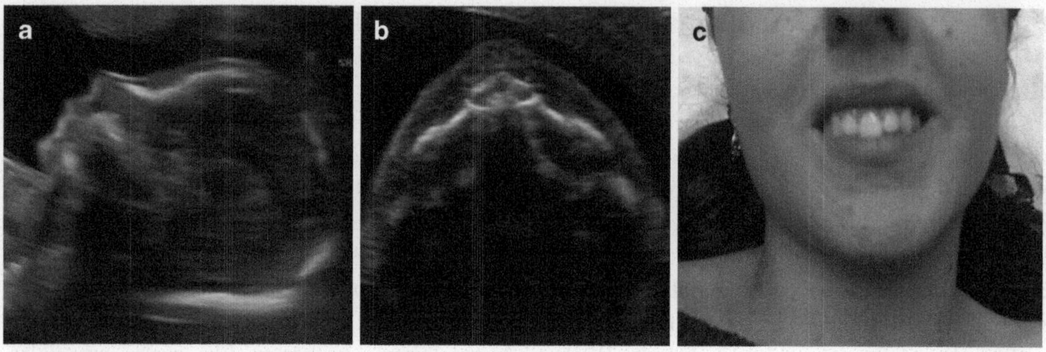

Fig. 20 Subtle cranio-facial anomalies with lobar holoprosencephaly. (**a**) The profile is flat; (**b**) there is one single median incisor tooth; (**c**) an adult with single median incisor tooth

7 Differential Diagnosis

Alobar holoprosencephaly with a large ventricular cavity and/or dorsal sac has an appearance similar to that of hydranencephaly. The demonstration of remmnants of the frontal cortex, the presence of a dorsal sac, fused thalami, and facial anomalies allow a clear distinction between these two entities, but, from a practical perspective, a diagnostic error would be anyhow uneventful given the very poor prognosis of both conditions.

Another condition that should be ruled out is severe hydrocephalus, where an acquired communication between ventricles and secondary disruption of the falx and of the cavum septi pellucidi occurs. The separation of the thalami and the absence of facial anomalies are suggestive of this condition instead of holoprosencephaly.

The diagnosis of lobar variants is more challenging; lobar holoprosencephaly must be distinguished from isolated absence of the septum pellucidum and other entities associated with it (schizencephaly, secondary disruption of the cerebral falx, septo-optic dysplasia) [34–41]. In our experience, coronal views are the most informative (Fig. 21), allowing to identify the three findings that are typical of lobar holoprosencephaly: incomplete cleavage of the hemispheres, absent or diminutive frontal horns, and fusion of the bodies of lateral ventricles. The attention must be focused on the anterior complex, in particular on the frontal horns which are well developed in the other mentioned conditions but are rudimental in holoprosencephaly [42, 43].

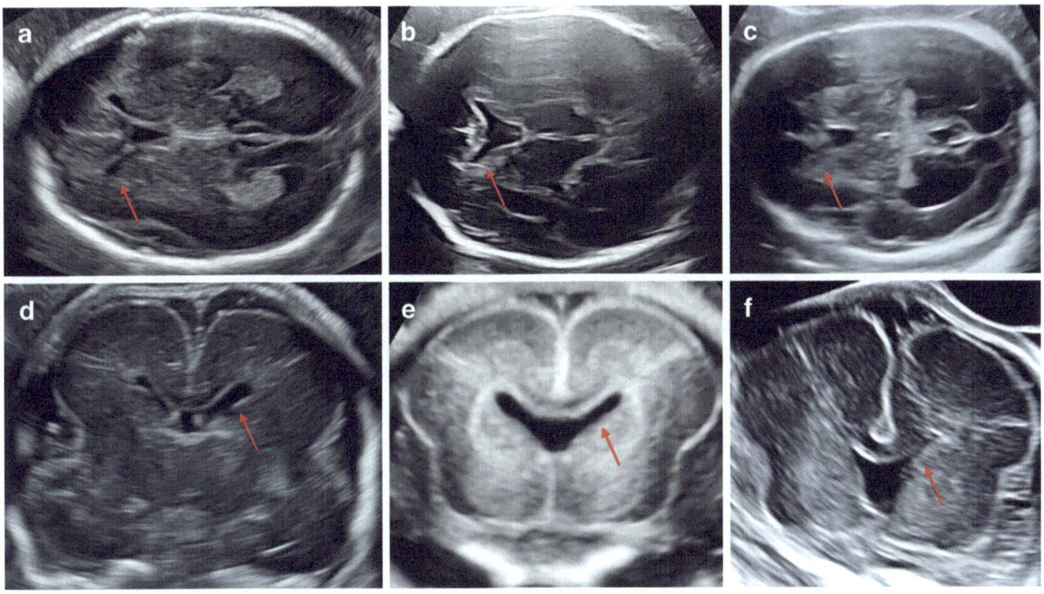

Fig. 21 Sagittal and coronal scan helping the differential diagnosis of lobar holoprosencephaly. (**a–d**) normal fetal brain with a present cavum septi pellucidi and well-developed frontal horns (arrows). (**b–e**) In case of isolated agenesis of cavum septi pellucidi (CSP), the frontal horns are well developed as well, but not separated by the membranes of SP. (**c–f**) Instead in case of lobar holoprosencephaly, frontal horns are hyphoplastic and the box-like structure resembling the CSP is the anterior part of the fused ventricle

8 Magnetic Resonance

The sonographic findings of alobar holoprosencephaly are obvious, and the diagnosis is usually straightforward. Fetal MRI in these cases is hardly necessary, but it may be helpful with types associated with lesser degree of anatomic derangement [44–46]. A clear cut differentiation among semilobar, lobar, and middle interhemispheric variant may however be difficult even with MRI.

However, MRI plays an important role in the detection of cortical folding abnormalities which could be associated with the less severe forms (Fig. 22).

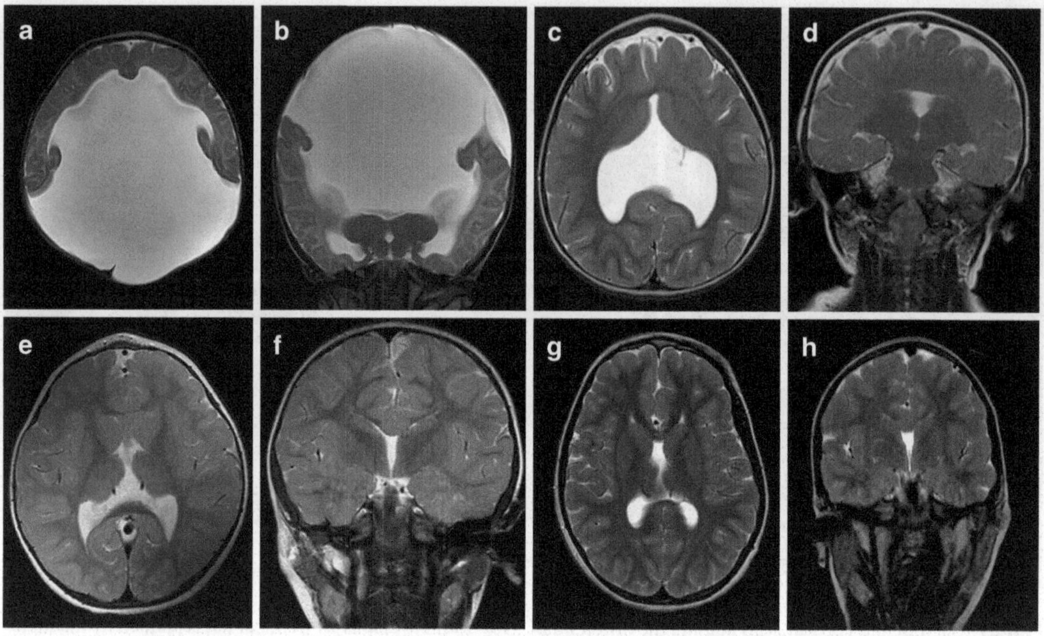

Fig. 22 Magnetic resonance imaging axial and coronal views of holoprosencephaly: (**a**, **b**) Alobar type: the brain mass is undivided and there is a large central ventricular cavity communicating superiorly with a dorsal sac. (Case courtesy of Dr. Ammar Haouimi, Radiopaedia.org, rID: 72035). (**c**, **d**) Semilobar type; the hemispheres are fused anteriorly and partly divided posteriorly; there is a single ventricular cavity from which two posterior horns originate. (Case courtesy of Dr. Ian Bickle, Radiopaedia.org, rID: 23218). (**e**, **f**) Lobar holoprosencephaly; the frontal lobes are incompletely divided superiorly; there is single ventricular cavity that however originates diminutive frontal horns and well-developed posterior horn. (Case courtesy of Assoc Prof Frank Gaillard, Radiopaedia.org, rID: 10511). (**g**, **h**) Middle variant of holoprosencephaly; in the axial and coronal planes, the findings are very similar to the lobar type. (Case courtesy of Prof Frank Gaillard, Radiopaedia.org, rID: 6690)

9 Prognosis

Alobar holoprosencephaly is lethal, and most fetuses affected miscarry spontaneously, albeit occasional cases with long survival have been described. In those with non-syndromic isolated alobar forms, the half would die within a few months of life and the remaining will suffer of extreme developmental delay [22, 47]. Semilobar holoprosencephaly is not necessarily lethal, but is associated with extremely severe neurologic compromise. Symptoms are evident since the neonatal period, with generalized hypotonia and frequent seizures, frequently unresponsive to medications, mental retardation, and feeding problems due to neurologically uncoordinated swallowing. Endocrine defects such as panhypopituitarism, growth hormone deficit, or diabetes insipidus are quite often associated with these conditions. Those cases with associated chromosomal abnormalities or syndromes have a worse outcome [48–50].

The prognosis of lobar holoprosencephaly is uncertain, and the available clinical data are limited. It has been reported that affected individuals may have a normal life span and well-developed language skills, but mental retardation and neurologic sequelae are common. Dysplasia of the aqueduct of Sylvius may be present, leading to obstructive hydrocephalus [21].

10 Obstetric Management and Options of Treatments

Genetic consultation is mandatory when holoprosencephaly is discovered by ultrasound; fetal karyotype assessment and chromosomal microarray analysis (CMA) should be offered to parents [10].

In recent days, when karyotype and CMA are normal, whole exome sequencing (WES, the sequencing of the protein-coding regions of genes) is proposed in some realities, even if not available in every setting and not always compatible with the timing of prenatal diagnosis [22].

Holoprosenephaly with normal chromosomes has an estimated recurrence risk in siblings of 6%, but this calculation is derived from sporadic events, while hereditary identified conditions have a recurrence risk of 25–50% [7]. It is important to recognize that in autosomal dominant cases, one of the parents may present with previously unrecognized mild features of holoprosencephaly as mild hypotelorism or a single incisor [8, 9], so the clinical analysis and the collection of family history are crucial.

Moreover, as the chance of a syndromic condition is quite high, a detailed ultrasound searching additional anomalies is required.

Termination of pregnancy can be offered to parents when legally permitted, as well as a pediatric, neuropediatric, and obstetric multidisciplinary counseling.

In continuing pregnancies, no modification of standard obstetriccare is required and a conservative management is recommended. Mode of delivery should be chosen according to standard obstetric indications, but the delivery should occur in a center with pediatric neurology experience.

References

1. Dubourg C, Bendavid C, Pasquier L, Henry C, Odent S, David V. Holoprosencephaly. Orphanet J Rare Dis. 2007;2:8.
2. Forrester MB, Merz RD. Epidemiology of holoprosencephaly in Hawaii, 1986-97. Paediatr Perinat Epidemiol. 2000;14(1):61–3.
3. Ong S, Tonks A, Woodward ER, Wyldes MP, Kilby MD. An epidemiological study of holoprosencephaly from a regional congenital anomaly register: 1995-2004. Prenat Diagn. 2007;27(4):340–7.
4. Matsunaga E, Shiota K. Holoprosencephaly in human embryos: epidemiologic studies of 150 cases. Teratology. 1977;16(3):261–72.
5. Volpe P, Campobasso G, De Robertis V, Rembouskos G. Disorders of prosencephalic development. Prenat Diagn. 2009;29(4):340–54.
6. Winter TC, Kennedy AM, Woodward PJ. Holoprosencephaly: a survey of the entity, with embryology and fetal imaging. Radiographics. 2015;35(1):275–90.
7. Cohen MM Jr. Perspectives on holoprosencephaly: part I. Epidemiology, genetics, and syndromology. Teratology. 1989;40(3):211–35.
8. Dubourg C, Kim A, Watrin E, de Tayrac M, Odent S, David V, Dupé V. Recent advances in understanding inheritance of holoprosencephaly. Am J Med Genet C Semin Med Genet. 2018;178(2):258–69.
9. Mercier S, Dubourg C, Garcelon N, Campillo-Gimenez B, Gicquel I, Belleguic M, Ratié L, Pasquier L, Loget P, Bendavid C, Jaillard S, Rochard L, Quélin C, Dupé V, David V, Odent S. New findings for phenotype-genotype correlations in a large European series of holoprosencephaly cases. J Med Genet. 2011;48(11):752–60.
10. Bendavid C, Rochard L, Dubourg C, Seguin J, Gicquel I, Pasquier L, Vigneron J, Laquerrière A, Marcorelles P, Jeanne-Pasquier C, Rouleau C, Jaillard S, Mosser J, Odent S, David V. Array-CGH analysis indicates a high prevalence of genomic rearrangements in holoprosencephaly: an updated map of candidate loci. Hum Mutat. 2009;30(8):1175–82.
11. Rizzo N, Pittalis MC, Pilu G, Orsini LF, Perolo A, Bovicelli L. Prenatal karyotyping in malformed fetuses. Prenat Diagn. 1990;10(1):17–23.
12. Rizzo N, Pittalis MC, Pilu G, Perolo A, Banzi C, Visentin A, Bovicelli L. Distribution of abnormal karyotypes among malformed fetuses detected by ultrasound throughout gestation. Prenat Diagn. 1996;16(2):159–63.
13. Solomon BD, Rosenbaum KN, Meck JM, Muenke M. Holoprosencephaly due to numeric chromosome abnormalities. Am J Med Genet C Semin Med Genet. 2010;154c(1):146–8.
14. Blaas HG, Eriksson AG, Salvesen KA, Isaksen CV, Christensen B, Møllerløkken G, Eik-Nes SH. Brains and faces in holoprosencephaly: pre- and postnatal description of 30 cases. Ultrasound Obstet Gynecol. 2002;19(1):24–38.
15. Lewis AJ, Simon EM, Barkovich AJ, Clegg NJ, Delgado MR, Levey E, Hahn JS. Middle interhemispheric variant of holoprosencephaly: a distinct cliniconeuroradiologic subtype. Neurology. 2002;59(12):1860–5.
16. Malinger G, Lev D, Kidron D, Heredia F, Hershkovitz R, Lerman-Sagie T. Differential diagnosis in fetuses with absent septum pellucidum. Ultrasound Obstet Gynecol. 2005;25(1):42–9.
17. Picone O, Hirt R, Suarez B, Coulomb A, Tachdjian G, Frydman R, Senat MV. Prenatal diagnosis of a possible new middle interhemispheric variant of holoprosencephaly using sonographic and magnetic resonance imaging. Ultrasound Obstet Gynecol. 2006;28(2):229–31.

18. Bronshtein M, Wiener Z. Early transvaginal sonographic diagnosis of alobar holoprosencephaly. Prenat Diagn. 1991;11(7):459–62.
19. Kousa YA, du Plessis AJ, Vezina G. Prenatal diagnosis of holoprosencephaly. Am J Med Genet C Semin Med Genet. 2018;178(2):206–13.
20. Pilu G, Romero R, Rizzo N, Jeanty P, Bovicelli L, Hobbins JC. Criteria for the prenatal diagnosis of holoprosencephaly. Am J Perinatol. 1987;4(1):41–9.
21. Pilu G, Sandri F, Perolo A, Giangaspero F, Cocchi G, Salvioli GP, Bovicelli L. Prenatal diagnosis of lobar holoprosencephaly. Ultrasound Obstet Gynecol. 1992;2(2):88–94.
22. Monteagudo A, Kuller JA, Craigo S, Fox NS, Norton ME, Rotmensch S, Ward A, Yeaton-Massey A. SMFM fetal anomalies consult series #3: intracranial anomalies. Am J Obstet Gynecol. 2020;223(6):B2–b46.
23. Sepulveda W, Wong AE. First trimester screening for holoprosencephaly with choroid plexus morphology ('butterfly' sign) and biparietal diameter. Prenat Diagn. 2013;33(13):1233–7.
24. Blaas HG. Holoprosencephaly at 10 weeks 2 days (CRL 33 mm). Ultrasound Obstet Gynecol. 2000;15(1):86–7.
25. Blaas HG, Eik-Nes SH, Vainio T, Isaksen CV. Alobar holoprosencephaly at 9 weeks gestational age visualized by two- and three-dimensional ultrasound. Ultrasound Obstet Gynecol. 2000;15(1):62–5.
26. Malinger G, Paladini D, Haratz KK, Monteagudo A, Pilu GL, Timor-Tritsch IE. ISUOG practice guidelines (updated): sonographic examination of the fetal central nervous system. Part 1: performance of screening examination and indications for targeted neurosonography. Ultrasound Obstet Gynecol. 2020;56(3):476–84.
27. Paladini D, Malinger G, Birnbaum R, Monteagudo A, Pilu G, Salomon LJ, Timor-Tritsch IE. ISUOG practice guidelines (updated): sonographic examination of the fetal central nervous system. Part 2: performance of targeted neurosonography. Ultrasound Obstet Gynecol. 2021;57(4):661–71.
28. Demyer W, Zeman W, Palmer CG. The face predicts the brain: diagnostic significance of median facial anomalies for holoprosencephaly (arhinencephaly). Pediatrics. 1964;34:256–63.
29. Montaguti E, Cariello L, Brunelli E, Youssef A, Livi A, Salsi G, Pilu G. Sonography of fetal holoprosencephaly: a guide to recognize the lesser varieties. J Matern Fetal Neonatal Med. 2022;35:9717–23.
30. Montaguti E, Brunelli E, Pilu G. A case of lobar holoprosencephaly: brain and facial typical features. Am J Obstet Gynecol. 2021;225(4):446–7.
31. Pilu G, Ambrosetto P, Sandri F, Tani G, Perolo A, Grisolia G, Ancora G. Intraventricular fused fornices: a specific sign of fetal lobar holoprosencephaly. Ultrasound Obstet Gynecol. 1994;4(1):65–7.
32. Visentin A, Pilu G, Falco P, Bovicelli L. The transfrontal view: a new approach to the visualization of the fetal midline cerebral structures. J Ultrasound Med. 2001;20(4):329–33.
33. Bernard JP, Drummond CL, Zaarour P, Molho M, Ville Y. A new clue to the prenatal diagnosis of lobar holoprosencephaly: the abnormal pathway of the anterior cerebral artery crawling under the skull. Ultrasound Obstet Gynecol. 2002;19(6):605–7.
34. Borkowski-Tillman T, Garcia-Rodriguez R, Viñals F, Branco M, Kradjen-Haratz K, Ben-Sira L, Lerman-Sagie T, Malinger G. Agenesis of the septum pellucidum: prenatal diagnosis and outcome. Prenat Diagn. 2020;40(6):674–80.
35. Falco P, Gabrielli S, Visentin A, Perolo A, Pilu G, Bovicelli L. Transabdominal sonography of the cavum septum pellucidum in normal fetuses in the second and third trimesters of pregnancy. Ultrasound Obstet Gynecol. 2000;16(6):549–53.
36. Malinger G, Lev D, Oren M, Lerman-Sagie T. Non-visualization of the cavum septi pellucidi is not synonymous with agenesis of the corpus callosum. Ultrasound Obstet Gynecol. 2012;40(2):165–70.
37. Pilu G, Tani G, Carletti A, Malaigia S, Ghi T, Rizzo N. Difficult early sonographic diagnosis of absence of the fetal septum pellucidum. Ultrasound Obstet Gynecol. 2005;25(1):70–2.
38. Ward A, Monteagudo A. Absent Cavum Septi Pellucidi. Am J Obstet Gynecol. 2020;223(6):B23–b6.
39. Webb EA, Dattani MT. Septo-optic dysplasia. Eur J Hum Genet. 2010;18(4):393–7.
40. Lee W, Comstock CH, Kazmierczak C, Wilson J, Gonçalves LF, Mody S, Yeo L, Romero R. Prenatal diagnostic challenges and pitfalls for schizencephaly. J Ultrasound Med. 2009;28(10):1379–84.
41. Lepinard C, Coutant R, Boussion F, Loisel D, Delorme B, Biquard F, Bonneau D, Guichet A, Descamps P. Prenatal diagnosis of absence of the septum pellucidum associated with septo-optic dysplasia. Ultrasound Obstet Gynecol. 2005;25(1):73–5.
42. Cagneaux M, Guibaud L. From cavum septi pellucidi to anterior complex: how to improve detection of midline cerebral abnormalities. Ultrasound Obstet Gynecol. 2013;42(4):485–6.
43. Winter TC, Kennedy AM, Byrne J, Woodward PJ. The cavum septi pellucidi: why is it important? J Ultrasound Med. 2010;29(3):427–44.
44. Griffiths PD, Jarvis D. In utero MR imaging of fetal holoprosencephaly: a structured approach to diagnosis and classification. AJNR Am J Neuroradiol. 2016;37(3):536–43.
45. Hahn JS, Barnes PD. Neuroimaging advances in holoprosencephaly: refining the spectrum of the midline malformation. Am J Med Genet C Semin Med Genet. 2010;154c(1):120–32.
46. Riddle A, Nagaraj U, Hopkin RJ, Kline-Fath B, Venkatesan C. Fetal magnetic resonance imaging (MRI) in Holoprosencephaly and associations with clinical outcome: implications for fetal counseling. J Child Neurol. 2021;36(5):357–64.
47. Damaj L, Bruneau B, Ferry M, Moutard ML, Garel C, Odent S, Adamsbaum C, Avni F, Tréguier C, Lazaro L. Pediatric outcome of children with the prenatal

diagnosis of isolated septal agenesis. Prenat Diagn. 2010;30(12–13):1143–50.
48. Hahn JS, Plawner LL. Evaluation and management of children with holoprosencephaly. Pediatr Neurol. 2004;31(2):79–88.
49. Kaliaperumal C, Ndoro S, Mandiwanza T, Reidy F, McAuliffe F, Caird J, Crimmins D. Holoprosencephaly: antenatal and postnatal diagnosis and outcome. Childs Nerv Syst. 2016;32(5):801–9.
50. Kauvar EF, Muenke M. Holoprosencephaly: recommendations for diagnosis and management. Curr Opin Pediatr. 2010;22(6):687–95.

Corpus Callosum Malformations

Ruben Ramirez Zegarra, Andrea Dall'Asta, Nicola Volpe, Elvira Di Pasquo, and Tullio Ghi

Abstract

Corpus callosum malformations represent one of the most common congenital malformations of the central nervous system detected prenatally. Several abnormalities can affect the corpus callosum including complete or partial agenesis as well as dysgenesis. These malformations may occur in isolation or be associated with a broad spectrum of cranial or extracranial anomalies or genetic disorders. Among the most prevalent brain malformations associated with this condition are malformations of cortical development, ventriculomegaly, and posterior fossa anomalies. Additionally, both chromosomal and single-gene disorders have been identified in fetuses affected by corpus callosum malformations. The initial diagnostic approach typically involves ultrasound and magnetic resonance imaging to identify and classify corpus callosum malformations, as well as to detect associated cerebral and/or extracerebral anomalies. Invasive genetic testing may also be employed to confirm or rule out the presence of any genetic syndromes. The prognosis of this condition varies widely, ranging from favorable neurodevelopmental outcomes to severe neurologic disability. Fetuses with isolated corpus callosum malformations generally have a good prognosis. However, the presence of additional cranial or extracranial malformations and genetic syndromes are usually indicators of poor prognosis. In this chapter, we offer a comprehensive overview of the complicated landscape of corpus callosum malformations, exploring their embryology, etiology, diagnostic modalities, prognostic considerations, and management strategies.

Keywords
Callosal anomalies · Neurosonography · Brain malformation · Midline anomalies · Callosal dysgenesis

1 Introduction

The corpus callosum is the major telencephalic commissure with the largest bundle of white matter that connects the right and left cerebral hemispheres. This interhemispheric communication

Supplementary Information The online version contains supplementary material available at https://doi.org/10.1007/978-3-031-70192-4_4.

R. Ramirez Zegarra · A. Dall'Asta · N. Volpe · E. Di Pasquo
Department of Medicine and Surgery, Obstetrics and Gynecology Unit, University of Parma, Parma, Italy
e-mail: andrea.dallasta@unipr.it

T. Ghi (✉)
Department of Woman and Child Health, Catholic University of Sacred Heart, Fondazione Policlinico Gemelli IRCCS, Rome, Italy
e-mail: tullio.ghi@unipr.it

P. Volpe, T. Ghi (eds.), *Fetal Neurosonography*, Ultrasound in Obstetrics and Gynecology, https://doi.org/10.1007/978-3-031-70192-4_4

network comprises around 200 million axons, representing 2–3% of all cortical fibers. Extending from the frontal lobe anteriorly to the quadrigeminal plate posteriorly, its principal role is the integration and transfer of motor, sensory, and cognitive information between both hemispheres [1, 2].

Corpus callosum malformations have been recognized for centuries, with the earliest documented case of completed agenesis of the corpus callosum (cACC) dating back to 1742 in Italy [3]. These anomalies are among the most common congenital malformations of the central nervous system detected in utero [4, 5]. Anomalies affecting the corpus callosum include complete (cACC) or partial agenesis of the corpus callosum (pACC) as well as dysgenesis of the corpus callosum (DCC) [1]. These malformations may manifest in isolation or alongside additional anatomical anomalies or genetic disorders.

Since the first report of prenatal diagnosis of a ACC in 1985 [6], advances in imaging modalities—such as ultrasound and magnetic resonance imaging (MRI)—have significantly enhanced our comprehension and characterization of these condition. To date, it is possible to accurately diagnose and classify these malformations in utero and detect additional intra- or extracranial anomalies. Similarly, progress in genetics have unveiled several genes associated with these conditions.

Predicting the prognosis of corpus callosum malformations is challenging, as this depends on the underlying etiology and/or the presence of additional malformations or genetic syndromes [7–11]. Furthermore, certain associated abnormalities can be only diagnosed later in pregnancy or after birth, further complicating the ability to predict antenatally neurodevelopmental outcomes.

In this chapter, we offer a comprehensive overview of the complicated landscape of corpus callosum malformations, exploring their embryology, etiology, diagnostic modalities, prognostic considerations, and management strategies. Our aim is to provide researchers and clinicians with valuable scientific evidence to enhance their understanding and management of these complex conditions.

2 Definition

The definition of corpus callosum malformations encompasses a broad spectrum of abnormalities, often described using varying terminology [12]. In this chapter, we will categorize corpus callosum malformations into three subtypes, as recently proposed [13]:

1. Complete Agenesis of the Corpus Callosum (cACC), which is featured by the total absence of all anatomical regions of the corpus callosum.
2. Partial Agenesis of the Corpus Callosum (pACC), which is featured by the absence of at least one anatomical region of the corpus callosum, usually the posterior region.
3. Dysgenesis of the Corpus Callosum (DCC), which is featured by the anatomical structure variations of the corpus callosum, which may include a "hypoplastic" or "thin," "hyperplastic" or "thick," and "dysplastic" corpus callosum configurations.

3 Embriology

The corpus callosum, alongside other telencephalic commissural structures such as the anterior and the hippocampal commissures, develops from the commissural plate during the embryonic development. At around 39 embryonic days, the upper part of the rostrally lying lamina terminalis (closure point of the anterior neuropore) thickens and becomes the commissural plate [14]. Over the subsequent days, this structure serves as a passive conduit for early axonal passage, primarily originating from the cingulate sulcus. With increasing fiber passage, the commissural plate continues to grow, and the first callosal fibers can be demonstrated at approximately 11 weeks of gestation [15].

At this stage, the progression of the corpus callosum development is a matter of debate, with two theories being proposed. The first states that the development of the corpus callosum initiates with the first pioneering callosal axons crossing the midline at the genu around 12–13 weeks of gestation. Subsequently, over the following weeks, there is an antero-posterior growth of the other corpus callosum regions—the body and the splenium. The last segment to develop is the rostrum, which appears at around 18–20 weeks of gestation [16, 17].

The second, more contemporary theory suggests that corpus callosum development is based on the fusion of two separate segments. Around 13–14 weeks of gestation, pioneering axons commence crossing the midline. The anterior segment, containing neocortical fibers from the anterior commissure begins to proliferate by 14–15 weeks; whereas the posterior segment, containing fibers from the hippocampal commissure starts to grow by 18–19 weeks of gestation. By 20 weeks of gestation, both segment have fused to form the complete corpus callosum [18, 19].

In case of callosal agenesis, due to the close embryological relationship among the corpus callosum and the other forebrain commissures—i.e., anterior commissure and hippocampal commissure—it is common for one or both to be absent as well. In most instances, the hippocampal commissure is also either missing or incomplete [1, 20–22].

4 Epidemiology

The prevalence of corpus callosum malformations ranges from 0.3% to 0.7% in the general population [4, 23]. In high-risk populations, like developmentally disabled children, the observed prevalence increases to approximately 2–3% [24]. The most frequent corpus callosum malformations appears to be cACC, followed by pACC and DCC [25–27]. However, recent prenatal studies utilizing high-resolution ultrasound probes suggest a higher prevalence of DCC than previously reported [28].

5 Etiology/Pathogenesis

Corpus callosum malformation is a highly heterogeneous condition, caused by a disruption at different developmental steps in the formation of the corpus callosum. Approximately, 70–75% of cases result from either developmental arrest caused by associated brain malformations or genetic disorders [7–11, 29]; or from disruptive events, such as congenital infections (e.g., cytomegalovirus and Zika virus), vascular incidents, or exogenous factors (e.g., maternal alcohol use during pregnancy and maternal metabolic diseases including diabetes and phenylketonuria) [30–33]. The remaining 25–30% of cases occur as isolated events with apparently unknown causes [27, 30].

In the majority of the cases of ACC, early neuronal axons fail to cross the midline due to the absence of the massa commissuralis; thus, preventing the formation of a normal corpus callosum. When this occurs, the early neuronal axons run antero-posteriorly, forming a large bundle of aberrant axons along the medial hemispheric walls, known as the bundles of Probst. This presentation is commonly referred to as Type 1 ACC. In other instances of ACC, disruption of developmental steps occurs earlier, resulting in commissural axons failing to form consequently, bundles of Probst are missing. This is commonly known as the Type 2 ACC [34, 35]. pACC and DCC occur often secondary to disruptive causes during corpus callosum development, such as additional brain malformations, infections, vascular accidents, or exogenous factors [36].

The reported prevalence of associated brain abnormalities ranges from approximately 45% to 75% and appears to be consistent across all subtypes of corpus callosum malformations [37, 38]. In cases of cACC, the most frequently observed brain abnormalities include malformations of cortical development, ventriculomegaly, and posterior fossa malformations [39]. pACC is often associated with ventriculomegaly and interhemispheric cysts [38], while DCC tends to be correlated with ventriculomegaly and cerebellar malformations [26] as well as macro- and microcephaly, and malformations of cortical development [40, 41]. Several malformations of cortical development have been described in cases with corpus callosum malformations, including gray matter heterotopia, polymicrogyria, focal cortical dysplasia, lissencephaly, and pachygyria [30, 42–44]. Additionally, other CNS malformations may include open spina bifida, as well as pericallosal and/or interhemispheric lipomas [30, 39, 45–47].

Extracranial malformations are detected in approximately 30% to 60% of cases of corpus callosum malformations, extending across various organ systems such as cardiac, gastrointestinal, genitourinary, musculoskeletal, and craniofacial systems [30, 37, 48, 49].

6 Genetic Background

Many genetic factors seem to contribute to the etiology of corpus callosum malformations [2]. Chromosomal anomalies are found in approximately 5% of cases with isolated corpus callosum malformations [50] and in 17– 30% of cases associated with additional cranial or extracranial malformations [23, 26, 37]. Common chromosomal anomalies include aneuploidies (mostly trisomy 21, 18 and 13, and mosaic trisomy 8) and chromosomal rearrangements such as deletions or duplications. While many cases of corpus callosum malformations are sporadic, recent studies have revealed an increasing number of submicroscopic copy number variations associated with this condition. Interestingly, around 9% of ACC cases present with "de novo" copy number variantions [51].

Approximately 20–35% of cases with identifiable genetic causes are linked to a wide array of single-gene disorders, including autosomal dominant or recessive and X-linked ihneritance [34, 52, 53]. Among the most prevalent genetic syndromes are the Aicardi (ACC, chorioretinal abnormalities, infantile seizures, and mental retardation), Andermann (ACC, progressive motor-sensory neuropathy and mental retardation), and Acrocallosal syndrome (ACC, polydactyly, craniofacial anomalies, mental retardation). Nevertheless, several other genetic syndromes have also been documented, including Walker-Warburg syndrome, Mowat -Wilson syndrome, tubulinopathies, and inborn errors of metabolism [54].

DCC has also been associated with certain genetic disorders. A hyperplastic corpus callosum has been observed in some genetic syndromes, including Cohen syndrome and megalencephaly-capillary malformation syndrome [55, 56]. Furthermore, a dysplastic corpus callosum is frequently found in children with pyridoxine-dependent epilepsy, a rare autosomal recessive epileptic encephalopathy characterized by seizures resistant to antiepileptic drugs. Typically, these seizures begin in the neonatal period and are managed through daily administration of pyridoxine [57].

The use of more advanced genetic testing techniques, such as chromosomal microarray and exome sequencing, has been shown to increase the diagnostic yield following a negative standard karyotype. The diagnostic yield of a chromosomal microarray analysis is around 11–12.5% [58, 59]. Exome sequencing appears to be the most informative genetic testing approach, with prenatally diagnosed cases of corpus callosum malformations manifesting pathogenic or likely pathogenic variants in at least 43% of instances. Notably, exome sequencing yields positive results in 55% of the cases associated with extracranial anomalies, 43% of cases with additional brain anomalies, and 32% of isolated cases [60]. This association may be even stronger for fetuses affected by DCC, wherein pathogenic or likely pathogenic variants are identified in 50% of isolated cases and up to 70% of cases with associated abnormalities [26].

All cases of corpus callosum malformations should be offered genetic counseling and invasive genetic testing, including standard karyotype and chromosomal microarray or—in the best case scenario—exome sequencing [61]. This is especially important for identifying etiology and assessing recurrence risk. De novo copy number variations and de novo single-gene pathogenic mutations pose a low risk of recurrence, estimated at 1%. If no genetic cause can be identified, the true recurrence risk remains uncertain but it is believed to be low.

7 Anatomy and Sonographic Findings of a Normal Corpus Callosum

The corpus callosum can be imaged prenatally using ultrasound and MRI, with each modality offering a different level of performance, contrast, and spatial resolution depending on the gestational age. While a transabdominal approach is often feasible, in cases where the fetus is in vertex presentation, high-resolution transvaginal ultrasound may provide images of superior quality. The corpus callosum is divided into four anatomical regions: the rostrum, genu, body, and splenium (Fig. 1).

Current international guidelines recommend examining the axial planes of the fetal brain for central nervous system malformations screening [62, 63] (Fig. 2). While the transventricular and the transthalamic planes may serve as screening planes for corpus callosum malformations, their accuracy is limited, especially in cases of pACC and DCC, as discussed later in this chapter. On the axial plane, attention should be particularly directed toward the structures of the anterior complex—which include, the callosal sulcus, the genu of the corpus callosum, the cavum septi pellucidi and, laterally, the anterior horns of the lateral ventricles (Fig. 2)—as the distortions in their anatomy may indicate corpus callosum malformations [64, 65]. Additionally, assessment of the shape and width of occipital horns of the lateral ventricles can be performed in this plane.

Traditionally, imaging of the corpus callosum was recommended from 19 weeks of gestation onward. But the introduction of a new spectrum of high-frequency ultrasound transducers has facilitated the visualization of the corpus callosum as early as 13–14 weeks of gestation [66, 67]. This coincides with the timeframe when the first pioneering callosal axons begin to cross the midline. Moreover, visualization of a small pericallosal artery branching from the anterior cerebral artery is feasible with 2D or 3D color Doppler as early as 11–13 weeks of gestation [68, 69] (Fig. 3).

The corpus callosum is best imaged in the midsagittal plane acquired through the anterior fontanelle, as this scanning section allows the visualization of its entire structure and length [70]. It appears as an anechoic to hypoechoic C-shaped band, located between the cingulate gyrus superiorly, and the cavum septi pellucidi and the cavum vergae inferiorly, delineated by two echogenic lines (Fig. 1, Video 1). Embryologically, all anatomic segments of the corpus callosum should be fully developed by 18–20 weeks of gestation; thus, diagnosing cACC or pACC before this timeframe may not be optimal. By applying color Doppler with low pulse repetition frequency, the two joint pericallosal arteries manifest outlining the upper border of the corpus callosum (Fig. 4). In the coronal

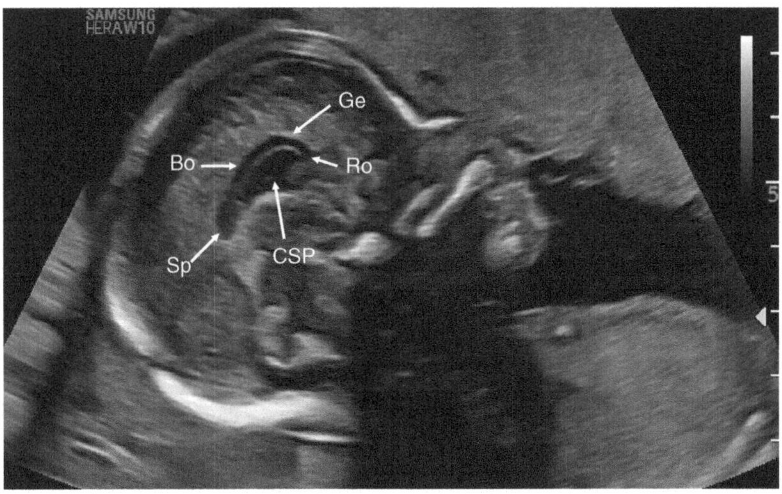

Fig. 1 Normal midtrimester anatomy of the midsagittal plane of the fetal brain demonstrating all anatomical regions of the corpus callosum: rostrum (Ro), genu (Ge), body (Bo), and splenium (Sp). *CSP* cavum septi pellucidi

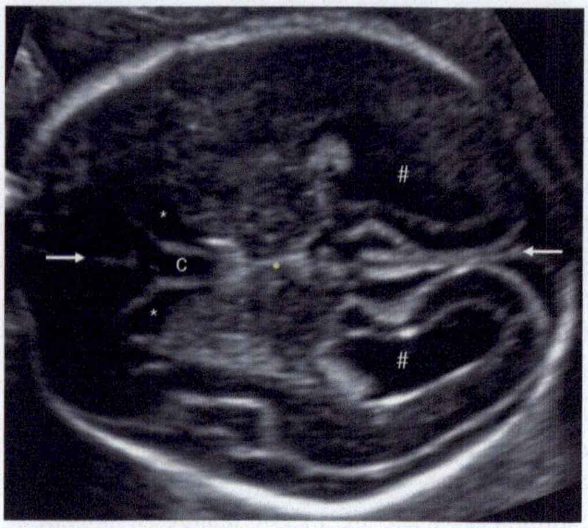

Fig. 2 Normal anatomy of the transventricular plane of the fetal brain at midtrimester ultrasound examination. The falx cerebri (thin arrows), the cavum septi pellucidi (C), the posterior (#) and anterior (*) horns of the lateral ventricles, should be visualized

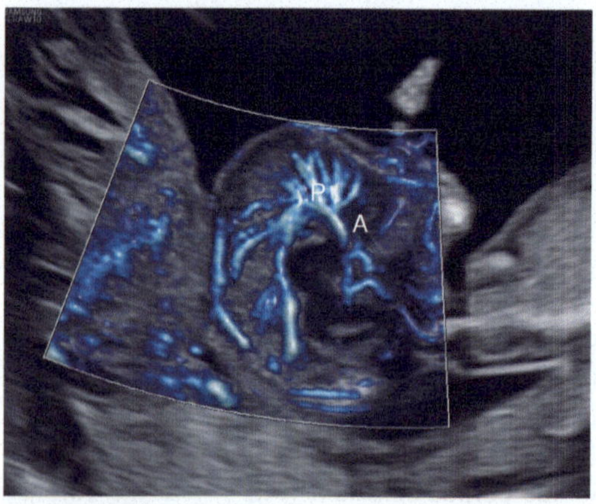

Fig. 3 Midsagittal view of normal fetal brain at 11–13 weeks using highly sensitive Doppler imaging (MV flow) to imagine the pericallosal artery (P) branching from the anterior cerebral artery (A)

plane, the corpus callosum is observed above the cavum septi pellucidi and appears as a thin hypoechoic horizontal band, bordered superiorly and inferiorly by two hyperechoic lines [70, 71] (Fig. 5).

The use of 3D ultrasound can aid in obtaining the midsagittal and coronal planes in cases where acquisition of these planes is technically difficult and transvaginal ultrasound is not feasible due to non-cephalic presenting fetus [72]. Multiplanar imaging from 3D ultrasound volumes may overcome issues related to suboptimal fetal positioning [73] and allow to reconstruct orthogonal volumes with no apparent significant drop in performance [74]. Using modern high-end equipment, it usually requires shorter acquisition times. However, image quality in 2D ultrasound scanning is superior to 3D ultrasound, especially when using 3D for reconstructing midsagittal planes from axial planes.

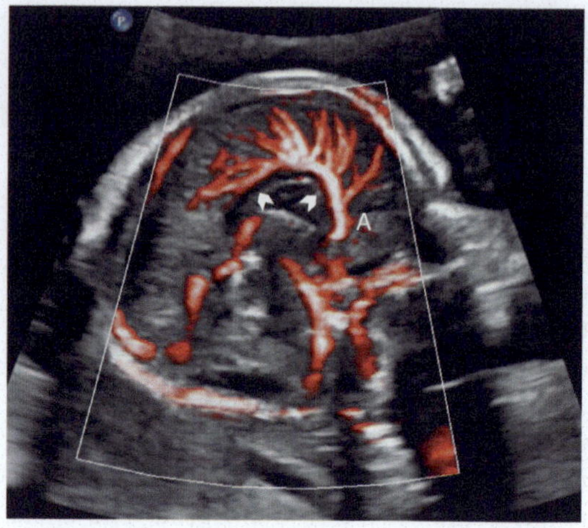

Fig. 4 Midsagittal view of normal fetal brain at 21 weeks of gestation using highly sensitive Doppler imaging to imagine the two joined pericallosal arteries (arrowheads) branching from the anterior cerebral artery (A)

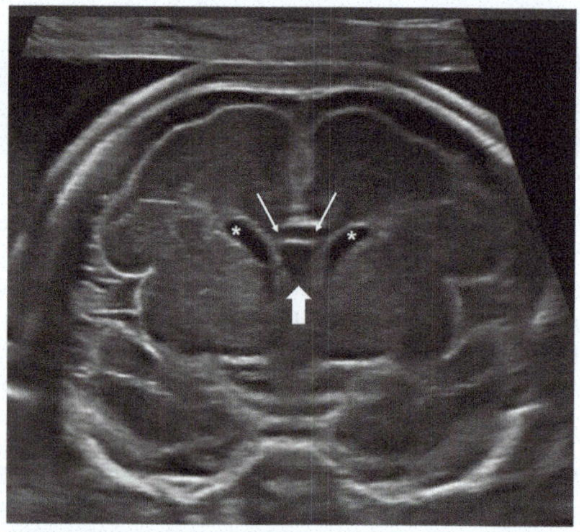

Fig. 5 Normal midtrimester anatomy of the coronal plane of the fetal brain showing the corpus callosum (thin arrows) above the cavum septi pellucidi (thick arrow). Note, also the normal shape of the frontal horns of the lateral ventricles (*)

Most international guidelines currently do not include the use of midsagittal or coronal planes in their recommendations for the standard examination of the fetal brain [62]. This could account for the suboptimal detection rates of prenatal ultrasound for corpus callosum malformations—especially in cases of pACC and DCC—reported in some studies [75].

8 Sonographic Findings

8.1 Complete Agenesis of the Corpus Callosum

8.1.1 Sonographic Findings at First Trimester

Prenatal diagnosis of corpus callosum malformations in the first trimester remains largely unexplored, primarily due to the limited data on the visualization of the corpus callosum before 14 weeks of gestation. However, advancements in ultrasound technology, especially the introduction of new high-resolution ultrasound machines, have made it possible to visualize the developing structures of the corpus callosum in the late first trimester [66, 67].

Non-visualization of the corpus callosum leading to suspect corpus callosum agenesis or dysgenesis may be feasible at 13–14 weeks of gestation, as shown in a recent study [66]. Furthermore, the lack of visualization of the pericallosal artery on color Doppler may represent an indirect sign of ACC in the first trimester [76]. Although these findings are promising, their diagnostic accuracy is yet to be evaluated in large studies before introducing them into clinical practice.

8.1.2 Sonographic Findings at Second Trimester or Later

Prenatal diagnosis of cACC is feasible and accurate from midtrimester onwards using transabdominal ultrasound with or without the adjunct of transvaginal ultrasound in the event of a cephalic presenting fetus [77, 78]. cACC is most commonly suspected in the presence of an indirect sign—i.e., the lack of visualization of the cavum septi pellucidi—on the transventricular or transthalamic planes. The diagnosis can be confirmed on the midsagittal plane, as well as on the transcaudate and transthalamic coronal planes.

In the transventricular plane, the classic distorted anatomy resulting from the absence of the corpus callosum has traditionally provided the indirect signs for suspecting cACC. However, these indirect findings may not always be present, potentially leading to false negative results [79]. The interhemispheric fissure is wide, and the roof of the third ventricle is displaced upwards, becoming visible on this plane (Fig. 6).

Disruption in the midline anatomy of the brain leads to the non-visualization of the cavum septi pellucidi, as this structure also originates from the commissural plate, from which the corpus callosum develops [80]. Furthermore, the frontal horns of the lateral ventricles are widely separated from the midline and run parallel to each other. The absence of posterior callosal axons, resulting in reduced white matter formation, contributes to an enlargement of the atria and occipital horns of the lateral ventricles, which present a characteristic "teardrop" shape (also called colpocephaly). Conversely, dilation of the frontal horns is limited by the compression of the superomedial borders by the bundles of Probst and the normally developed caudate nuclei at their lateral borders (Fig. 6, Video 1). Moreover, ventriculomegaly may also manifest from midtrimester onwards, since a progressive dilatation of the posterior horns of the lateral ventricles starting from the late second trimester is frequently observed. Based on a published study, ventriculomegaly is visualized in approximately in one-fourth of fetuses with cACC before 24 weeks of gestation, becoming more evident later in pregnancy (Fig. 7, Video 2) [79].

When cACC is suspected, referral ultrasound assessment for fetal neurosonography is indicated and includes the multiplanar evaluation of the fetal brain preferably using the transvaginal approach in cephalic presenting fetus [81]. In the midsagittal plane, a definitive diagnosis is achieved when the corpus callosum is completely absent (Fig. 8, Video 2). In the third trimester, the cerebral sulci exhibit a radial disposition of the

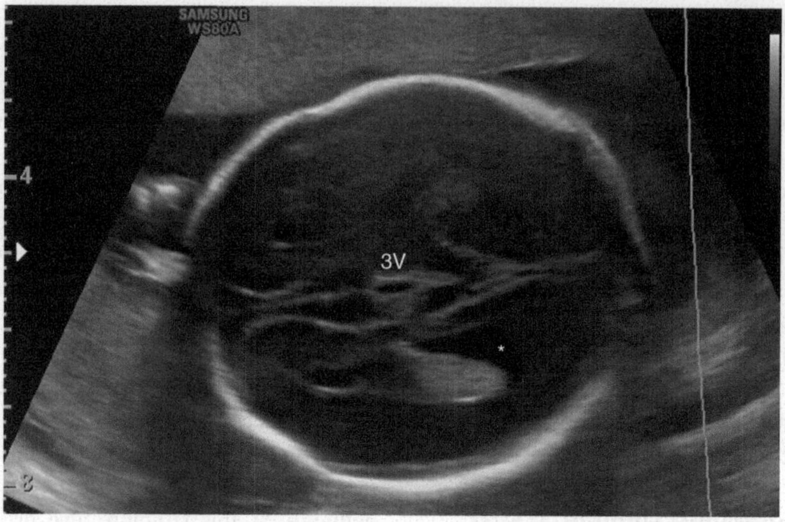

Fig. 6 Indirect signs of agenesis of the corpus callosum on the transventricular plane at midtrimester ultrasound. The interhemispheric fissure is wide, the cavum septi pellucidi is absent, and the third ventricle (3 V) is visualized due to the upward displacement of its roof. Note the frontal horns of the lateral ventricles widely separated from the midline and running paralell to each other, and the tear-drop shape (colpocephaly) of the posterior horn of the lateral ventricle (*)

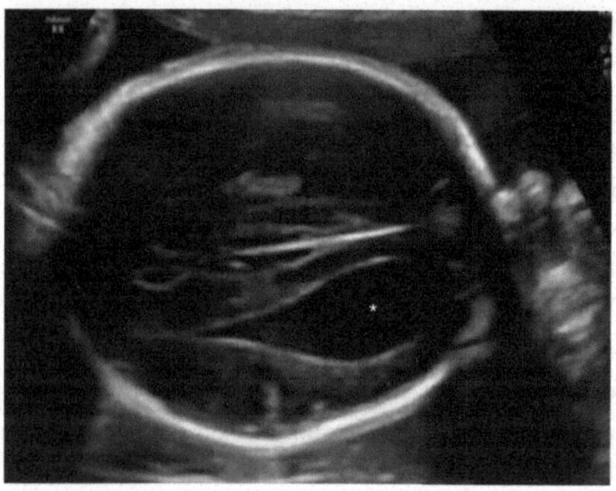

Fig. 7 Transventricular plane of a fetus with complete agenesis of the corpus callosum and ventriculomegaly. Note the wide interhemispheric fissure and the dilated, tear-drop shaped occipital horn of the lateral ventricle (*)

internal aspect of the hemispheres due to the absence of the corpus callosum.

Using color Doppler, the abnormal course of the anterior cerebral artery can be observed, ascending linearly with the pericallosal artery missing (Fig. 9). The course of the anterior cerebral artery may be also quantified by measuring the furthest distance between the anterior border of the tela choroidea to the ascending branch of the anterior cerebral artery—i.e., the tela-choroidea-to-anterior-cerebral-artery distance. In cases of cACC, this distance is significantly shorter measuring around 4 mm [82].

In the coronal plane, the absence of the corpus callosum and the cavum septi pellucidi leads to the upward displacement of the roof of the third ventricle into the interhemispheric space, reaching the falx cerebri which appears interrupted. Furthermore, the lateral ventricles assume a comma-shaped or a bullhorn-shaped appearance due to the lateral displacement of the medial borders of the frontal horns caused by the presence of the Probst bundles (Fig. 10, Video 3).

8.2 Partial Agenesis of the Corpus Callosum

Diagnosing pACC is more challenging compared to cACC. Relying solely on the transventricular plane to identify indirect signs of ACC, such as absent cavum septi pellucidi, colpocephaly, and ventriculomegaly, proves insufficient in pACC cases [79, 83]. Moreover, the presence of some portions of the corpus callosum on the midsagit-

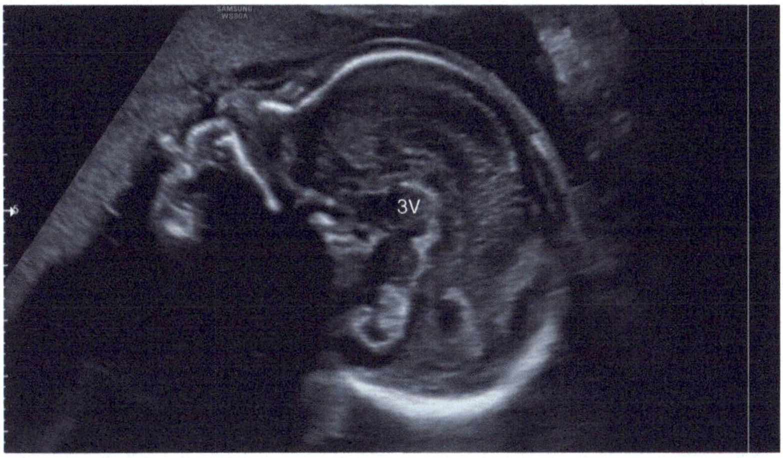

Fig. 8 Midsagittal view of a 24-week fetus affected by completed agenesis of the corpus callosum. Note the absence of the corpus callosum and cavum septi pellucidi above the third ventricle (3 V)

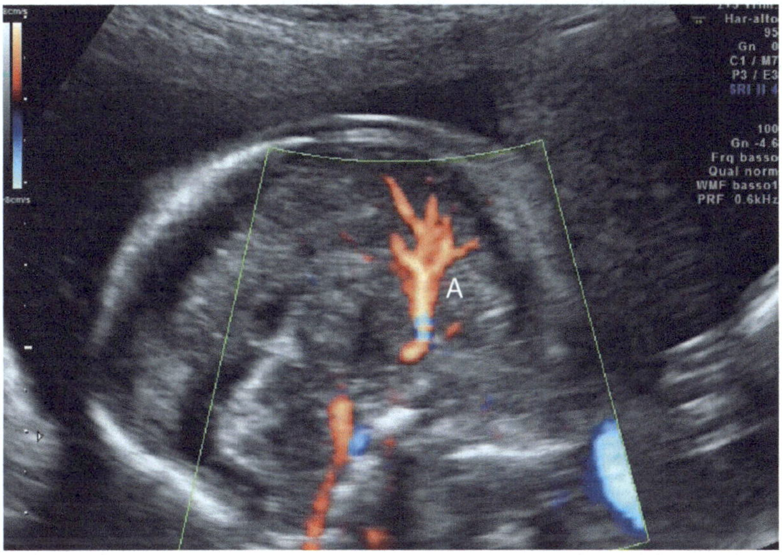

Fig. 9 Midsagittal view of the brain of a 22-week fetus with complete agenesis of the corpus callosum using color Doppler. Note the anterior cerebral artery (A) ascending with no evidence of a branching pericallosal artery

tal and coronal planes, albeit with abnormal features, may lead to misinterpretation of the sonographic findings.

In the transventricular plane, the cavum septi pellucidi may be absent or exhibit a triangular shape, although more often, it presents with an abnormal rectangular shape (wider and shorter) [38, 84, 85]. A length-to-width ratio of the cavum septi pellucidi below the fifth percentile or less than 1.5 may be useful as a screening tool for identifying cases with pACC [85].

In the midsagittal plane, the corpus callosum typically appears shorter. In the event of a primarily abnormal development, the most commonly missing portion is represented by the splenium with or without the posterior part of the body (Fig. 1a, Video 4); however, the absence of the rostrum and the genu may also occur (Fig. 11) [38]. Using color Doppler, the pericallosal artery can be visualized following the anterior part of the corpus callosum until reaching its most posterior segment, where it takes an upward, posterior and oblique direction [83]. The above-mentioned tela-choroidea-to-anterior-cerebral-artery distance can also be used to determine the abnormal course of the anterior cerebral artery. In cases with pACC, this distance is significantly shorter compared to normal cases [82].

A "short" but completely formed corpus callosum, typically defined as falling below the third or fifth percentile in length, can sometimes be mistaken for pACC. This confusion often arises when relying on available nomograms to diagnose a "short" corpus callosum [86–88]. However, the adoption of of callosal length nomograms alone has not been demonstrated to improve the differentiation between normal and abnormal callosal development. More specifically, there is currently no established threshold of callosal length reliably predicting adverse neurodevelopmental outcomes [89]. Indeed, evidence from the literature suggests that fetuses with a "short" corpus callosum are not necessarily associated with genetic disorders [26] or adverse neurodevelopmental outcomes [90].

Therefore, the term "short" corpus callosum should be abandoned and no longer used to describe a corpus callosum malformation. Instead, emphasis should be placed on the correct visualization of all anatomical segments of the corpus callosum, rather than solely measuring its length [13].

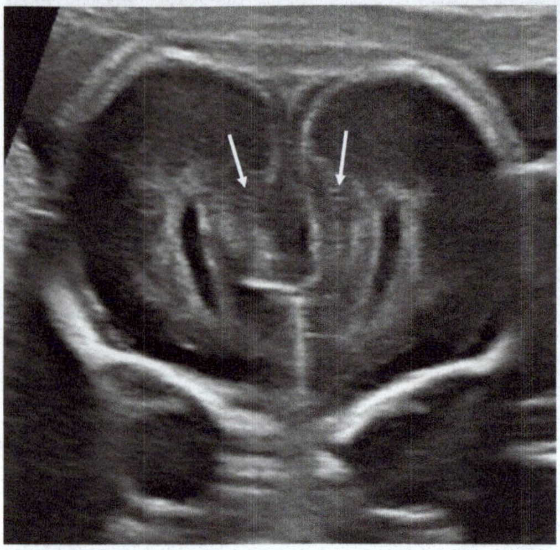

Fig. 10 Coronal view of the brain of a 23-week fetus with complete agenesis of the corpus callosum. Note the absence of the corpus callosum and cavum septi pellucidi, and the presence of bullhorn-shaped frontal horns of the lateral ventricles due to the lateral displacement of the medial borders caused by the Probst bundles (arrows)

8.3 Dysgenesis of the Corpus Callosum

The sonographic diagnosis of DCC poses even greater challenge compared to the previously described anomalies mainly because of the often unremarkable axial views of the fetal brain [83]. However, while the corpus callosum is imaged on the midsagittal plane, it usually demonstrates an abnormal shape.

Similar to pACC, the use of nomograms has been proposed to aid in identifying DCC [86, 87]. However, caution is advised when relying on nomograms, as they have demonstrated inadequacies and significant heterogeneity in defining thresholds.

Hyperplasia or increased thickness of the corpus callosum is commonly defined as a callosal thickness above two standard deviations above the mean values of the reference charts [87];

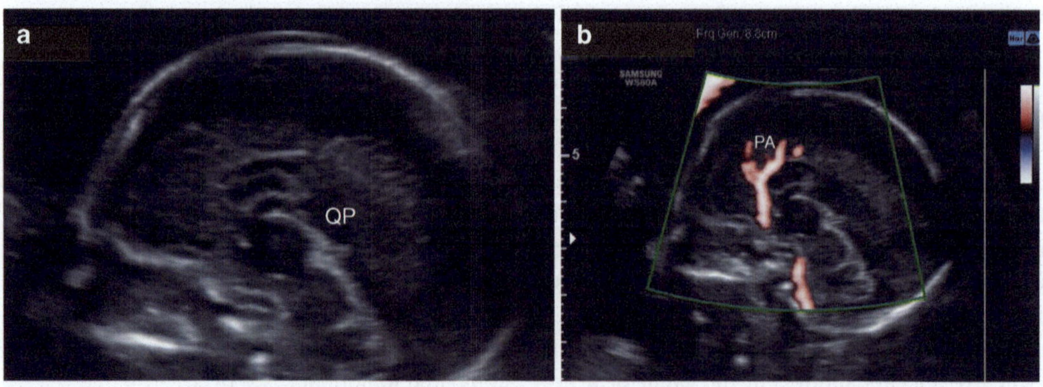

Fig. 11 Two ultrasound images on the midsagittal view of the brain of two fetuses with hyperplastic or "thick" corpus callosum (white arrows)

however, qualitative assessment has also been reported. The abnormal shape may affect all anatomical segments of the corpus callosum, or it may only be confined to the anterior and posterior parts [40, 91] (Fig. 12). The increased thickness of the corpus callosum is amenable to be spotted at second trimester but in some of these cases, this finding has been demonstrated to normalize at late gestation.

A hypoplastic or thin corpus callosum is characterized by callosal thickness below the tenth percentile for gestational age according to reference charts [83]. The body and splenium are the most commonly affected regions.

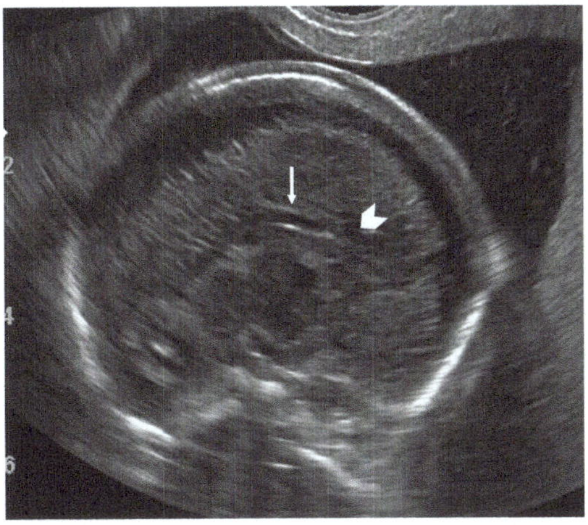

Fig. 12 Midsagittal view of a fetal brain with partial agenesis of the corpus callosum. Note that the rostrum and part of the genu are missing (arrowhead), whereas the body and splenium are normally formed (arrow)

A dysplastic corpus callosum exhibits an abnormal shape and structure (Fig. 13) and usually coexists with hypoplasia of the corpus callosum. Prenatal diagnosis of this condition is rare unless associated cranial or extracranial malformations are present alongside [92].

9 Differential Diagnosis

The sonographic diagnosis of corpus callosum malformations is achieved when the corpus callosum cannot be visualized or has an abnormal shape in the midsagittal plane of the fetal brain. Contrarily, indirect signs on the transventricular plane might require differentiation from other entities. When a corpus callosum malformation is suspected, expert multiplanar neurosonography is indicated to confirm this abnormality or rule out cerebral anomalies potentially associated with this condition.

Non-visualization of the cavum septi pellucidi is one of the most common findings associated with corpus callosum malformations, but it can also present with other brain abnormalities, such as septal agenesis, septo-optic dysplasia, holoprosencephaly, schizencephaly, poroencephaly/hydranencephaly, basilar encephaloceles, and severe hydrocephalus [80]. Of note, the examiner is to be familiar with the normal

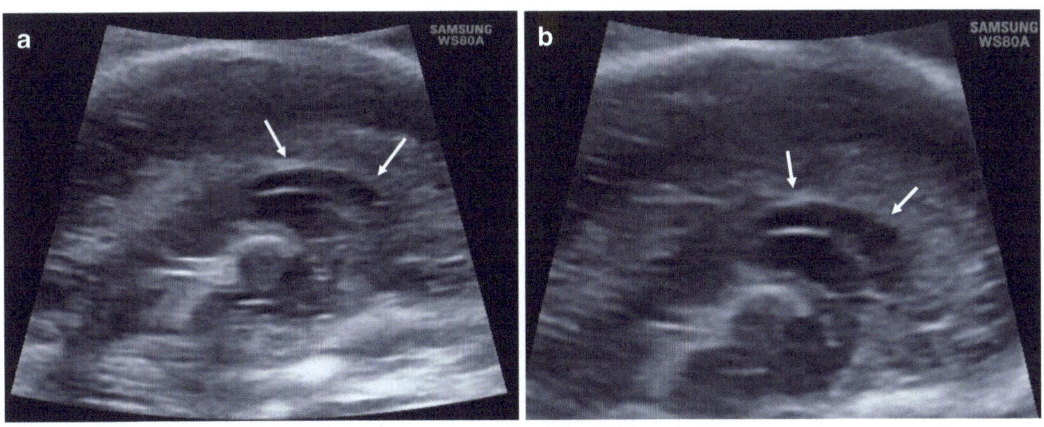

Fig. 13 Ultrasound images of two fetuses affected by agenesis of the corpus callosum and malformations of the cortical development

sonographic appearance of the CSP on the axial plane as in some circumstances of cACC small interhemispheric cysts may mimic the appearance of the cavum septi pellucidi. Furthermore, the columns of the fornix—usually visualized caudal to the transthalamic plane—might be mistakenly interpreted as the cavum septi pellucidi [93].

10 MRI

The MRI findings in cases affected by corpus callosum malformations are similar to those observed on ultrasound. They include the racing car sign (top-down view of the lateral ventricles running parallel, resembling a Formula One car), the "moose head" appearance (anterior to posterior views of the frontal horns resemble a moose's head), the "sunray appearance" (midline views show gyri radiating outwards from the ventricles), colpocephaly, bundles of Probst, and an upward-displaced third ventricle [54]. For a better description of these findings, please see the chapter "Prenatal MR Imaging of Brain Malformations" of this book.

The utility of adding MRI to the antenatal work-up of fetuses with sonographic diagnosis of corpus callosum malformations has been the subject of extensive debate. It is now acknowledged that if expert multiplanar neurosonography is performed, MRI may not be required to confirm the diagnosis of cACC [94, 95]. However, MRI may seems more accurate than ultrasound in confirming pACC and DCC [96].

Moreover, MRI enables the detection of additional brain abnormalities not usually seen with ultrasound, such as malformations of cortical development and posterior fossa abnormalities. In cases of apparently isolated complete ACC at ultrasound, antenatal MRI detects approximately 8–10% of associated abnormalities while an additional 4–5% is noted at postnatal MRI. For sonographically isolated pACC, antenatal MRI reveals 12% of additional brain abnormalities, with an additional 12 to 16% only identified postnatally [50, 97, 98]. Therefore, MRI should be used as a complementary tool to ultrasound in the assessment and characterization of corpus callosum malformations.

There is no consensus regarding the optimal timing for MRI, but it is common practice to schedule it at third trimester. This is due to the fact that certain associated brain abnormalities—particularly malformations of cortical development—may often become evident later in pregnancy, and could be missed if MRI is performed earlier. It is important to remember that neurodevelopmental outcomes are significantly worse with additional brain abnormalities Hence, MRI should be considered an important component of the prenatal assessment of corpus callosum malformations.

11 Prognosis

The prognosis of fetuses with corpus callosum malformations depends largely on the presence of associated cranial (Figs. 14 and 15) or extracranial malformations or genetic conditions [7–11]. Non-isolated cases usually exhibit poor neurodevelopmental outcomes [99]. However, it remains unclear which specific additional findings are indicative of worse prognosis, as many are non-specific in predicting poor neurodevelopmental outcomes [100]. Furthermore, accurately identifying before birth isolated cases of corpus callosum malformations is challenging, as many associated abnormalities may be only detected postnatally.

Corpus callosum malformations are associated with a broad spectrum of adverse neurodevelopmental outcomes, ranging from mild behavioral problems to severe neurological impairment. Children affected by these conditions typically display core deficits across three domains: reduced interhemispheric transfer of sensory-motor information, decreased cognitive processing speed, and difficulties in complex reasoning and novel problem-solving [101]. Additional symptoms may include gross and fine motor control impairments, visual problems, delayed speech development, seizures or epilepsy, feeding issues, and impaired hand-eye coordination [54]. Behavioral (attention deficits)

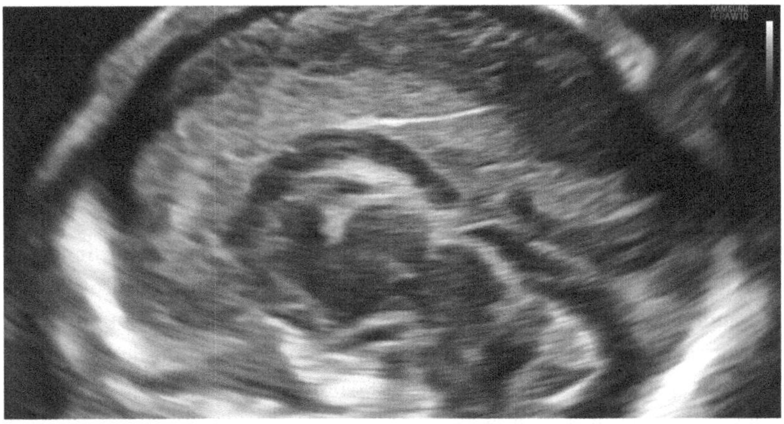

Fig. 14 Ultrasound image of a fetus exhibiting a dysgenetic corpus callosum. Note the abnormal shape and structure

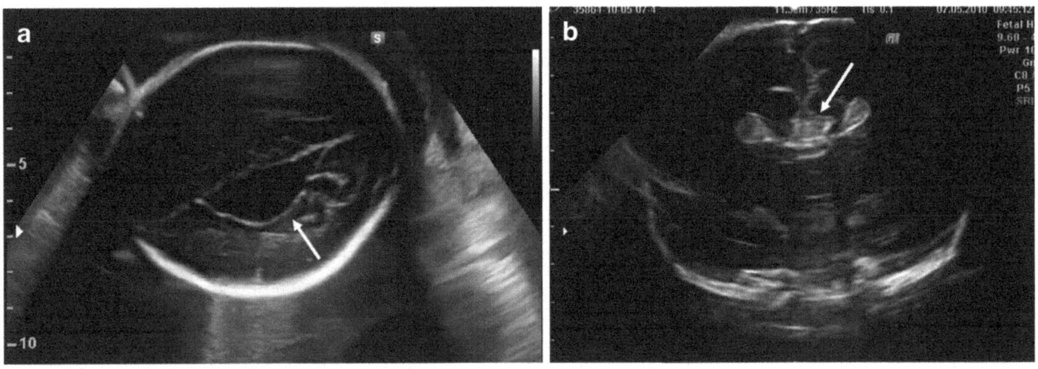

Fig. 15 Ultrasound images of two different fetuses with agenesis of the corpus callosum and (**a**) interhemispheric cyst (arrow) and (**b**) pericallosal lipoma (arrow) respectively

and social differences often observed in autism spectrum disorders may also be present [102, 103]. Furthermore, corpus callosum malformations have been associated with schizophrenia [104, 105].

Even when the intelligence quotient is within the normal range, children with isolated conditions may experience subtle deficits across various neurodevelopmental domains, which often become apparent later in life [106, 107]. Their intellectual abilities typically range within the "low-average" to "average" compared to the general population. Moreover, they may encounter difficulties in "higher" language functions, complex information processing, memory skills, and in specific academic areas, such as mathematics [108].

Truly isolated cACC (no additional brain malformations identified postnatally) is associated with favorable prognosis in most cases. Approximately, 75–85% of these cases exhibit normal or subtle neurodevelopment outcomes, with 16% experiencing borderline/moderate impairment, and 8% severe disability [50, 97, 109]. According to the literature, the prognosis of pACC does not seem to be different than that of cACC [50, 110–112], despite some reports suggesting otherwise [9, 97]. Isolated pACC is associated with normal neurodevelopmental outcomes in 70% of cases, whereas 15% and 13% are associated with borderline to moderate and severe neurodevelopmental outcomes, respectively. Nevertheless, around 12–15% of cases—prenatally diagnosed as "isolated" pACC—exhibit additional abnormalities upon postnatal imaging [50].

Assessing the prognosis of a hypoplastic/thin corpus callosum is difficult due to the limited number of studies focusing on this specific malformation. The variability in neurodevelopmental outcomes in affected children mainly depends on the presence of associated cranial or extracranial abnormalities [83, 113]. Isolated cases of hypoplastic corpus callosum demonstrate neurodevelopmental outcomes similar to those with ACC [83]. Some studies have suggested a correlation between hypoplastic CC and autism [114].

The prognosis for fetuses with hyperplastic or "thick" corpus callosum is usually unfavorable given the presence of multiple brain abnormalities, with outcomes ranging from neonatal seizures, schizophrenia, and mental retardation to early neonatal demise [40]. However, if a hyperplastic/"thick" corpus callosum is an isolated or transient finding, a favorable outcome is expected [91]. The neurodevelopmental prognosis for a dysplastic corpus callosum depends on the associated abnormalities [18, 115].

The presence of mild ventriculomegaly in the context of colpocephaly is frequently observed in fetuses with corpus callosum malformations and generally does not impact negatively on the prognosis unless the callosal anomaly is not isolated [116, 117]. However while a subtle increase in the ventricular width is typical noted post-diagnosis during pregnancy [118], progression to severe ventriculomegaly may signal poorer outcomes [119].

Prenatal counseling for cases involving corpus callosum malformations should account for additional brain malformations, genetic disorders, family history of developmental problems, congenital infection result, and fetal growth pattern [120]. Counseling for cases with isolated findings is challenging, as prenatal imaging may not always differentiate between isolated and non-isolated cases, given that 5–15% of additional brain abnormalities are diagnosed postnatally, depending on the condition [50]. Serial follow-up during pregnancy using ultrasound (and at times MRI) is essential to detect cranial and extracranial malformations that may not be evident during the second trimester scan. Prenatal counseling should also emphasize the need of a long-term follow-up, especially for isolated cases, as various degrees of neurologic and neuropsychological impairment may only manifest later in life, particularly during school age [7].

12 Options of Treatment

To date, there is no specific treatment available for any malformation of the corpus callosum. The treatment of affected individual is usually symptom-dependent, involving various interventions such as antiepileptic medications, special education, physiotherapy, surgical procedures to address associated abnormalities (e.g., ventriculoperitoneal shunt for associated hydrocephalus), speech and visual rehabilitation, as well as psychological and psychiatric therapies [54].

In cases where additional cranial or extracranial abnormalities or genetic disorders are present, according to the local legislations many parents may opt for termination of pregnancy due to the associated unfavorable prognosis [28, 121].

13 Obstetric Management

Prenatal management typically involves a targeted ultrasound examination at midtrimester to assess the fetal organ systems comprehensively—including fetal neurosonography—as part of the initial workout. This approach facilitates the identification of other associated abnormalities that may require prenatal or postnatal intervention. Additionally, regular follow-up ultrasound scans (and in selected cases fetal MRI) should be routinely performed to identify any late-manifesting brain abnormalities [61]. Furthermore, prenatal genetic testing—i.e., standard karyotype, chromosomal microarray, and/or exome sequencing—should be routinely offered whether available during initial prenatal counseling.

Surveillance of fetuses affected by any corpus callosum malformation should be conducted by an interdisciplinary team comprising maternal-fetal medicine experts, midwives, clinical geneticists, neuroradiologists, pediatricians, pediatric neurologists, and neonatologists.

Obstetric management, including mode and site of delivery, largely depends on the associated abnormalities of the affected fetuses. In the majority of the cases, vaginal delivery is appropriate. Postnatally, MRI should be performed to confirm prenatal imaging findings. Subsequently, a postnatal multidisciplinary follow-up for the affected children should be organized in collaboration with neonatologists and pediatric neurologists to promptly identify neuropsychological disorders that may benefit from supportive therapy [122].

References

1. Raybaud C, Girard N. Malformations of the Telencephalic commissures. In: Pediatric neuroradiology: brain. Berlin, Heidelberg: Springer; 2005. p. 41–69. https://doi.org/10.1007/3-540-26398-5_3.
2. Palmer EE, Mowat D. Agenesis of the corpus callosum: a clinical approach to diagnosis. Am J Med Genet C Semin Med Genet. 2014;166C(2):184–97. https://doi.org/10.1002/ajmg.c.31405.
3. Bianchi GB. Storia del mostro di due corpi. Torino. Published online 1749.
4. Morris JK, Wellesley DG, Barisic I, Addor MC, Bergman JEH, Braz P, Cavero-Carbonell C, Draper ES, Gatt M, Haeusler M, Klungsoyr K, Kurinczuk JJ, Lelong N, Luyt K, Lynch C, O'Mahony MT, Mokoroa O, Nelen V, Neville AJ, Pierini A, Randrianaivo H, Rankin J, Rissmann A, Rouget F, Schaub B, Tucker DF, Verellen-Dumoulin C, Wiesel A, Zymak-Zakutnia N, Lanzoni M, Garne E. Epidemiology of congenital cerebral anomalies in Europe: a multicentre, population-based EUROCAT study. Arch Dis Child. 2019;104(12):1181–7. https://doi.org/10.1136/archdischild-2018-316733.
5. Raybaud C, Levrier O, Brunel H, Girard N, Farnarier P. MR imaging of fetal brain malformations. Childs Nerv Syst. 2003;19(7–8):455–70. https://doi.org/10.1007/s00381-003-0769-2.
6. Comstock CH, Culp D, González J, Boal DB. Agenesis of the corpus callosum in the fetus: its evolution and significance. J Ultrasound Med. 1985;4(11):613–6. https://doi.org/10.7863/jum.1985.4.11.613.
7. Romaniello R, Arrigoni F, De Salvo P, Bonaglia MC, Panzeri E, Bassi MT, Parazzini C, Righini A, Borgatti R. Long-term follow-up in a cohort of children with isolated corpus callosum agenesis at fetal MRI. Ann Clin Transl Neurol. 2021;8(12):2280–8. https://doi.org/10.1002/acn3.51484.
8. Folliot-Le Doussal L, Chadie A, Brasseur-Daudruy M, Verspyck E, Saugier-Veber P, Marret S, Perinatal Network of Haute-Normandie. Neurodevelopmental outcome in prenatally diagnosed isolated agenesis of the corpus callosum. Early Hum Dev. 2018;116:9–16. https://doi.org/10.1016/j.earlhumdev.2017.10.004.
9. Yeh HR, Park HK, Kim HJ, Ko TS, Won HS, Lee MY, Shim JY, Yum MS. Neurodevelopmental outcomes in children with prenatally diagnosed corpus callosal abnormalities. Brain and Development. 2018;40(8):634–41. https://doi.org/10.1016/j.braindev.2018.04.012.
10. Tang PH, Bartha AI, Norton ME, Barkovich AJ, Sherr EH, Glenn OA. Agenesis of the corpus callosum: an MR imaging analysis of associated abnormalities in the fetus. AJNR Am J Neuroradiol. 2009;30(2):257–63. https://doi.org/10.3174/ajnr.A1331.
11. Romaniello R, Marelli S, Giorda R, Bedeschi MF, Bonaglia MC, Arrigoni F, Triulzi F, Bassi MT, Borgatti R. Clinical characterization, genetics, and long-term follow-up of a large cohort of patients with agenesis of the corpus callosum. J Child Neurol. 2017;32(1):60–71. https://doi.org/10.1177/0883073816664668.
12. Mahallati H, Sotiriadis A, Celestin C, Millischer AE, Sonigo P, Grevent D, O'Gorman N, Bahi-Buisson N, Attié-Bitach T, Ville Y, Salomon LJ. Heterogeneity in defining fetal corpus callosal pathology: systematic review. Ultrasound Obstet Gynecol. 2021;58(1):11–8. https://doi.org/10.1002/uog.22179.
13. Salomon LJ, Paladini D. Fetal corpus callosum anomalies: from disease of classification to classification of disease. Ultrasound Obstet Gynecol. 2023;64:151–4. https://doi.org/10.1002/uog.27564.
14. Development of the telencephalon (first cerebral vesicle). https://embryology.ch/en/organogenesis/nervous-system/. Accessed 6 Feb 2024.
15. Loeser JD, Alvord EC. Agenesis of the corpus callosum. Brain. 1968;91(3):553–70. https://doi.org/10.1093/brain/91.3.553.
16. Rakic P, Yakovlev PI. Development of the corpus callosum and cavum septi in man. J Comp Neurol. 1968;132(1):45–72. https://doi.org/10.1002/cne.901320103.
17. Barkovich AJ, Norman D. Anomalies of the corpus callosum: correlation with further anomalies of the brain. AJR Am J Roentgenol. 1988;151(1):171–9. https://doi.org/10.2214/ajr.151.1.171.
18. Raybaud C. The corpus callosum, the other great forebrain commissures, and the septum pellucidum: anatomy, development, and malformation. Neuroradiology. 2010;52(6):447–77. https://doi.org/10.1007/s00234-010-0696-3.
19. Paul LK. Developmental malformation of the corpus callosum: a review of typical callosal development and examples of developmental disorders with callosal involvement. J Neurodev Disord. 2011;3(1):3–27. https://doi.org/10.1007/s11689-010-9059-y.
20. Cesaretti C, Nanni M, Ghi T, Parazzini C, Conte G, Contro E, Grisolia G, Righini A. Variability of forebrain commissures in callosal agenesis: a prenatal

MR imaging study. AJNR Am J Neuroradiol. 2016;37(3):521–7. https://doi.org/10.3174/ajnr.A4570.

21. Raybaud C, Girard N. Anatomic MRI study of commissural agenesis and dysplasia of the telencephalon (agenesis of the corpus callosum and related anomalies). Clinical correlations and morphogenetic interpretation. Neurochirurgie. 1998;44(1 Suppl):38–60. http://www.ncbi.nlm.nih.gov/pubmed/9757324
22. Contro E, Nanni M, Bellussi F, Salsi G, Grisolia G, Sanz-Cortès M, Righini A, Rizzo N, Pilu G, Ghi T. The hippocampal commissure: a new finding at prenatal 3D ultrasound in fetuses with isolated complete agenesis of the corpus callosum. Prenat Diagn. 2015;35(9):919–22. https://doi.org/10.1002/pd.4645.
23. Glass HC, Shaw GM, Ma C, Sherr EH. Agenesis of the corpus callosum in California 1983-2003: a population-based study. Am J Med Genet A. 2008;146A(19):2495–500. https://doi.org/10.1002/ajmg.a.32418.
24. Jeret JS, Serur D, Wisniewski K, Fisch C. Frequency of agenesis of the corpus callosum in the developmentally disabled population as determined by computerized tomography. Pediatr Neurosci. 1985;12(2):101–3. https://doi.org/10.1159/000120229.
25. Rüland AM, Berg C, Gembruch U, Geipel A. Prenatal diagnosis of anomalies of the corpus callosum over a 13-year period. Ultraschall Med. 2016;37(6):598–603. https://doi.org/10.1055/s-0034-1399699.
26. Nguyen T, Heide S, Guilbaud L, Valence S, Vande PS, Blondiaux E, Keren B, Quenum-Miraillet G, Jouannic JM, Mandelbrot L, Picone O, Guet A, Tsatsaris V, Milh M, Girard N, Vincent M, Nizon M, Poirsier C, Vivanti A, Benachi A, des Portes V, Guibaud L, Patat O, Spentchian M, Frugère L, Héron D, Garel C. Abnormalities of the corpus callosum. Can prenatal imaging predict the genetic status? Correlations between imaging phenotype and genotype. Prenat Diagn. 2023;43(6):746–55. https://doi.org/10.1002/pd.6382.
27. Pashaj S, Merz E. Detection of fetal corpus callosum abnormalities by means of 3D ultrasound. Ultraschall Med. 2016;37(2):185–94. https://doi.org/10.1055/s-0041-108565.
28. Rodríguez MA, Echevarría M, Perdomo L, Gómez-Chiari M, García S, Prats P, Serra B, Albaiges G. Prevalence of corpus callosum pathology in an unselected population. Should assessment of the corpus callosum be included in the routine 20 weeks scan? Prenat Diagn. 2024; https://doi.org/10.1002/pd.6510.
29. Fratelli N, Papageorghiou AT, Prefumo F, Bakalis S, Homfray T, Thilaganathan B. Outcome of prenatally diagnosed agenesis of the corpus callosum. Prenat Diagn. 2007;27(6):512–7. https://doi.org/10.1002/pd.1719.
30. Alby C, Malan V, Boutaud L, Marangoni MA, Bessières B, Bonniere M, Ichkou A, Elkhartoufi N, Bahi-Buisson N, Sonigo P, Millischer AE, Thomas S, Ville Y, Vekemans M, Encha-Razavi F, Attié-Bitach T. Clinical, genetic and neuropathological findings in a series of 138 fetuses with a corpus callosum malformation. Birth Defects Res A Clin Mol Teratol. 2016;106(1):36–46. https://doi.org/10.1002/bdra.23472.
31. Sowell ER, Mattson SN, Thompson PM, Jernigan TL, Riley EP, Toga AW. Mapping callosal morphology and cognitive correlates: effects of heavy prenatal alcohol exposure. Neurology. 2001;57(2):235–44. https://doi.org/10.1212/wnl.57.2.235.
32. Levy HL, Lobbregt D, Barnes PD, Poussaint TY. Maternal phenylketonuria: magnetic resonance imaging of the brain in offspring. J Pediatr. 1996;128(6):770–5. https://doi.org/10.1016/s0022-3476(96)70328-1.
33. de Fatima Vasco Aragao M, van der Linden V, Brainer-Lima AM, Coeli RR, Rocha MA, Sobral da Silva P, Durce Costa Gomes de Carvalho M, van der Linden A, Cesario de Holanda A, Valenca MM. Clinical features and neuroimaging (CT and MRI) findings in presumed Zika virus related congenital infection and microcephaly: retrospective case series study. BMJ. 2016;353:i1901. https://doi.org/10.1136/bmj.i1901.
34. Schell-Apacik CC, Wagner K, Bihler M, Ertl-Wagner B, Heinrich U, Klopocki E, Kalscheuer VM, Muenke M, von Voss H. Agenesis and dysgenesis of the corpus callosum: clinical, genetic and neuroimaging findings in a series of 41 patients. Am J Med Genet A. 2008;146A(19):2501–11. https://doi.org/10.1002/ajmg.a.32476.
35. Sztriha L. Spectrum of corpus callosum agenesis. Pediatr Neurol. 2005;32(2):94–101. https://doi.org/10.1016/j.pediatrneurol.2004.09.007.
36. Dávila-Gutiérrez G. Agenesis and dysgenesis of the corpus callosum. Semin Pediatr Neurol. 2002;9(4):292–301. https://doi.org/10.1053/spen.2002.32505.
37. Santo S, D'Antonio F, Homfray T, Rich P, Pilu G, Bhide A, Thilaganathan B, Papageorghiou AT. Counseling in fetal medicine: agenesis of the corpus callosum. Ultrasound Obstet Gynecol. 2012;40(5):513–21. https://doi.org/10.1002/uog.12315.
38. De Keersmaecker B, Jansen K, Aertsen M, Naulaers G, De Catte L. Outcome of partial agenesis of corpus callosum. Am J Obstet Gynecol. 2023;8:456.e1–9. https://doi.org/10.1016/j.ajog.2023.10.007.
39. Hetts SW, Sherr EH, Chao S, Gobuty S, Barkovich AJ. Anomalies of the corpus callosum: an MR analysis of the phenotypic spectrum of associated malformations. AJR Am J Roentgenol. 2006;187(5):1343–8. https://doi.org/10.2214/AJR.05.0146.
40. Lerman-Sagie T, Ben-Sira L, Achiron R, Schreiber L, Hermann G, Lev D, Kidron D, Malinger G. Thick

fetal corpus callosum: an ominous sign? Ultrasound Obstet Gynecol. 2009;34(1):55–61. https://doi.org/10.1002/uog.6356.
41. Rypens F, Sonigo P, Aubry MC, Delezoide AL, Cessot F, Brunelle F. Prenatal MR diagnosis of a thick corpus callosum. AJNR Am J Neuroradiol. 1996;17(10):1918–20. http://www.ncbi.nlm.nih.gov/pubmed/8933878
42. Vola EA, Griffiths PD, Parazzini C, Palumbo G, Scola E, Severino M, Pinelli L, D'Errico I, Di Maurizio M, Pecco N, Rossi A, Triulzi F, Righini A. Complete agenesis of corpus callosum and unilateral cortical formation anomalies detected on fetal MR imaging: a phenotype strongly associated with the male fetuses. Eur Radiol. 2023;33(3):2258–65. https://doi.org/10.1007/s00330-022-09173-9.
43. Ramirez Zegarra R, Casati D, Volpe N, Lanna M, Dall'Asta A, Chiarelli A, Ormitti F, Percesepe A, Montaguti E, Labadini C, Salsi G, di Pasquo E, Bonasoni MP, Quarello E, Pilu G, Grisolia G, Righini A, Ghi T. The "cortical invagination sign": a midtrimester sonographic marker of unilateral cortical focal dysgyria in fetuses with complete agenesis of the corpus callosum. Am J Obstet Gynecol MFM. 2023;5(12):101198. https://doi.org/10.1016/j.ajogmf.2023.101198.
44. Tarui T, Madan N, Farhat N, Kitano R, Ceren Tanritanir A, Graham G, Gagoski B, Craig A, Rollins CK, Ortinau C, Iyer V, Pienaar R, Bianchi DW, Grant PE, Im K. Disorganized patterns of sulcal position in fetal brains with agenesis of corpus callosum. Cereb Cortex. 2018;28(9):3192–203. https://doi.org/10.1093/cercor/bhx191.
45. Kunpalin Y, Deprest J, Papastefanou I, Bredaki E, Sacco A, Russo F, Richter J, Jansen K, Ourselin S, De Coppi P, David AL, Ushakov F, De Catte L. Incidence and patterns of abnormal corpus callosum in fetuses with isolated spina bifida aperta. Prenat Diagn. 2021;41(8):957–64. https://doi.org/10.1002/pd.5945.
46. Atallah A, Lacalm A, Massoud M, Massardier J, Gaucherand P, Guibaud L. Prenatal diagnosis of pericallosal curvilinear lipoma: specific imaging pattern and diagnostic pitfalls. Ultrasound Obstet Gynecol. 2018;51(2):269–73. https://doi.org/10.1002/uog.17400.
47. Ickowitz V, Eurin D, Rypens F, Sonigo P, Simon I, David P, Brunelle F, Avni FE. Prenatal diagnosis and postnatal follow-up of pericallosal lipoma: report of seven new cases. AJNR Am J Neuroradiol. 2001;22(4):767–72. http://www.ncbi.nlm.nih.gov/pubmed/11290497
48. Kitova TT, Kitov B, Milkov D, Gaigi S. Postnatally diagnosed agenesis of corpus callosum in fetuses. Fetal Pediatr Pathol. 2014;33(4):239–43. https://doi.org/10.3109/15513815.2014.915366.
49. Kidron D, Shapira D, Ben Sira L, Malinger G, Lev D, Cioca A, Sharony R, Lerman ST. Agenesis of the corpus callosum. An autopsy study in fetuses. Virchows Arch. 2016;468(2):219–30. https://doi.org/10.1007/s00428-015-1872-y.
50. D'Antonio F, Pagani G, Familiari A, Khalil A, Sagies TL, Malinger G, Leibovitz Z, Garel C, Moutard ML, Pilu G, Bhide A, Acharya G, Leombroni M, Manzoli L, Papageorghiou A, Prefumo F. Outcomes associated with isolated agenesis of the corpus callosum: a meta-analysis. Pediatrics. 2016;138(3):e20160445. https://doi.org/10.1542/peds.2016-0445.
51. Sajan SA, Fernandez L, Nieh SE, Rider E, Bukshpun P, Wakahiro M, Christian SL, Rivière JB, Sullivan CT, Sudi J, Herriges MJ, Paciorkowski AR, Barkovich AJ, Glessner JT, Millen KJ, Hakonarson H, Dobyns WB, Sherr EH. Both rare and de novo copy number variants are prevalent in agenesis of the corpus callosum but not in cerebellar hypoplasia or polymicrogyria. PLoS Genet. 2013;9(10):e1003823. https://doi.org/10.1371/journal.pgen.1003823.
52. Edwards TJ, Sherr EH, Barkovich AJ, Richards LJ. Clinical, genetic and imaging findings identify new causes for corpus callosum development syndromes. Brain. 2014;137(Pt 6):1579–613. https://doi.org/10.1093/brain/awt358.
53. Bedeschi MF, Bonaglia MC, Grasso R, Pellegri A, Garghentino RR, Battaglia MA, Panarisi AM, Di Rocco M, Balottin U, Bresolin N, Bassi MT, Borgatti R. Agenesis of the corpus callosum: clinical and genetic study in 63 young patients. Pediatr Neurol. 2006;34(3):186–93. https://doi.org/10.1016/j.pediatrneurol.2005.08.008.
54. Tsai P, Shinar S. Agenesis of the corpus callosum: what to tell expecting parents? Prenat Diagn. 2023;43(12):1527–35. https://doi.org/10.1002/pd.6447.
55. Conway RL, Pressman BD, Dobyns WB, Danielpour M, Lee J, Sanchez-Lara PA, Butler MG, Zackai E, Campbell L, Saitta SC, Clericuzio CL, Milunsky JM, Hoyme HE, Shieh J, Moeschler JB, Crandall B, Lauzon JL, Viskochil DH, Harding B, Graham JM. Neuroimaging findings in macrocephaly-capillary malformation: a longitudinal study of 17 patients. Am J Med Genet A. 2007;143A(24):2981–3008. https://doi.org/10.1002/ajmg.a.32040.
56. Kivitie-Kallio S, Norio R. Cohen syndrome: essential features, natural history, and heterogeneity. Am J Med Genet. 2001;102(2):125–35. https://doi.org/10.1002/1096-8628(20010801)102:2<125::aid-ajmg1439>3.0.co;2-0.
57. Oesch G, Maga AM, Friedman SD, Poliachik SL, Budech CB, Wright JN, Bok LA, Gospe SM. Geometric morphometrics reveal altered corpus callosum shape in pyridoxine-dependent epilepsy. Neurology. 2018;91(1):e78–86. https://doi.org/10.1212/WNL.0000000000005748.
58. de Wit MC, Boekhorst F, Mancini GM, Smit LS, Groenenberg IAL, Dudink J, de Vries FAT, Go ATJI, Galjaard RJH. Advanced genomic testing may aid in counseling of isolated agenesis of the corpus callosum on prenatal ultrasound. Prenat Diagn.

2017;37(12):1191–7. https://doi.org/10.1002/pd.5158.

59. She Q, Fu F, Guo X, Tan W, Liao C. Genetic testing in fetuses with isolated agenesis of the corpus callosum. J Matern Fetal Neonatal Med. 2021;34(14):2227–34. https://doi.org/10.1080/14767058.2019.1660769.
60. Mustafa HJ, Barbera JP, Sambatur EV, Pagani G, Yaron Y, Baptiste CD, Wapner RJ, Brewer CJ, Khalil A. Diagnostic yield of exome sequencing in prenatal agenesis of corpus callosum: a systematic review and meta-analysis. Ultrasound Obstet Gynecol. 2023;63:312–20. https://doi.org/10.1002/uog.27440.
61. Society for Maternal-Fetal Medicine (SMFM), Rotmensch S, Monteagudo A. Agenesis of the corpus callosum. Am J Obstet Gynecol. 2020;223(6):B17–22. https://doi.org/10.1016/j.ajog.2020.08.179.
62. Salomon LJ, Alfirevic Z, Berghella V, Bilardo CM, Chalouhi GE, Da Silva CF, Hernandez-Andrade E, Malinger G, Munoz H, Paladini D, Prefumo F, Sotiriadis A, Toi A, Lee W. ISUOG practice guidelines (updated): performance of the routine mid-trimester fetal ultrasound scan. Ultrasound Obstet Gynecol. 2022;59(6):840–56. https://doi.org/10.1002/uog.24888.
63. AIUM practice parameter for the performance of detailed second- and third-trimester diagnostic obstetric ultrasound examinations. J Ultrasound Med. 2019;38(12):3093–100. https://doi.org/10.1002/jum.15163.
64. Viñals F, Correa F, Gonçalves-Pereira PM. Anterior and posterior complexes: a step towards improving neurosonographic screening of midline and cortical anomalies. Ultrasound Obstet Gynecol. 2015;46(5):585–94. https://doi.org/10.1002/uog.14735.
65. Cagneaux M, Guibaud L. From cavum septi pellucidi to anterior complex: how to improve detection of midline cerebral abnormalities. Ultrasound Obstet Gynecol. 2013;42(4):485–6. https://doi.org/10.1002/uog.12505.
66. Weissbach T, Massarwa A, Hadi E, Lev S, Haimov A, Katorza E, Brenner-Weissmann A, Krampl-Bettelheim E, Kasprian G, Sharon R, Achiron R, Weisz B, Kivilevitch Z, Kassif E. Early fetal corpus callosum: demonstrating normal growth and detecting pathologies in early pregnancy. AJNR Am J Neuroradiol. 2023;44(2):199–204. https://doi.org/10.3174/ajnr.A7757.
67. Birnbaum R, Barzilay R, Brusilov M, Wolman I, Malinger G. The early pattern of human corpus callosum development: a transvaginal 3D neurosonographic study. Prenat Diagn. 2020;40(10):1239–45. https://doi.org/10.1002/pd.5735.
68. Conturso R, Contro E, Bellussi F, Youssef A, Pacella G, Martelli F, Rizzo N, Pilu G, Ghi T. Demonstration of the pericallosal artery at 11-13 weeks of gestation using 3D ultrasound. Fetal Diagn Ther. 2015;37(4):305–9. https://doi.org/10.1159/000366156.
69. Vasciaveo L, Rizzo G, Khalil A, Alameddine S, Di Girolamo R, Candia M, De Lucia G, Mappa I, Liberati M, Nappi L, D'Antonio F. Assessment of pericallosal artery at 11-14 weeks of gestation: cohort study and meta-analysis. J Clin Ultrasound. 2022;50(7):984–8. https://doi.org/10.1002/jcu.23191.
70. Volpe N, Ramirez Zegarra R, Ghi T. Second-trimester anatomy of the fetal brain. In: Visual Encyclopedia of Ultrasound in Obstetrics and Gynecology (VISUOG). 2022. https://www.isuog.org/education/visuog/obstetrics/normal-sonograms/second-and-third-trimester/fetal-brain-anatomy.html
71. Youssef A, Ghi T, Pilu G. How to image the fetal corpus callosum. Ultrasound Obstet Gynecol. 2013;42(6):718–20. https://doi.org/10.1002/uog.12367.
72. Pashaj S, Merz E. 3-dimensional ultrasound: how can the fetal corpus callosum be demonstrated correctly? Ultraschall Med. 2021;42(3):278–84. https://doi.org/10.1055/a-1365-8611.
73. Pilu G, Segata M, Ghi T, Carletti A, Perolo A, Santini D, Bonasoni P, Tani G, Rizzo N. Diagnosis of midline anomalies of the fetal brain with the three-dimensional median view. Ultrasound Obstet Gynecol. 2006;27(5):522–9. https://doi.org/10.1002/uog.2751.
74. Muscatello A, Accurti V, Conte V, Franchi V, Colagrande I, Carta A, Patacchiola F, Palermo P, Carta G. Comparison between two- and three-dimensional ultrasound in visualization of corpus callosum during second trimester routine scan: our experience. Fetal Diagn Ther. 2013;33(3):201–2. https://doi.org/10.1159/000346399.
75. Griffiths PD, Brackley K, Bradburn M, Connolly DJA, Gawne-Cain ML, Griffiths DI, Kilby MD, Mandefield L, Mooney C, Robson SC, Vollmer B, Mason G. Anatomical subgroup analysis of the MERIDIAN cohort: failed commissuration. Ultrasound Obstet Gynecol. 2017;50(6):753–60. https://doi.org/10.1002/uog.17502.
76. Díaz-Guerrero L, Giugni-Chalbaud G, Sosa-Olavarría A. Assessment of pericallosal arteries by color Doppler ultrasonography at 11-14 weeks: an early marker of fetal corpus callosum development in normal fetuses and agenesis in cases with chromosomal anomalies. Fetal Diagn Ther. 2013;34(2):85–9. https://doi.org/10.1159/000351657.
77. Rydberg C, Tunón K. Detection of fetal abnormalities by second-trimester ultrasound screening in a non-selected population. Acta Obstet Gynecol Scand. 2017;96(2):176–82. https://doi.org/10.1111/aogs.13037.
78. Fadda GM, Capobianco G, Balata A, Litta P, Ambrosini G, D'Antona D, Cosmi E, Dessole S. Routine second trimester ultrasound screening for prenatal detection of fetal malformations in Sassari University Hospital, Italy: 23 years of experience in

42,256 pregnancies. Eur J Obstet Gynecol Reprod Biol. 2009;144(2):110–4. https://doi.org/10.1016/j.ejogrb.2009.02.045.
79. Paladini D, Pastore G, Cavallaro A, Massaro M, Nappi C. Agenesis of the fetal corpus callosum: sonographic signs change with advancing gestational age. Ultrasound Obstet Gynecol. 2013;42(6):687–90. https://doi.org/10.1002/uog.12506.
80. Barkovich AJ, Norman D. Absence of the septum pellucidum: a useful sign in the diagnosis of congenital brain malformations. AJR Am J Roentgenol. 1989;152(2):353–60. https://doi.org/10.2214/ajr.152.2.353.
81. Paladini D, Malinger G, Birnbaum R, Monteagudo A, Pilu G, Salomon LJ, Timor-Tritsch IE. ISUOG practice guidelines (updated): sonographic examination of the fetal central nervous system. Part 2: performance of targeted neurosonography. Ultrasound Obstet Gynecol. 2021;57(4):661–71. https://doi.org/10.1002/uog.23616.
82. Karl K, Chaoui R. Tela-choroidea-to-anterior-cerebral-artery distance (TACAD): novel marker on color Doppler to identify fetuses with complete or partial agenesis of corpus callosum. Ultrasound Obstet Gynecol. 2023;62(5):701–6. https://doi.org/10.1002/uog.26275.
83. Ghi T, Carletti A, Contro E, Cera E, Falco P, Tagliavini G, Michelacci L, Tani G, Youssef A, Bonasoni P, Rizzo N, Pelusi G, Pilu G. Prenatal diagnosis and outcome of partial agenesis and hypoplasia of the corpus callosum. Ultrasound Obstet Gynecol. 2010;35(1):35–41. https://doi.org/10.1002/uog.7489.
84. Shen O, Gelot AB, Moutard ML, Jouannic JM, Sela HY, Garel C. Abnormal shape of the cavum septi pellucidi: an indirect sign of partial agenesis of the corpus callosum. Ultrasound Obstet Gynecol. 2015;46(5):595–9. https://doi.org/10.1002/uog.14776.
85. Karl K, Esser T, Heling KS, Chaoui R. Cavum septi pellucidi (CSP) ratio: a marker for partial agenesis of the fetal corpus callosum. Ultrasound Obstet Gynecol. 2017;50(3):336–41. https://doi.org/10.1002/uog.17409.
86. Achiron R, Achiron A. Development of the human fetal corpus callosum: a high-resolution, cross-sectional sonographic study. Ultrasound Obstet Gynecol. 2001;18(4):343–7. https://doi.org/10.1046/j.0960-7692.2001.00512.x.
87. Malinger G, Zakut H. The corpus callosum: normal fetal development as shown by transvaginal sonography. AJR Am J Roentgenol. 1993;161(5):1041–3. https://doi.org/10.2214/ajr.161.5.8273605.
88. Tsur A, Weisz B, Rosenblat O, Shai D, Derazne E, Stevenson DK, Achiron R, Katorza E. Personalized charts for the fetal corpus callosum length. J Matern Fetal Neonatal Med. 2019;32(23):3931–8. https://doi.org/10.1080/14767058.2018.1479389.
89. Corroenne R, Grevent D, Kasprian G, Stirnemann J, Ville Y, Mahallati H, Salomon LJ. Corpus callosal reference ranges: systematic review of methodology of biometric chart construction and measurements obtained. Ultrasound Obstet Gynecol. 2023;62(2):175–84. https://doi.org/10.1002/uog.26187.
90. Meidan R, Bar-Yosef O, Ashkenazi I, Yahal O, Berkenstadt M, Hoffman C, Tsur A, Achiron R, Katorza E. Neurodevelopmental outcome following prenatal diagnosis of a short corpus callosum. Prenat Diagn. 2019;39(6):477–83. https://doi.org/10.1002/pd.5460.
91. Shinar S, Har-Toov J, Lerman-Sagie T, Malinger G. Thick corpus callosum in the second trimester can be transient and is of uncertain significance. Ultrasound Obstet Gynecol. 2016;48(4):452–7. https://doi.org/10.1002/uog.15678.
92. Leombroni M, Khalil A, Liberati M, D'Antonio F. Fetal midline anomalies: diagnosis and counselling part 1: corpus callosum anomalies. Eur J Paediatr Neurol. 2018;22(6):951–62. https://doi.org/10.1016/j.ejpn.2018.08.007.
93. Callen PW, Callen AL, Glenn OA, Toi A. Columns of the fornix, not to be mistaken for the cavum septi pellucidi on prenatal sonography. J Ultrasound Med. 2008;27(1):25–31. https://doi.org/10.7863/jum.2008.27.1.25.
94. Santirocco M, Rodó C, Illescas T, Vázquez É, Garrido M, Higueras T, Arévalo S, Maiz N, Carreras E. Accuracy of prenatal ultrasound in the diagnosis of corpus callosum anomalies. J Matern Fetal Neonatal Med. 2021;34(3):439–44. https://doi.org/10.1080/14767058.2019.1609931.
95. Zhang Y. Prenatal ultrasound for the diagnosis of the agenesis of corpus callosum: a meta-analysis. J Matern Fetal Neonatal Med. 2023;36(2):2228454. https://doi.org/10.1080/14767058.2023.2228454.
96. Manevich-Mazor M, Weissmann-Brenner A, Bar Yosef O, Hoffmann C, Mazor RD, Mosheva M, Achiron RR, Katorza E. Added value of fetal MRI in the evaluation of fetal anomalies of the corpus callosum: a retrospective analysis of 78 cases. Ultraschall Med. 2018;39(5):513–25. https://doi.org/10.1055/s-0043-113820.
97. Sotiriadis A, Makrydimas G. Neurodevelopment after prenatal diagnosis of isolated agenesis of the corpus callosum: an integrative review. Am J Obstet Gynecol. 2012;206(4):337.e1–5. https://doi.org/10.1016/j.ajog.2011.12.024.
98. Sileo FG, Di Mascio D, Rizzo G, Caulo M, Manganaro L, Bertucci E, Masmejan S, Liberati M, D'Amico A, Nappi L, Buca D, Van Mieghem T, Khalil A, D'Antonio F. Role of prenatal magnetic resonance imaging in fetuses with isolated agenesis of corpus callosum in the era of fetal neurosonography: A systematic review and meta-analysis. Acta Obstet Gynecol Scand. 2021;100(1):7–16. https://doi.org/10.1111/aogs.13958.
99. Bayram AK, Kütük MS, Doganay S, Özgün MT, Gümüş H, Başbuğ M, Kumandaş S, Canpolat M, Per H. An analysis of 109 fetuses with prenatal diagnosis

of complete agenesis of corpus callosum. Neurol Sci. 2020;41(6):1521–9. https://doi.org/10.1007/s10072-019-04224-4.
100. Goodyear PW, Bannister CM, Russell S, Rimmer S. Outcome in prenatally diagnosed fetal agenesis of the corpus callosum. Fetal Diagn Ther. 2001;16(3):139–45. https://doi.org/10.1159/000053898.
101. Brown WS, Paul LK. The neuropsychological syndrome of agenesis of the corpus callosum. J Int Neuropsychol Soc. 2019;25(3):324–30. https://doi.org/10.1017/S135561771800111X.
102. Lau YC, Hinkley LBN, Bukshpun P, Strominger ZA, Wakahiro MLJ, Baron-Cohen S, Allison C, Auyeung B, Jeremy RJ, Nagarajan SS, Sherr EH, Marco EJ. Autism traits in individuals with agenesis of the corpus callosum. J Autism Dev Disord. 2013;43(5):1106–18. https://doi.org/10.1007/s10803-012-1653-2.
103. Badaruddin DH, Andrews GL, Bölte S, Schilmoeller KJ, Schilmoeller G, Paul LK, Brown WS. Social and behavioral problems of children with agenesis of the corpus callosum. Child Psychiatry Hum Dev. 2007;38(4):287–302. https://doi.org/10.1007/s10578-007-0065-6.
104. David AS, Wacharasindhu A, Lishman WA. Severe psychiatric disturbance and abnormalities of the corpus callosum: review and case series. J Neurol Neurosurg Psychiatry. 1993;56(1):85–93. https://doi.org/10.1136/jnnp.56.1.85.
105. Motomura N, Satani S, Inaba M. Monozygotic twin cases of the agenesis of the corpus callosum with schizophrenic disorder. Psychiatry Clin Neurosci. 2002;56(2):199–202. https://doi.org/10.1046/j.1440-1819.2002.00944.x.
106. Bernardes da Cunha S, Carneiro MC, Miguel Sa M, Rodrigues A, Pina C. Neurodevelopmental outcomes following prenatal diagnosis of isolated corpus callosum agenesis: a systematic review. Fetal Diagn Ther. 2021;48(2):88–95. https://doi.org/10.1159/000512534.
107. des Portes V, Rolland A, Velazquez-Dominguez J, Peyric E, Cordier MP, Gaucherand P, Massardier J, Massoud M, Curie A, Pellot AS, Rivier F, Lacalm A, Clément A, Ville D, Guibaud L. Outcome of isolated agenesis of the corpus callosum: A population-based prospective study. Eur J Paediatr Neurol. 2018;22(1):82–92. https://doi.org/10.1016/j.ejpn.2017.08.003.
108. Siffredi V, Anderson V, Leventer RJ, Spencer-Smith MM. Neuropsychological profile of agenesis of the corpus callosum: a systematic review. Dev Neuropsychol. 2013;38(1):36–57. https://doi.org/10.1080/87565641.2012.721421.
109. Lanna M, Scelsa B, Cutillo G, Amendolara M, Doneda C, Balestriero M, Faiola S, Casati D, Spaccini L, Cetin I. Long-term outcome of consecutive case series of congenital isolated agenesis of corpus callosum. Ultrasound Obstet Gynecol. 2022;60(4):494–8. https://doi.org/10.1002/uog.24898.
110. Shwe WH, Schlatterer SD, Williams J, du Plessis AJ, Mulkey SB. Outcome of agenesis of the corpus callosum diagnosed by fetal MRI. Pediatr Neurol. 2022;135:44–51. https://doi.org/10.1016/j.pediatrneurol.2022.07.007.
111. Moutard ML, Kieffer V, Feingold J, Lewin F, Baron JM, Adamsbaum C, Gélot A, Isapof A, Kieffer F, de Villemeur TB. Isolated corpus callosum agenesis: a ten-year follow-up after prenatal diagnosis (how are the children without corpus callosum at 10 years of age?). Prenat Diagn. 2012;32(3):277–83. https://doi.org/10.1002/pd.3824.
112. Volpe P, Paladini D, Resta M, Stanziano A, Salvatore M, Quarantelli M, De Robertis V, Buonadonna AL, Caruso G, Gentile M. Characteristics, associations and outcome of partial agenesis of the corpus callosum in the fetus. Ultrasound Obstet Gynecol. 2006;27(5):509–16. https://doi.org/10.1002/uog.2774.
113. Bayram E, Topcu Y, Yis U, Cakmaci H, Kurul SH. Comparison of cranial magnetic resonance imaging findings and clinical features in patients with corpus callosum abnormalities. Neuropediatrics. 2014;45(1):30–5. https://doi.org/10.1055/s-0033-1349228.
114. Casanova MF, El-Baz A, Elnakib A, Switala AE, Williams EL, Williams DL, Minshew NJ, Conturo TE. Quantitative analysis of the shape of the corpus callosum in patients with autism and comparison individuals. Autism. 2011;15(2):223–38. https://doi.org/10.1177/1362361310386506.
115. Hyun Yoo J, Hunter J. Imaging spectrum of pediatric corpus callosal pathology: a pictorial review. J Neuroimaging. 2013;23(2):281–95. https://doi.org/10.1111/j.1552-6569.2011.00681.x.
116. Li Y, Estroff JA, Khwaja O, Mehta TS, Poussaint TY, Robson CD, Feldman HA, Ware J, Levine D. Callosal dysgenesis in fetuses with ventriculomegaly: levels of agreement between imaging modalities and postnatal outcome. Ultrasound Obstet Gynecol. 2012;40(5):522–9. https://doi.org/10.1002/uog.11098.
117. Noguchi R, Abe K, Hamada H, Ogura T, Obata M, Miyazono Y, Yoshikawa H. Outcomes of patients with prenatally diagnosed agenesis of the corpus callosum in conjunction with ventriculomegaly. Arch Gynecol Obstet. 2014;290(2):237–42. https://doi.org/10.1007/s00404-014-3196-6.
118. Masmejan S, Blaser S, Keunen J, Seaward G, Windrim R, Kelly E, Ryan G, Baud D, Van Mieghem T. Natural history of ventriculomegaly in fetal agenesis of the corpus callosum. J Ultrasound Med. 2020;39(3):483–8. https://doi.org/10.1002/jum.15124.
119. Garel C, Moutard ML. Main congenital cerebral anomalies: how prenatal imaging aids counseling. Fetal Diagn Ther. 2014;35(4):229–39. https://doi.org/10.1159/000358519.
120. Hart AR, Vasudevan C, Griffiths PD, Foulds N, Piercy H, de Lacy P, Boxall S, Howe D, Vollmer

B. Antenatal counselling for prospective parents whose fetus has a neurological anomaly: part 2, risks of adverse outcome in common anomalies. Dev Med Child Neurol. 2022;64(1):23–39. https://doi.org/10.1111/dmcn.15043.

121. Ballardini E, Marino P, Maietti E, Astolfi G, Neville AJ. Prevalence and associated factors for agenesis of corpus callosum in Emilia Romagna (1981-2015). Eur J Med Genet. 2018;61(9):524–30. https://doi.org/10.1016/j.ejmg.2018.06.004.

122. Scelsa B. Fetal neurology: from prenatal counseling to postnatal follow-up. Diagnostics (Basel, Switzerland). 2022;12(12):3083. https://doi.org/10.3390/diagnostics12123083.

Anomalies of the Cavum Septi Pellucidi (CSP)

Giulia Biancotto and Dario Paladini

Abstract

In this chapter, we describe the sonographic features of major anomalies of the Cavum Septi Pellucidi (CSP). These anomalies include the isolated septal agenesis, the septo-optic dysplasia, and the lobar holoprosencephaly. Callosal agenesis is also associated with the non-visualization of the CSP. The prenatal differential diagnosis of these conditions is challenging, and it is thoroughly described in this chapter.

Keywords

Fetus · CSP · Septal agenesis · Septo-optic dysplasia · Corpus callosum agenesis · Lobar holoprosencephaly · Ultrasound · Neurosonography

The septum pellucidum is a cerebral structure composed by two juxtaposed laminae of white matter, located between the medial edge of the frontal horns and the bodies of the lateral ventricles [1]. It contains also hypothalamic and hippocampal fibers diverging from the forniceal columns and it is considered as part of the limbic system [2, 3]. During fetal life, the septal folds are separated by a fluid-filled cavity, the cavum septi pellucidi (CSP), an anatomical landmark which can be easily identified during the second-trimester ultrasound examination. The rostral and superior margins of the CSP are represented by the corpus callosum, while the body of the fornices represents the posterior and inferior limits. Occasionally, the CSP develops a posterior recess between the splenium and the hippocampal commissure, known as the *cavum vergae.*

According to Rakic and Yakovlev [4], who conducted a series of anatomical examinations on cadavers, the *lamina reuniens* plays a key role in the developmental events leading to the formation of the corpus callosum and the CSP as well as other structures of the telencephalon. Indeed, at 8 weeks of gestation, the *lamina reuniens* contributes to the formation of the two folds of the septum pellucidum, while the CSP developed later (10–12 weeks) by cavitation, as a subcallosal pocket of the *sulcus medianus telencephali medii* [5].

On ultrasound, the CSP appears as an anechoic space, interrupting the midline in the anterior part of the fetal brain. Its shape is variable and has been reported as squared, or, less frequently, triangular [6, 7]. The CSP is easily visualized on the three planes of the fetal brain [8] (Fig. 1).

Although the development of the CSP begins as early as the 10–12 weeks of gestation, this structure is reliably visualized on ultrasound

G. Biancotto · D. Paladini (✉)
Fetal Medicine and Surgery Unit, Istituto IRCCS G. Gaslini, Genoa, Italy

P. Volpe, T. Ghi (eds.), *Fetal Neurosonography*, Ultrasound in Obstetrics and Gynecology,
https://doi.org/10.1007/978-3-031-70192-4_5

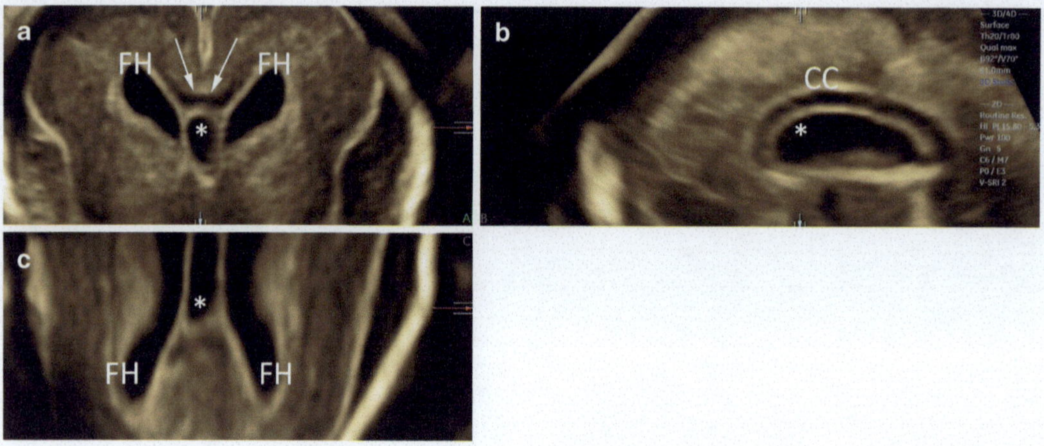

Fig. 1 CSP. Multiplanar imaging of the fetal brain at 20 gestational weeks. The volume was acquired through the anterior fontanelle. An asterisk is positioned where the reference marker dot would be, to highlight its position, identifying the CSP. (**a**) on the coronal transcaudate plane, the CSP is clearly evident, surrounded by the frontal horns (FH) of the lateral ventricles and surmounted by the corpus callosum (arrows), visible in cross-section; (**b**) on the reconstructed midsagittal plane, the CSP is shown below the whole length of the corpus callosum (CC); (**c**) on the reconstructed axial plane, the CSP is visible in between the two frontal horns (FH) of the lateral ventricles

between 18 and 37 weeks of gestation—when its development is complete; hence, failure to demonstrate this structure before 16 weeks and later than 37 is to be considered a normal finding. Indeed, a study conducted by Falco et al. showed that the CSP was seen in 40% of cases at 15 weeks, 82% between 16 and 17 weeks, 100% between 18 and 37 weeks, and 79% from 38 to 21 weeks [9]. As pregnancy progresses, the CSP undergoes slight variations in shape and size [10], while the septal layers progressively fuse to each other along the midline, with the generation of a single septum pellucidum. This is the reason why in the majority of cases, the CSP cannot be detected at ultrasound scan after 37 weeks of gestation.

Initially, in the 1980s, the CSP was used merely as an ultrasound indicator for the correct plane of measurement of the biparietal diameter; later, it was noted how a large CSP was associated with aneuploidies [11]. At the same time, the scientific community became aware of the fact that non-visualization of the CSP represents a strong marker of callosal agenesis. Therefore, the CSP has been included among the structures that should be observed in the routine second-trimester anomaly scan [12, 13]. We therefore identify two possible scenarios at mid trimester ultrasound screening for CNS anomalies:

1. The CSP is present and apparently normal (both in size and shape). In this case, no further diagnostic investigation is indicated.
2. The CSP is abnormal (either not visualized or with unusual appearance). In this case, fetal neurosonography is mandatory [14].

1 Non-visualization of the CSP

Non-visualization of the CSP represents an indication to fetal neurosonography. In fact, this finding can be associated with complete agenesis of corpus callosum (cACC). A thorough evaluation of the corpus callosum on the midsagittal plane of the fetal head and the search for other signs of cACC are therefore mandatory in these cases.

Of note, non-visualization of the CSP on the axial plane does not always underlies a cACC. In fact, on some occasions, the CSP is poorly visualized due to a reduced or even virtual amount of fluid within the septal leaflets (Fig. 2a and b). In these cases, if a normal corpus callosum can be

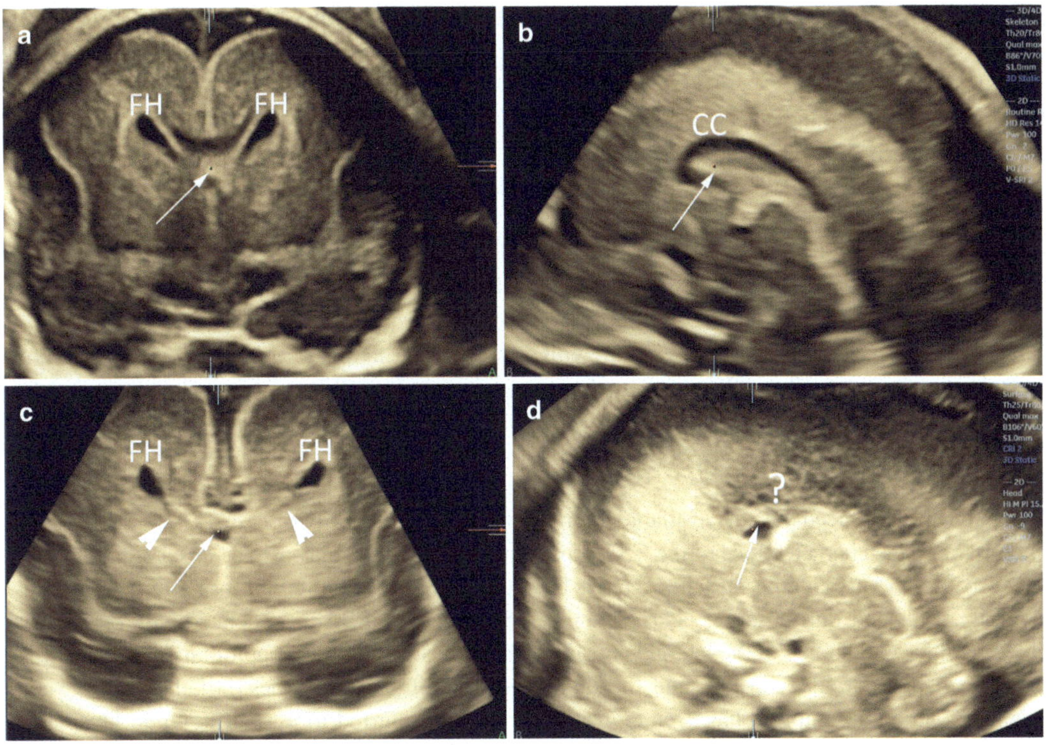

Fig. 2 Non-visualization of the CSP is not synonymous with complete agenesis of corpus callosum (cACC). (**a**, **b**) virtual CSP with normal corpus callosum (20 gestational weeks); (**c**, **d**) cACC (20 gestational weeks). (**a**) on the coronal, transcaudate plane, the CSP (arrow) cannot be visualized. However, the frontal horns of the lateral ventricles (FH) show a normal configuration and the corpus callosum is visible in cross-section as a hypoechoic structure in between the two frontal horns; (**b**) on the midsagittal plane, the whole corpus callosum (CC) is seen, with a normal aspect. All 4 components are visible (rostrum, genu, body, splenium); (**c**) in this case, on the coronal transcaudate plane again the CSP cannot be demonstrated (arrow). The frontal horns (FH) are seen, but they are distorted in their inferior portion (arrowheads). Furthermore, the cross-section of the corpus callosum is not visible (compare with [A]); (**d**) on the midsagittal plane, the corpus callosum is not visible (?) as per cACC. Only a small remnant of the CSP (arrow) can be seen

demonstrated (Fig. 2b), the neurological outcome is highly likely to be normal [5]. In other cases of non-visualization of the CSP, hyperechoic tissue and strands inside the CSP might be observed. The pathophysiology of these conditions has not been fully understood. It seems that these findings might be due to a fetal development arrest or with subsequent collection of substances or blood within it, rather than to an early CSP obliteration [5]. Also in these cases, a favorable outcome can be expected. Therefore, if the presence of a normal corpus callosum could be demonstrated on transvaginal neurosonography, a virtual/poorly defined CSP may be considered a not relevant finding.

Of note, "*absence of the septum pellucidum*" is not a synonym for "*absence of the CSP*." Indeed, the former identifies a developmental anomaly in which the two leaflets of the septum pellucidum have not developed causing a wide communication between the two frontal horns; the latter corresponds to the non-visualization of the CSP, which has been addressed above.

Of note, in addition to cACC, also other severe anomalies such as congenital hydrocephalus, holoprosencephaly (HPE) and secondary disruptive or compressive processes (hydrocephalus, hydranencephaly, and schizencephaly/porencephaly) can be associated with a non-visualized CSP [15].

2 Abnormal Appearance of the CSP

In normal conditions, the antero-posterior diameter of the CSP is greater than the latero-lateral one [7]. Hence, if a smaller or square-shaped CSP is seen (Fig. 3), fetal neurosonography should be performed because this appearance of the CSP may be due to partial agenesis of the corpus callosum [16]. On the other hand, a prominent CSP has been found in association with aneuploidies (trisomy 18 in 92%, trisomy 13 in 37%, and trisomy 21 in 42% of cases), 22q11 microdeletion (67% of cases), and neurodevelopmental delay [11, 17, 18].

Lastly, as evidenced by the available literature, not only the characteristics of the CSP itself but also of the surrounding structures must be carefully evaluated during target neurosonography (i.e., the frontal horns of the lateral ventricle, the genu of the corpus callosum, and the falx). The term "anterior complex" has been coined to identify the group of these structure [6]. The reason why the anterior complex, rather than the CSP only, should be assessed, relies on the fact that some severe genetic conditions, such as hemimegalencephaly and tubulinopathies, can be associated with only subtle distortion of the anterior complex and they might be missed if only the CSP is evaluated [6].

3 Septal Agenesis (SA; Agenesis of the Septum Pellucidum)/Septo-Optic Dysplasia (SOD)

3.1 Definition

Septal agenesis (SA) is a rare cerebral anomaly characterized by the absence of the laminae that form the septum pellucidum. It is defined *partial* if only one lamina is missing, *complete* if both are absent [19]. When SA is isolated (i.e., neither associated with other major malformations nor with severe ventriculomegaly), the prognosis is usually good, with normal neurologic development in the majority of cases.

However, SA may also be observed in the context of more severe malformation complexes. Specifically, if SA is associated with optic nerve hypoplasia and/or hypopituitarism, as well as with additional anomalies [20], the resulting condition is referred to as "Septo-Optic Dysplasia" (SOD) or De Morsier syndrome. Of note, the antenatal diagnosis of SOD is extremely challenging [19, 21–23].

SA/SOD can coexist with cerebral malformations, such as lobar HPE, cACC, severe ventriculomegaly, and bilateral cortical malformations ("SOD-plus syndrome"), including schizencephaly (SCZ) and polymicrogyria (PMG) [15, 23, 24].

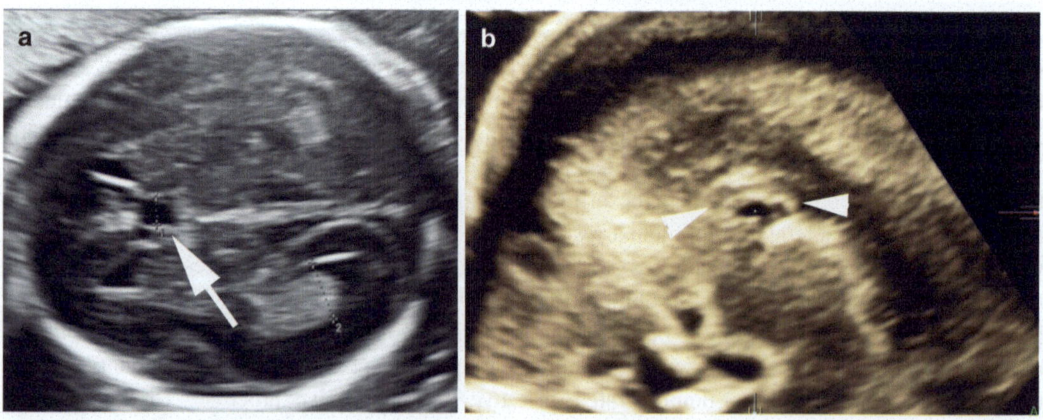

Fig. 3 Partial agenesis of the corpus callosum (pACC). In most cases, a CSP is present, though distorted. It may be smaller but especially shorter than normal. (**a**) on the axial transventricular plane, the CSP (arrow) is indeed visible, but is rather small, and squared; (**b**) on transvaginal neurosonography, the midsagittal plane demonstrates an incomplete and dysraphic corpus callosum (arrowheads) consistent with a diagnosis of pACC

3.2 Epidemiology

The actual incidence of isolated SA is unknown. The prevalence of SA in the general population was reported to be 2–3 cases per 100,000 births [15]. In the EUROCAT registry, between 2005 and 2014, the prevalence of SOD was reported to be 1.9–2.5/100,000 births [25].

3.3 Etiology/Pathogenesis

The etiology of SA and SOD has not been fully elucidated. It is likely to be multifactorial, involving both environmental factors such as drug and alcohol abuse, young maternal age, vascular insults, exposure to teratogens, viral infections [26, 27], as well as genetic factors [21, 27].

3.4 Genetic Background

SOD is mostly sporadic, even though numerous cases of familial clusters have been described and mutations in genes that play key roles in brain development, including HESX1, SOX2, SOX3, OTX2, TCF7L1 [28, 29], have been identified. Both recessive and dominant inheritance are described [30].

3.5 Sonographic Findings

SA should be suspected when the laminae of the septum pellucidum are not visible, and the frontal horns of the lateral ventricles appear to communicate on the midline (Fig. 4a). The frontal horns may present a squared appearance with the tip pointing downward. The corpus callosum is usually present, although it might be thin in some cases [22, 23, 31].

3.6 Differential Diagnosis

As already noted, the differential diagnosis between SA and SOD in the fetus is challenging, and it is not always achievable before birth. Various markers that may play a role in the differential diagnosis have been proposed: the estriol levels in maternal urine and serum, the fetal blood levels of growth hormone, adrenocorticotropic hormone, and prolactin [22], the size of the optic chiasm (OC) (decussation, optic tracts posteriorly, and optic nerves anteriorly) in the third trimester of pregnancy, with the assistance of MRI and 3D ultrasound [22, 32–34]. However, in instances where SA is diagnosed, no antenatal markers have been identified which can be used to reliably exclude SOD and patients

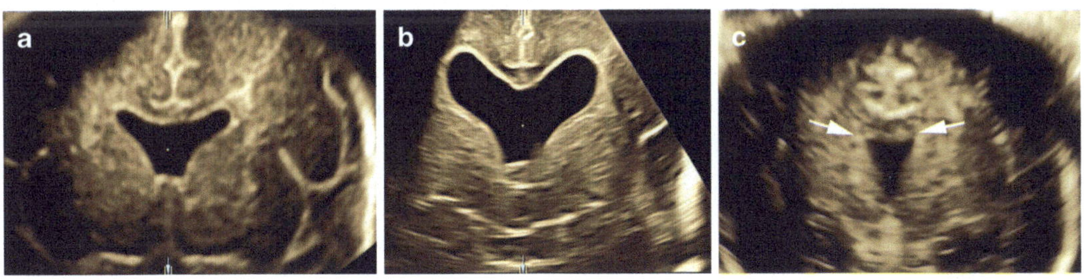

Fig. 4 (**a**) Septal agenesis (30 gestational weeks). On the coronal, transcaudate plane, the absence of the septal leaflets with communication between the two frontal horns is visible; (**b**) Another case of septal agenesis (27 gestational weeks) associated with ventriculomegaly. Note on the coronal transcaudate plane the rounder, enlarged aspect of the frontal horns. The absence of the septal leaflets is also clearly evident; (**c**) Lobar holoprosencephaly (32 gestational weeks). Note the absence of septal leaflets. However, in lobar holoprosencephaly, the amount of cerebro-spinal fluid within the frontal horns is often reduced, so that they become thread-like and difficult to spot (arrows). The diagnosis of lobar holoprosencephaly was confirmed by the identification of partial fusion of the frontal lobes (not visible on this image)

should be informed about the possibility of a postnatal diagnosis of this condition.

In general, the diagnosis of SOD can be strongly suspected in the presence of major cortical malformations. Some authors claim that the size of the fetal OC is highly predictive of the risk of optic nerve hypoplasia, and several nomograms of the normal fetal optic tracts and nerves have been published [32, 34]. However, OC cannot be used to rule out or in SOD in case of SA [34–36]. The definitive diagnosis of SOD can only be confirmed after birth, by demonstrating optic nerve hypoplasia through instrumental investigations (such as CT or MRI), and by performing pituitary functional test and neuro-ophthalmological assessment.

Lobar HPE represents another condition in which the septum pellucidum cannot be demonstrated [23]. However, the diagnosis of SA is favored by the presence of normal (or pointed) shape of the frontal horns (even if fused), normal interhemispheric fissure separating the frontal lobes (vs frontal lobe fusion in HPE), normal corpus callosum, and anterior cerebral arteries. MRI might help in the diagnosis of less straightforward cases by demonstrating the lack of separation of the frontal lobes in lobar HPE. In addition, a rounder aspect of the frontal horns seems to be present in lobar HPE while a more pointed one is associated with SA.

A condition frequently associated with SA is schizencephaly (SCZ). Indeed, it is crucial to carefully look for the presence of cortical clefts, more often bilateral, but sometimes small and unilateral [24, 37].

3.7 MRI

MRI is a valuable diagnostic tool complementary to ultrasound for better characterization of SA anomaly. It can be employed to assess the size of the OC to exclude optic nerve hypoplasia although this is not always possible. Additionally, MRI can aid the search for possible associated cortical anomalies, such as PMG and closed-lipped SCZ.

3.8 Prognosis

The association with other cerebral and/or extracerebral anomalies represents the most significant prognostic factor although low levels of maternal estriol also seem to be correlated with unfavorable outcomes [22].

Of note, additional anomalies are reported to be identified only after birth in about 10% of SA cases defined as apparently isolated in utero [19]. Children with isolated SA generally present favorable neurological outcomes although there is an overall risk of approximately 19% for SOD and a risk of about 7% of severe neurological disability [38–41].

The outcome of SOD is variable. In 40% of cases, visual disturbances are present, from blindness to nearly normal vision [42]. Optic nerve hypoplasia can be unilateral or bilateral (in 57% and 32% of cases, respectively) with significant visual impairment in 23% of patients. Regarding the endocrine impairments, hypopituitarism is present in 62–80% of patients, and although growth hormone deficiency (leading to short stature in childhood) is the most common endocrine anomaly, additional hormonal deficiencies (thyroid-stimulating, adrenocorticotropic, and gonadotropin-releasing hormones) can develop. In 80% of cases with visual and endocrine impairment, developmental delay was found [42]. The prognosis is very poor if SOD is associated with cortical malformations; in fact, in these cases, seizures and/or spastic motor deficits, intellectual deficits, and other neurological manifestations may be present.

3.9 Treatment Options

Postnatal treatment is symptomatic. Patients with SOD should be closely followed-up by a multidisciplinary team. Children may benefit from developmental programs for individuals with visual disabilities and physical and occupational therapies. Hormonal deficiencies can be treated with hormone replacement therapies.

On the contrary, no treatment is indicated for isolated SA.

3.10 Obstetric Management

Since the risk of aneuploidy and genetic imbalances is low, karyotype and CGH array are not indicated. However, if an invasive procedure is carried out, it is highly advisable to carry out an exome sequencing. Although the risk of recurrence is low, a family history of SOD is an indication for fetal neurosonography in the second trimester, to exclude recurrence.

References

1. Barany L, Meszaros C, Ganslandt O, Buchfelder M, Kurucz P. Neural and vascular architecture of the septum pellucidum: an anatomical study and considerations for safe endoscopic septum pellucidotomy. J Neurosurg. 2020;133(3):902–11.
2. Tortori-Donati P, Rossi A. Pediatric neuroradiology [Internet]. Berlin, Heidelberg: Springer Berlin Heidelberg; 2005. [cited 2023 Nov 14]. https://doi.org/10.1007/b137533.
3. Pauling KJ, Bodensteiner JB, Hogg JP, Schaefer GB. Does selection bias determine the prevalence of the cavum septi pellucidi? Pediatr Neurol. 1998;19(3):195–8.
4. Rakic P, Yakovlev PI. Development of the corpus callosum and cavum septi in man. J Comp Neurol. 1968;132(1):45–72.
5. Malinger G, Lev D, Oren M, Lerman-Sagie T. Non-visualization of the cavum septi pellucidi is not synonymous with agenesis of the corpus callosum. Ultrasound Obstet Gynecol. 2012;40(2): 165–70.
6. Viñals F, Correa F, Gonçalves-Pereira PM. Anterior and posterior complexes: a step towards improving neurosonographic screening of midline and cortical anomalies. Ultrasound Obstet Gynecol. 2015;46(5):585–94.
7. Karl K, Esser T, Heling KS, Chaoui R. Cavum septi pellucidi (CSP) ratio: a marker for partial agenesis of the fetal corpus callosum. Ultrasound Obstet Gynecol. 2017;50(3):336–41.
8. Malinger G, Paladini D, Haratz KK, Monteagudo A, Pilu GL, Timor-Tritsch IE. ISUOG practice guidelines (updated): sonographic examination of the fetal central nervous system. Part 1: performance of screening examination and indications for targeted neurosonography. Ultrasound Obstet Gynecol. 2020;56(3):476–84.
9. Falco P, Gabrielli S, Visentin A, Perolo A, Pilu G, Bovicelli L. Transabdominal sonography of the cavum septum pellucidum in normal fetuses in the second and third trimesters of pregnancy. Ultrasound Obstet Gynecol. 2000;16(6):549–53.
10. Jou HJ, Shyu MK, Wu SC, Chen SM, Su CH, Hsieh FJ. Ultrasound measurement of the fetal cavum septi pellucidi. Ultrasound Obstet Gynecol. 1998;12(6):419–21.
11. Chaoui R, Heling K, Zhao Y, Sinkovskaya E, Abuhamad A, Karl K. Dilated cavum septi pellucidi in fetuses with microdeletion 22q11. Prenat Diagn. 2016;36(10):911–5.
12. Winter TC, Kennedy AM, Byrne J, Woodward PJ. The cavum septi pellucidi: why is it important? J Ultrasound Med. 2010;29(3):427–44.
13. Salomon LJ, Alfirevic Z, Berghella V, Bilardo C, Hernandez-Andrade E, Johnsen SL, et al. Practice guidelines for performance of the routine mid-trimester fetal ultrasound scan. Ultrasound in Obstet Gynecol. 2011;37(1):116–26.
14. Paladini D, Malinger G, Birnbaum R, Monteagudo A, Pilu G, Salomon LJ, et al. ISUOG practice guidelines (updated): sonographic examination of the fetal central nervous system. Part 2: performance of targeted neurosonography. Ultrasound Obstet Gynecol. 2021;57(4):661–71.
15. Barkovich AJ, Norman D. Absence of the septum pellucidum: a useful sign in the diagnosis of congenital brain malformations. AJR Am J Roentgenol. 1989;152(2):353–60.
16. Shen O, Gelot AB, Moutard ML, Jouannic JM, Sela HY, Garel C. Abnormal shape of the cavum septi pellucidi: an indirect sign of partial agenesis of the corpus callosum. Ultrasound Obstet Gynecol. 2015;46(5):595–9.
17. Ding H, Zhao D, Cai A, Wei Q. Dilated cavum septi pellucidi as sole prenatal ultrasound defect: case-base analysis of fetal outcomes. Eur J Obstet Gynecol Reprod Biol. 2019;237:85–8.
18. Abele H, Babiy-Pachomow O, Sonek J, Hoopmann M, Schaelike M, Kagan KO. The cavum septi pellucidi in euploid and aneuploid fetuses. Ultrasound Obstet Gynecol. 2013;42(2):156–60.
19. Di Pasquo E, Kuleva M, Arthuis C, Morganelli G, Ormitti F, Millischer AE, et al. Prenatal diagnosis and outcome of fetuses with isolated agenesis of septum pellucidum: cohort study and meta-analysis. Ultrasound Obstet Gynecol. 2022;59(2):153–61.
20. Benson JC, Nascene D, Truwit C, McKinney AM. Septo-optic dysplasia: assessment of associated findings with special attention to the olfactory sulci and tracts. Clin Neuroradiol. 2019;29(3):505–13.
21. Volpe P, Campobasso G, De Robertis V, Rembouskos G. Disorders of prosencephalic development. Prenat Diagn. 2009;29(4):340–54.
22. Lepinard C, Coutant R, Boussion F, Loisel D, Delorme B, Biquard F, et al. Prenatal diagnosis of absence of the septum pellucidum associated with septo-optic dysplasia. Ultrasound Obstet Gynecol. 2005;25(1):73–5.
23. Malinger G, Lev D, Kidron D, Heredia F, Hershkovitz R, Lerman-Sagie T. Differential diagnosis in fetuses with absent septum pellucidum. Ultrasound Obstet Gynecol. 2005;25(1):42–9.

24. Raybaud C, Girard N, Lévrier O, Peretti-Viton P, Manera L, Farnarier P. Schizencephaly: correlation between the lobar topography of the cleft(s) and absence of the septum pellucidum. Childs Nerv Syst. 2001;17(4–5):217–22.
25. Garne E, Rissmann A, Addor MC, Barisic I, Bergman J, Braz P, et al. Epidemiology of septo-optic dysplasia with focus on prevalence and maternal age—a EUROCAT study. Eur J Med Genet. 2018;61(9):483–8.
26. McMahon CL, Braddock SR. Septo-optic dysplasia as a manifestation of valproic acid embryopathy. Teratology. 2001;64(2):83–6.
27. Kelberman D, Dattani MT. Septo-optic dysplasia—novel insights into the aetiology. Horm Res. 2008;69(5):257–65.
28. Thomas PQ, Dattani MT, Brickman JM, McNay D, Warne G, Zacharin M, et al. Heterozygous HESX1 mutations associated with isolated congenital pituitary hypoplasia and septo-optic dysplasia. Hum Mol Genet. 2001;10(1):39–45.
29. Fernández-Marmiesse A, Pérez-Poyato MS, Fontalba A, Marco de Lucas E, Martínez MT, Cabero Pérez MJ, et al. Septo-optic dysplasia caused by a novel FLNA splice site mutation: a case report. BMC Med Genet. 2019;20(1):112.
30. Wales J, Quarrell O. Evidence for possible Mendelian inheritance of septo-optic dysplasia. Acta Paediatr. 1996;85(3):391–2.
31. Pilu G, Sandri F, Cerisoli M, Alvisi C, Salvioli GP, Bovicelli L. Sonographic findings in septo-optic dysplasia in the fetus and newborn infant. Am J Perinatol. 1990;7(4):337–9.
32. Bault JP. Visualization of the fetal optic chiasma using three-dimensional ultrasound imaging. Ultrasound Obstet Gynecol. 2006;28(6):862–4.
33. Bault JP, Salomon LJ, Guibaud L, Achiron R. Role of three-dimensional ultrasound measurement of the optic tract in fetuses with agenesis of the septum pellucidum. Ultrasound Obstet Gynecol. 2011;37(5):570–5.
34. Paladini D, Birnbaum R, Donarini G, Maffeo I, Fulcheri E. Assessment of fetal optic chiasm: an echoanatomic and reproducibility study. Ultrasound Obstet Gynecol. 2016;48(6):727–32.
35. Viñals F, Ruiz P, Correa F, Gonçalves PP. Two-dimensional visualization and measurement of the fetal optic chiasm: improving counseling for antenatal diagnosis of agenesis of the septum pellucidum. Ultrasound Obstet Gynecol. 2016;48(6):733–8.
36. Haratz KK, Melcer Y, Leibovitz Z, Feit H, Lerman-Sagie T, Lev D, et al. Ultrasound nomograms of the fetal optic nerve sheath diameter. Ultraschall Med. 2019;40(4):476–80.
37. Malinger G, Kidron D, Schreiber L, Ben-Sira L, Hoffmann C, Lev D, et al. Prenatal diagnosis of malformations of cortical development by dedicated neurosonography. Ultrasound Obstet Gynecol. 2007;29(2):178–91.
38. Damaj L, Bruneau B, Ferry M, Moutard ML, Garel C, Odent S, et al. Pediatric outcome of children with the prenatal diagnosis of isolated septal agenesis. Prenat Diagn. 2010;30(12–13):1143–50.
39. Borkowski-Tillman T, Garcia-Rodriguez R, Viñals F, Branco M, Kradjen-Haratz K, Ben-Sira L, et al. Agenesis of the septum pellucidum: prenatal diagnosis and outcome. Prenat Diagn. 2020;40(6):674–80.
40. Celentano C, Prefumo F, Liberati M, Tartaro A, Gallo G, Lattanzio G, et al. Prenatal diagnosis of septal agenesis with normal pituitary function. Prenat Diagn. 2006;26(11):1075–7.
41. Belhocine O, André C, Kalifa G, Adamsbaum C. Does asymptomatic septal agenesis exist? A review of 34 cases. Pediatr Radiol. 2005;35(4):410–8.
42. Shinar S, Blaser S, Chitayat D, Selvanathan T, Chau V, Shannon P, et al. Long-term postnatal outcome of fetuses with prenatally suspected septo-optic dysplasia. Ultrasound Obstet Gynecol. 2020;56(3):371–7.

Cystic Posterior Fossa Anomalies

Cystic Posterior Fossa, From the Second to the First Trimester

Ilaria Fantasia, Claudiana Olivieri, Mariachiara Bosco, and Paolo Volpe

Abstract

The prenatal diagnosis of cystic malformation of the posterior fossa represents a critical aspect of antenatal care, offering valuable insights into the early identification and management of these congenital anomalies. The diagnosis of these malformations has traditionally been performed in the second trimester of pregnancy. However, the introduction of high-frequency probes has allowed to explore in detail the anatomy of the posterior cranial fossa already from the first trimester of pregnancy, opening new perspectives on the diagnostic classification of these pathologies and on prenatal counseling.

This chapter reviews current methodologies and technologies employed in the prenatal assessment of cystic posterior fossa malformations, emphasizing the role of advanced imaging modalities such as ultrasound and fetal neurosonography. The diagnostic challenges associated with distinguishing between different types of cystic malformations, such as Dandy–Walker malformation, vermian hypoplasia, Blake's pouch cyst, mega cisterna magna, and arachnoid cysts, are discussed.

Moreover, we will describe the new markers for cystic malformation of posterior fossa that may allow the identification of these anomalies already from the first trimester and the natural evolution of the pathology from the first to the second trimester, with related sonographic appearance. As prenatal diagnostic techniques advance, we emphasize the importance of understanding the relevance of emerging technologies to enhance the precision and effectiveness of diagnosing fetal cystic posterior fossa malformations.

Keywords

Anomaly scan · Cerebellum · Embryology · Fetal central nervous system · Fourth ventricle · Neurosonography

1 Introduction

The term cystic posterior fossa (CPF) anomalies includes a group of abnormalities characterized, on the axial transcerebellar view, by the presence of an apparent cerebrospinal fluid (CSF) collection in the posterior fossa. This sonographic appearance may arise from the incomplete

I. Fantasia · C. Olivieri · P. Volpe (✉)
Fetal Medicine Unit, Di Venere Hospital Bari, Bari, Italy

M. Bosco
Unit of Obstetrics and Gynecology, Department of Surgery, Dentistry, Pediatrics and Gynecology, University of Verona, AOUI Verona, Verona, Italy
e-mail: mariachiara.bosco@univr.it

P. Volpe, T. Ghi (eds.), *Fetal Neurosonography*, Ultrasound in Obstetrics and Gynecology,
https://doi.org/10.1007/978-3-031-70192-4_6

closure of the fourth ventricle (4th V), distension of the cisterna magna (CM), or the presence of true arachnoid cysts. CPF anomalies include Blake's pouch cyst (BPC), vermian hypoplasia (VH), Dandy–Walker malformation (DWM), megacisterna magna (MCM), and arachnoid cysts (AC). Despite sharing a similar sonographic appearance, these abnormalities are associated with distinct prognosis in terms of postnatal outcomes [1]. Unfortunately, although possible in some cases, a precise diagnosis using ultrasound and/or magnetic resonance imaging is challenging and primarily relying on subjective criteria.

Understanding the anatomical development of the posterior fossa is key for a correct identification and interpretation of sonographic signs that may indicate the presence of cystic anomalies in the posterior fossa.

Evidence from embryologic studies shows that the development of the posterior fossa is complex and dynamic throughout gestation and the various structures have different embryologic origins. Indeed, the walls of the metencephalon form the cerebellum, and the metencephalic cavity constitutes the upper (cranial) portion of the 4th V. The lower (caudal) portion of the 4th V, where the choroid plexus extend (as an invagination of the tela choroidea), originates from the cranial portion of the myelencephalon [2]. From the early fetal stages, the cerebellum and its vermis grow, and by 18–20 weeks' gestation, the cerebellar vermis has "closed" the 4th V [1, 3, 4]. At this gestational age, the 4th V appears as a midline cavity without communication with the cisterna magna. Indeed, the classical ultrasound image suspicious for PFC anomalies reveals, on the axial transcerebellar view, a fluid collection in the posterior fossa and/or a 4th V opening posteriorly and apparently communicating with the cisterna magna (Fig. 1). However, it is important to note that this sonographic marker cannot be considered diagnostic of PCF anomalies at any gestational age due to the progressive development of the posterior fossa. In fact, in the late first trimester, the fourth ventricle is notably large, with a relatively small cerebellum on top of it (Fig. 2a). Over the subsequent weeks, the cerebellum grows progressively enclosing the 4th V (Fig. 2b). Typically, by 18–19 weeks, the vermis has "closed" the 4th V. In fact, at this gestational age, on midsagittal view of the posterior fossa, it is possible to evaluate the position of the vermis through the measurement of the brainstem (or tegmentum)-vermis angle, which is always <18° in normal cases. Therefore, the demonstration of an opening after 18–19 weeks may be indicative

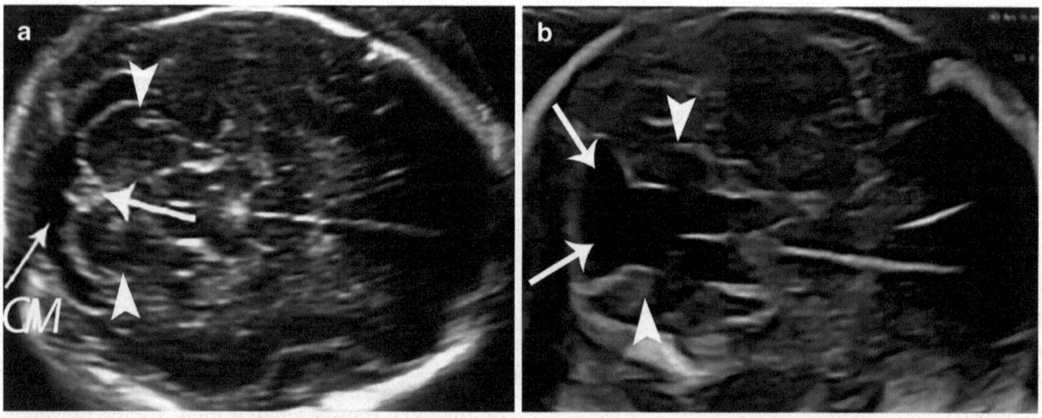

Fig. 1 (**a**) Axial transcerebellar view of the fetal head at 20 weeks showing in (**a**) the two cerebellar hemispheres (arrowheads), the vermis (arrow), and the cisterna magna (CM). (**b**) In this image, the two cerebellar hemispheres are visible (arrowheads), there is a cleft of the cerebellar vermis with an open fourth ventricle and a fluid collection in the posterior fossa (arrows)

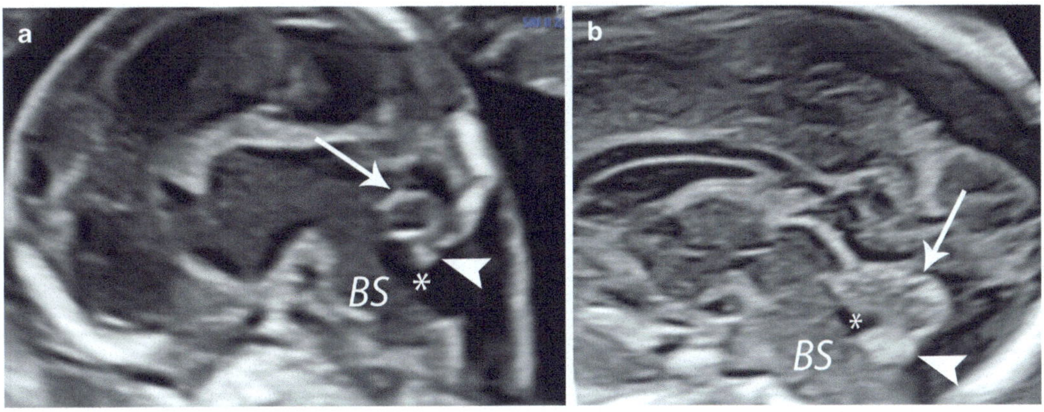

Fig. 2 Midsagittal view of the posterior fossa obtained with a transvaginal approach through the posterior fontanelle. (**a**) At 13 weeks, a small vermis (arrow) is on the top of a narrow fourth ventricle and the choroid plexus of the fourth ventricle is placed along the caudal portion of the vermis (*). (**b**) At 20 weeks, the fourth ventricle is completely closed by the vermis (arrow) and the choroid plexus of the fourth ventricle is still visible along its caudal portion (arrowhead) closing completely the fourth ventricle (*). *BS* brainstem

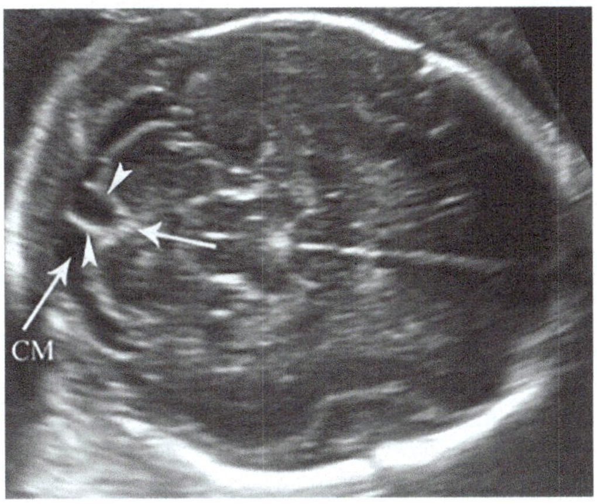

Fig. 3 Axial view of the posterior fossa showing the remnants of the Blake's pouch (arrowheads) immediately below the inferior portion of the vermis (arrow). *CM* cisterna magna

of a cystic posterior fossa anomaly [1, 3–5]. Additionally, a small finger-like appendage of the 4th V, known as the Blake's pouch (BP), is often observed protruding into the cisterna magna, caudal to the cerebellum [1, 3, 4, 6] (Fig. 3).

In cases where the closure of the fourth ventricle fails, two main processes may be implicated: impaired vermian development, preventing the correct closure of the 4th V at its inferior extent, and/or inadequate fenestration of the caudal part of the fourth ventricular roof (including the BP), which leads to a consequent cranial elevation of the vermis. The failed closure of the 4th V is distinctive of DWM, BPC, and VH (Fig. 4). Conversely, this process is not implicated in the pathogenesis of megacisterna magna (MCM) and of true arachnoid loculations (arachnoid cyst). Indeed, in these cases, the fluid collection in the posterior fossa is associated with anomalies of the CM and the subarachnoid space rather than of the cerebellum and 4th V. Indeed, in MCM and AC, the vermis is normal and the 4th V is properly closed (Fig. 5).

The complex nature of the embryologic development of the posterior fossa, the close relationship of the implicated anatomical structures and the wide spectrum of abnormalities with possible intermediate forms has made the prenatal differential diagnosis of cystic posterior fossa anomalies extremely challenging [7, 8].

The detection of CPF anomalies has been traditionally obtained in the second trimester [9]. Therefore, we here report the sonographic evaluation of the posterior fossa in the midtrimester, at anomaly scan. However, sonographic signs indicative for CPF anomalies can be detected at earlier gestational ages [10–12], as we will report later in this chapter.

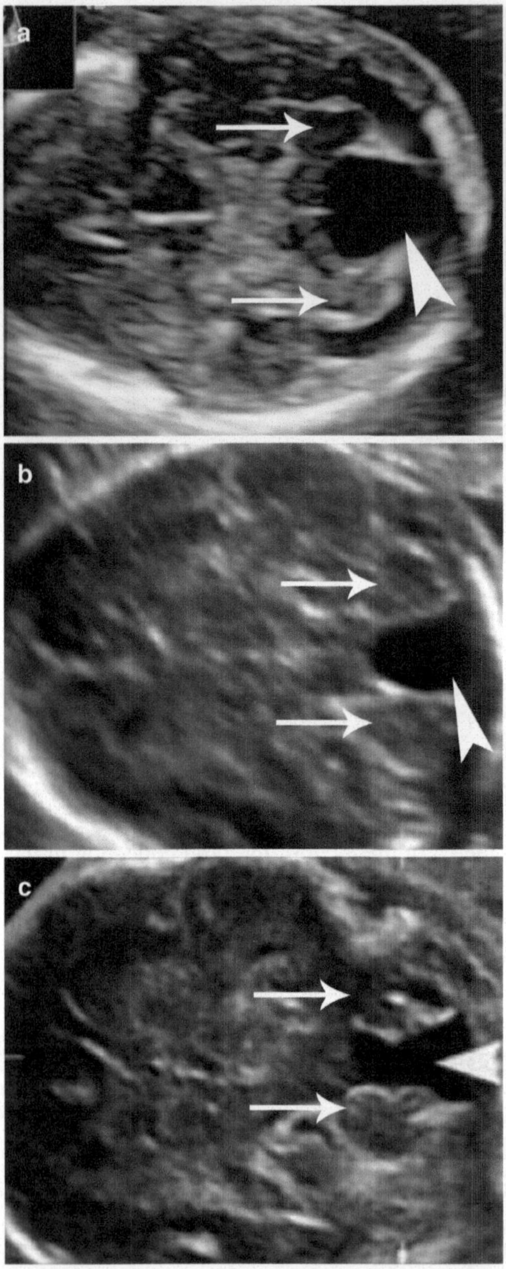

Fig. 4 Axial view of the posterior fossa showing the different appearance of the cerebellar hemispheres (arrows) and of the open fourth ventricle (arrowheads) because of the upward rotation of the vermis in Dandy–Walker malformation (**a**), in vermian hypoplasia (**b**) and in Blake's pouch cyst (**c**)

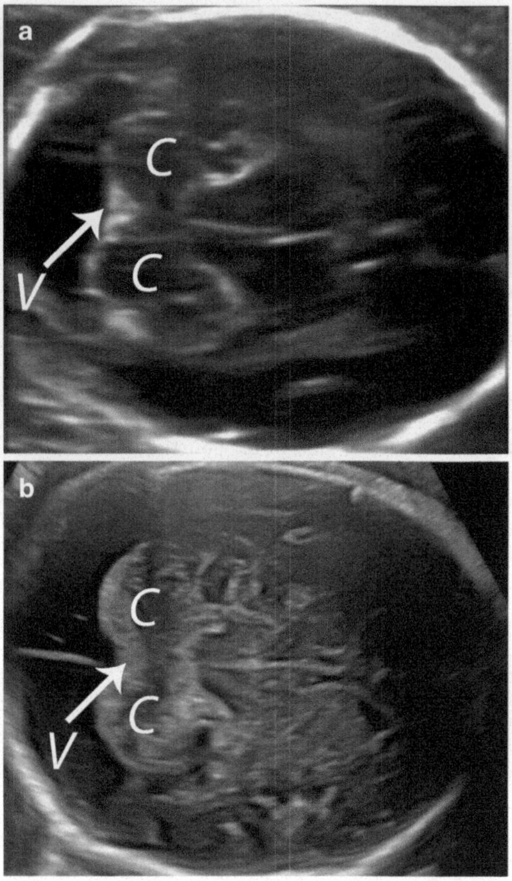

Fig. 5 Axial view of the posterior fossa showing the two cerebellar hemispheres (C), a normally positioned of the vermis with normal size (arrow) and a collection of fluid of the posterior fossa in a case of megacisterna magna (**a**) and arachnoid cyst (**b**). *V* vermis

1.1 Sonographic Evaluation of the Posterior Fossa in the Midtrimester

For an adequate assessment of the posterior fossa and its malformations, a multiplanar evaluation of the fetal brain is needed, with specific attention to the midsagittal plane. This plane allows a detailed visualization of the posterior fossa and its anatomical landmarks (Fig. 6) Various direct and indirect signs must be considered to perform

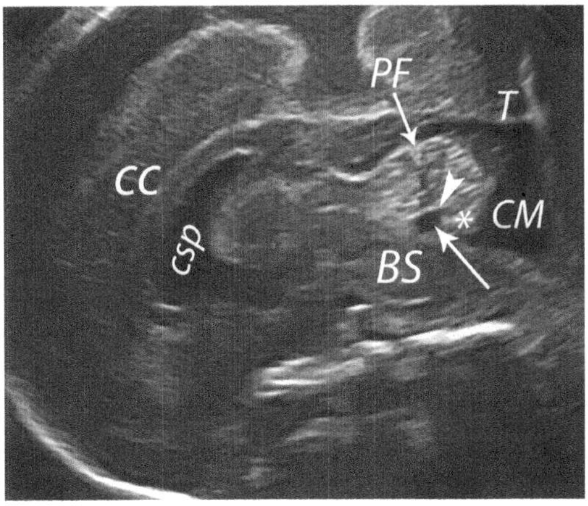

Fig. 6 Anatomical components of the posterior fossa and its anatomical landmarks (midsagittal view of the posterior fossa, posterior transvaginal approach): by drawing a line through the primary fissure (PF) and the fastigium (arrowheads), it is possible to divide the vermis in its anterior and posterior part. *CC* corpus callosum, *CSP* cavum septi pellucidi, *BS* brainstem, *T* tentorium, *CM* cisterna magna, * choroid plexus of the fourth ventricle

a comprehensive evaluation of the anatomical defect, including:

- Vermian biometry, position, and morphology.
- Fastigial point and vermian fissures.
- Size of the posterior fossa.
- Position of the torcular herophili/tentorium.
- Morphology of the cyst and its relationship with the fourth ventricle and subarachnoid spaces.
- Presence of an upward vermian rotation.
- Presence of ventriculomegaly (VM).

The assessment of the size, integrity, and position of the cerebellar vermis has an important role in helping differential diagnosis (Fig. 6); however, a correct characterization of the cerebellar vermis is challenging given its dynamic development throughout gestation and the difficult identification of its anatomical components.

However, advancements in ultrasound technology, with the introduction of high-frequency transabdominal (TA) and transvaginal (TV) probes, have allowed a more accurate study of the anatomy of the vermis. In this regard, recent findings have shown that the choroid plexus of the fourth ventricle (4th V-CP) has consistently been interpreted as the lower (caudal) portion of the vermis, rather than being recognized as a distinct structure. Consequently, the closure of the 4th V is determined not only by the vermis but also by the 4th V-CP [12] (Figs. 2 and 6). This finding has a major impact on the characterization of cystic anomalies of the posterior fossa. The correct identification of the choroid plexus not only impacts on the precise assessment of vermian size, but also plays a crucial role in guiding the differential diagnosis of these conditions.

1.2 The Fourth Ventricle-Choroid Plexus (4th V-CP)

The rudimentary 4th V-CP appears in the caudal part of the fourth ventricular roof around 44 postovulatory days. This plexus anatomically separates the thin ependymal roof of the fourth ventricle in two segments: a more cranial portion, connected to the cerebellar vermis at its upper end [the anterior membranous area (AMA)] and a more caudal portion [the posterior membranous area (PMA)] [2, 12–14]. The understanding of the relationship between these structures is crucial as it is thought that DWM derives from an abnormal development of the AMA while BPC represents an abnormal development of the PMA. (Diagram 1).

Research has shown that sonographic identification of the 4th V-CP is feasible from 12 weeks' gestation onwards. This can be achieved by assessing the coronal and midsagittal views of the fetal head, both in normal fetuses and in those with PCF anomalies (Figs. 7 and 8). The approach can be either with a high-resolution TA and/or a TV probe through the posterior fontanelle or using a multiplanar 3D reconstruction [12]. In normal fetuses, the 4th V-CP appears as an echogenic oval-shaped structure attached to the lower portion of the vermis and to the adjacent cerebellar hemispheres (Figs. 2, 6 and 7). This structure gradually occupies the space caudal to the 4th-V, between the vermis and the brainstem, "closing" the cavity at 18–19 weeks of gestation [12] (Fig. 2).

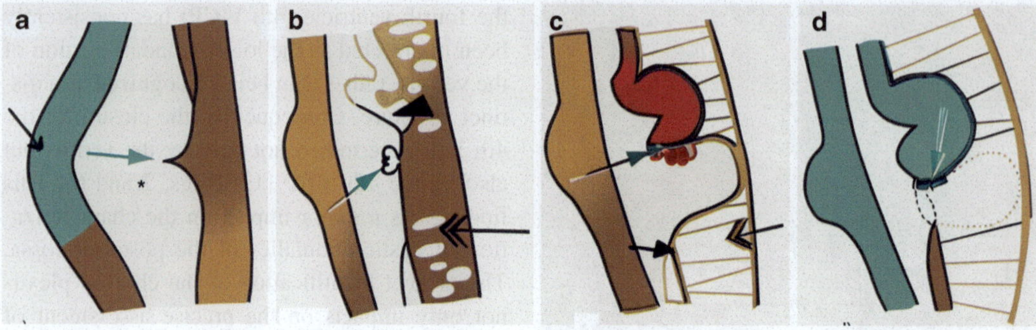

Diagram 1 (**a**) During formation of the dorsal pontine flexure (black arrow), a transverse crease (green arrow) forms in the roof of the rhombencephalic vesicle (*), dividing it into anterior (cranial) and posterior (caudal) membranous areas. (**b**) The vermis (black arrowhead) develops from the rhombic lip at the superior margin of the anterior membranous area. Choroid plexus develops in the crease (green arrow). Cavitation starts in the overlying meninx primitiva (double arrow) to form the subarachnoid space. (**c**) As the cerebellum grows inferiorly, the posterior membranous area bulges out between the vermis (green arrow) and the nucleus gracilis (black arrow), forming Blake's pouch. The subarachnoid space remains trabeculated by pia-arachnoid septations (double arrow). (**d**) Blake's pouch fenestrates (dotted line), and the neck of Blake's pouch becomes the foramen of Magendie (dashed line). The choroid plexus (green arrow) now appears to be in the cisterna magna

An analysis of previously published studies has revealed that the 4th V-CP, in the second trimester, has been consistently misinterpreted as the caudal portion of the cerebellar vermis. This has two main implications: firstly, by including the 4th V-CP in the measurement of the vermis, the reference ranges of the vermis size published so far might have overestimated its true size; secondly, without a correct identification of the 4th V-CP, the size of the 4th V-CP itself cannot be assessed and a small CP, which can be another cause of an open 4th V at 20–22 weeks, might be missed, as described later.

A second way of integrating the assessment of the 4th V-CP into the examination of the posterior fossa involves the evaluation of its position within the 4th V. To achieve this, it is essential to include the coronal view in addition to the midsagittal one. On the coronal plane, it is possible to visualize both the medial and the lateral segments of the 4th V-CP within the fourth ventricle. The medial segments, also referred to as longitudinal or vertical limbs, and the lateral segments, known as horizontal or transverse limbs, can be distinguished. In the midsagittal plane, only the vertical limbs are visible, and they appear to be connected to inferior part of the vermis, corresponding to the medial part of the 4th V-CP (Fig. 7).

The assessment of 4th V-CP position may yield important information for the differential diagnosis of fetal cystic posterior fossa abnormalities, particularly those characterized by an open fourth ventricle like DWM and BPC, each carrying distinct prognostic implications [12, 15]. In DWM, the abnormal persistence of the AMA, located superiorly to the choroid plexus of the fourth ventricle (4th V-CP), results in the expanding AMA intervening between the hypoplastic vermis and the 4th V-CP. This leads to ballooning of the fourth ventricular roof, which displaces the CP infero-laterally [12, 15, 16]. Therefore, in DWM, the 4th V-CP appears infero-

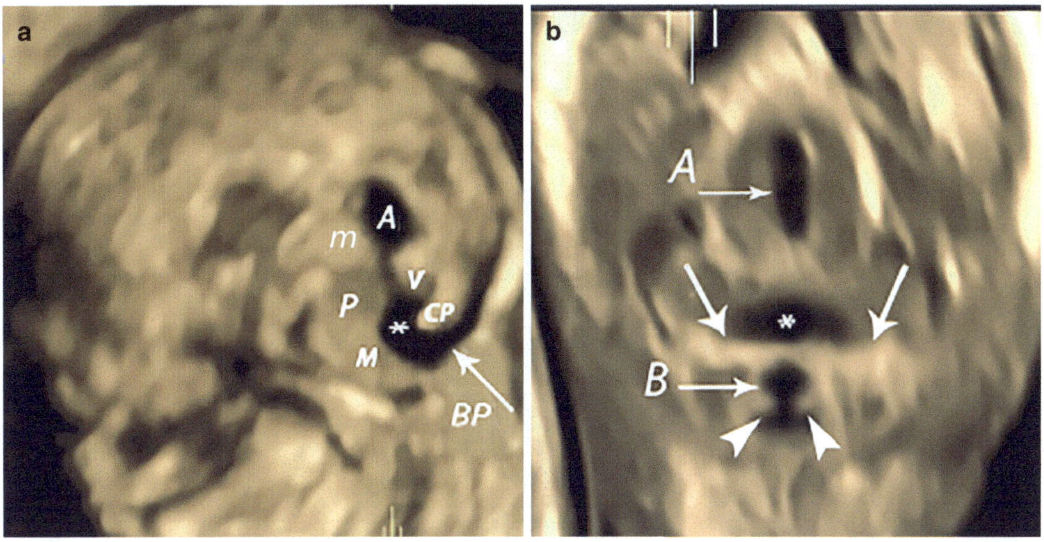

Fig. 7 Anatomy of the fourth ventricular choroid plexus and related anatomical structure at 13 weeks' gestation. Three-dimensional volume dataset acquired laterally with a 6–12 MHz transvaginal volumetric transducer. Multiplanar imaging in the midsagittal (**a**) and in the coronal plane (**b**). (**a**) On the midsagittal plane, the downward and oblique direction of the vertical limbs of the choroid plexus is shown (CP). As evident, the choroid plexus lies just caudal to the developing vermis (V) and cranial to the Blake's pouch (BP), at the level of the roof of the fourth ventricle (*). Note also the prominent Sylvian aqueduct (A). (**b**) On the coronal plane, the diverging vertical limbs (arrowheads) embracing the superolateral part of the Blake's pouch inlet (B) and the proximal part of the horizontal limbs (arrows) are shown. Note also the prominent Sylvian aqueduct (A). *m* midbrain; *P* pons, *M* medulla

laterally displaced on ultrasound, outside the cyst and distant from the vermian margin (Fig. 8). The PMA, located inferiorly to the CP, forms the Blake's pouch, which is a normally transient evagination of the 4th V. BPC represents a persistence of this evagination and derives from abnormal or delayed development of the PMA; as such, in BPC the 4th V-CP is situated to the superolateral aspects of the cyst, just beneath the vermis (Fig. 8). For this reason, recognizing the location of the 4th V-CP in both normal and abnormal conditions is crucial for accurately interpreting findings of cystic posterior fossa anomalies at ultrasound.

Of note, the above-mentioned structures are more easily identified in the first trimester than in the second. This is due to the relatively less prominent size of the vermis compared to the 4th V-CP, enhancing the feasibility of assessing the posterior fossa in the first trimester [12, 17].

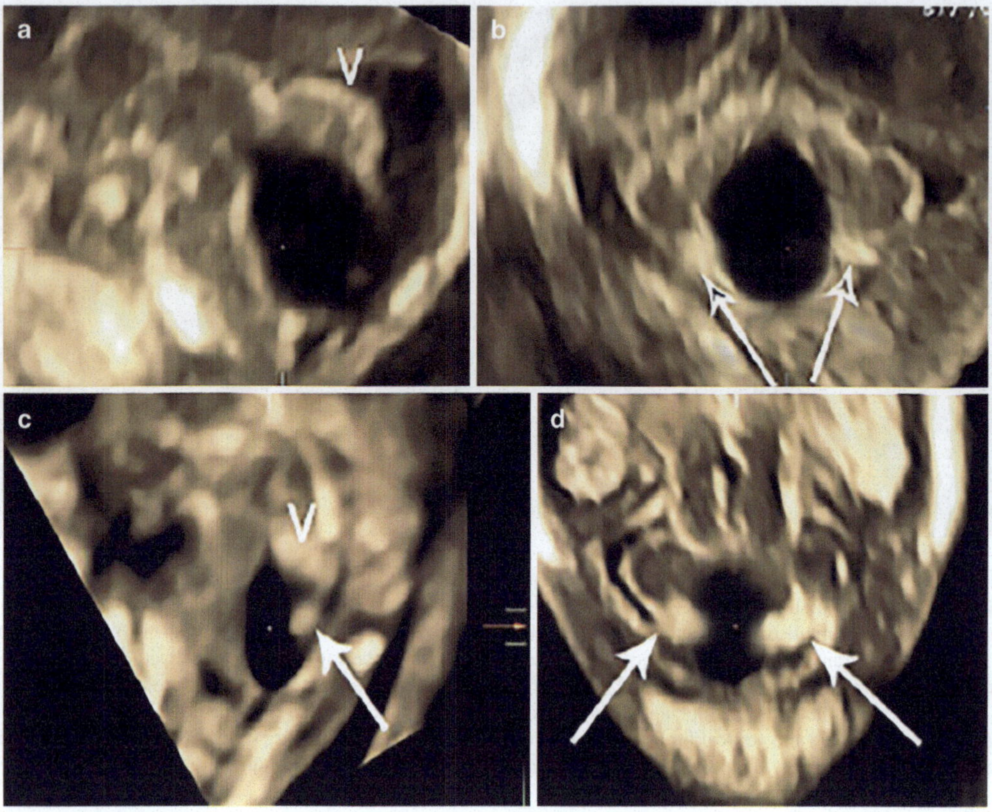

Fig. 8 Position of the choroid plexus of the fourth ventricle in posterior fossa anomalies at 13 weeks. Three-dimensional ultrasound images obtained using multiplanar image correlation with volume contrast imaging. (A) and (B) show the appearance of the posterior fossa in a fetus with Dandy–Walker malformation: the vermis (V) is rotated upward, and the choroid plexus of the fourth ventricle is not visible in the midsagittal plane (**a**) while it can be seen infero-laterally displaced and outside the cyst (arrows) in the coronal plane (**b**). (**c** and **d**) show the appearance of the posterior fossa in a fetus with a Blake pouch's cyst: in the midsagittal plane (**c**), the choroid plexus of the fourth ventricle is visible just beneath the vermis (arrows) and in the coronal plane (**d**), the choroid plexus of the fourth ventricle is located superolaterally and inside the cyst (arrows)

2 Dandy–Walker Malformation

Dandy–Walker malformation (DWM) is the most severe abnormality of the posterior fossa and refers to the association of various defects of the posterior fossa such as:

1. Hypoplasia or partial agenesis of the vermis.
2. Cystic dilatation of the 4th V filling the posterior fossa and extending into the cisterna magna.
3. Upward displacement of the tentorium and torcula herophili.
4. Upward rotation of the vermis.

2.1 Etiology and Pathogenesis

The incidence is approximately 25,000–30,000 live births. It has been suggested that DWM can be classified among mesenchymal-neuroepithelial signaling defects. Notably, several cerebellar growth factors are derived from the overlying leptomeninges [7, 8]. Consequently, abnormalities of the cerebellar leptomeninges may result in abnormalities of the cerebellum itself and the adjacent CSF spaces as it happens in DMW. Indeed, it is believed that an abnormal development of AMA is closely associated with the pathogenesis of DWM.

2.2 Ultrasound Findings

The suspicion of DWM arises from the observation of a triangular or square-shaped open 4th V that appears to communicate with the cisterna magna in the axial plane of the fetal head on the transcerebellar view (Fig. 9). Additionally, there is enlargement of the posterior cranial fossa. The median sagittal view is crucial to assess the presence, integrity, and position of the vermis as well as the position of the torcular/tentorium. Typically, the vermis is small, and its configuration may be either normal, indicating hypoplasia, or abnormal (with the absence of fastigium and/or fissures), indicating dysplasia and/or partial agenesis [1, 4, 18] (Fig. 9). The brainstem-vermis (BV) angle typically is >45° because of the upward rotation of the small vermis [4]. In addition, superior displacement of the torcular/tentorium is observed in the majority of cases (Fig. 9).

2.3 Differential Diagnosis

The DWM must be distinguished from other cystic anomalies of the posterior fossa. An accurate differential diagnosis requires the evaluation of multiple parameters:

- The presence of an apparent communication between the 4th V and cisterna magna (open 4th V) associated with an upwardly rotated but intact vermis is indicative of BPC (Fig. 10). In such cases, the rotation of the vermis is typically less pronounced, and the BV angle is usually less than 45°;

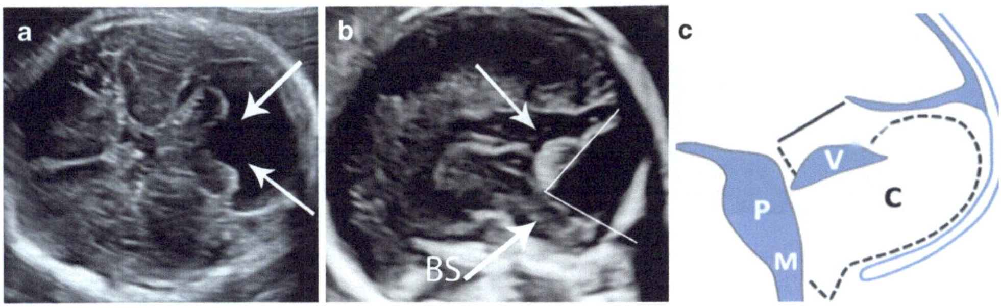

Fig. 9 Sonographic appearance of Dandy–Walker malformation at 19 weeks' gestation. (**a**) Axial view of the posterior fossa showing a cerebellar cleft and a collection of fluid in the posterior fossa (arrows). (**b**) Midsagittal view of the posterior fossa showing an upward displacement of the small vermis (arrow) and an open fourth ventricle communicating with the cisterna magna. The brainstem-to-vermis angle exceeds 45°. (**c**) Schematic representation of the same findings. *BS* brainstem, *T* tentorium, *P* pons, *M* medulla, *C* cyst, *V* vermis

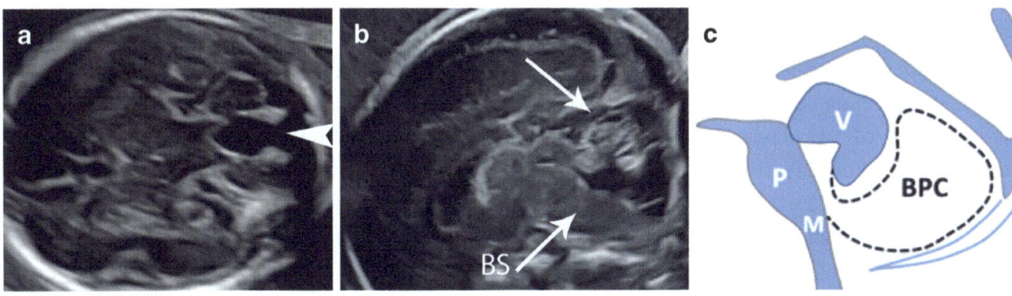

Fig. 10 Sonographic appearance of a case of Blake's pouch cyst at 22 weeks' gestation. (**a**) Axial view of the posterior fossa showing an hourglass opening of the fourth ventricle (arrowhead). (**b**) Sagittal view of the posterior fossa showing upward displacement of a normal vermis (arrow) and an open fourth ventricle, communicating with the cisterna magna. The upward rotation of the vermis is mild; *BS* brain stem. (**c**) Schematic diagram of the same finding. *P* pons, *M* medulla, *BPC* Blake pouch cyst, *V* vermis

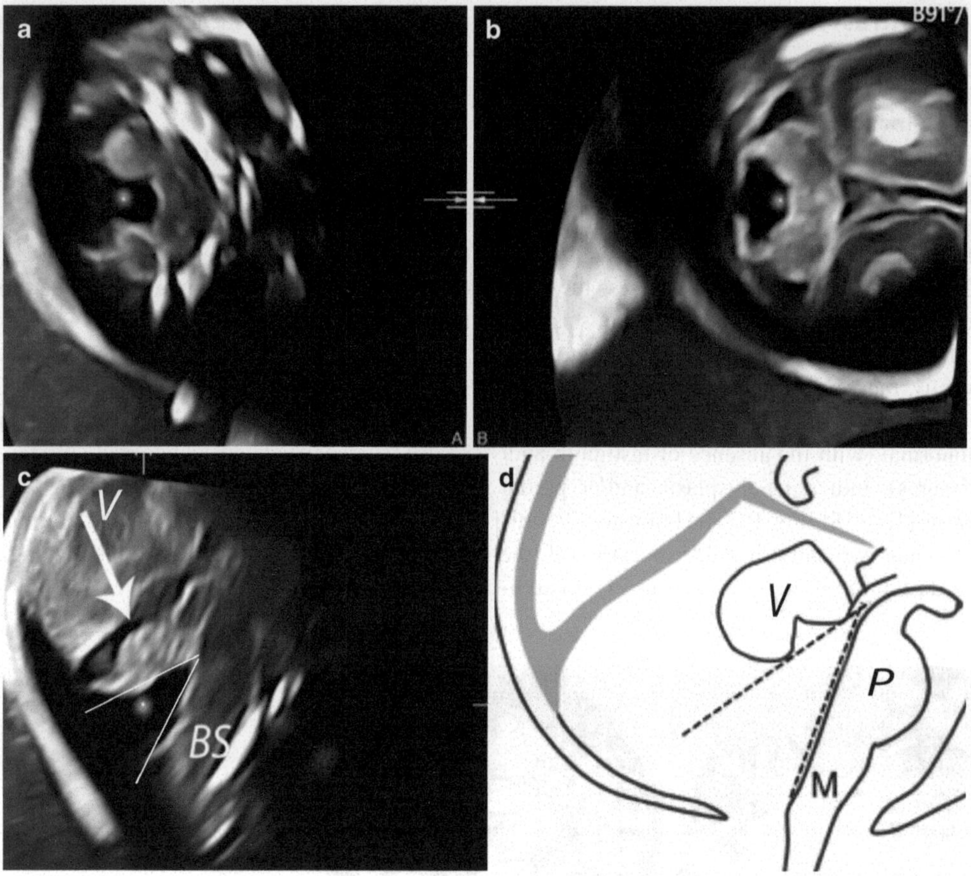

Fig. 11 Sonographic appearance of vermian hypoplasia at 20 weeks' gestation. Three-dimensional ultrasound images, obtained using multiplanar image correlation, showing in (**a**) the presence of a collection of fluid in the posterior fossa with an open fourth ventricle in the axial section; in (**b**) the coronal view the presence of a communication between the fourth ventricle and the cisterna magna is visible; in (**c**) the small vermis (V) is seen in the midsagittal section with a brainstem-to-vermis angle superior than normal, but not exceeding 45°; in (**d**) a schematic drawing of the midsagittal section. *P* pons, *M* medulla oblongata

- The presence of an apparent communication between the 4th V and cisterna magna (open 4th V) associated with a hypoplastic vermis, a normally inserted tentorium/torcular herophili, and no expansion of the posterior fossa is indicative of VH. The rotation of the vermis in VH generally does not exceed 45° (Fig. 11); [4].
- The presence of an enlarged cisterna magna with an intact cerebellum and a closed 4th V is indicative of MCM (Fig. 12).

Table 1 summarizes the differences in these parameters which aid the differential diagnosis.

However, as mentioned earlier, intermediate forms of DWM can occur, where not all typical elements of DWM are present, making the differential diagnosis particularly challenging. Indeed, the severity of fluid space enlargement and rhombencephalic malformations may vary significantly. When the vermis is marginally small and the posterior fossa is not enlarged or only slightly enlarged, the diagnosis becomes complex. At this stage, the differential diagnosis includes vermian hypoplasia and a Blake's pouch cyst causing vermian compression/distortion. Although imaging plays a crucial role in discrimination, there is considerable phenotypical overlap. In such cases, the position of the 4th V-CP

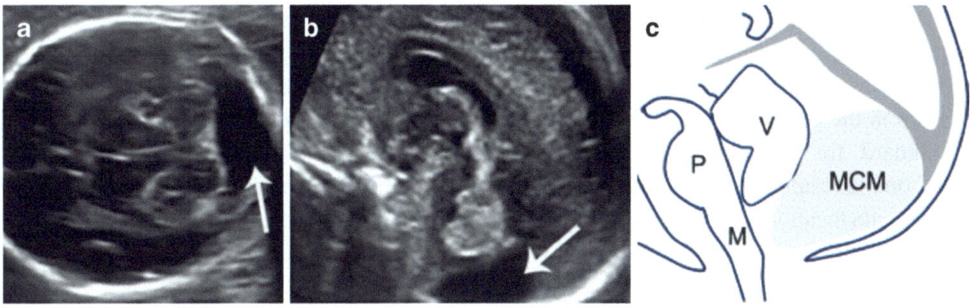

Fig. 12 Sonographic appearance of megacisterna magna at 21 weeks' gestation. (**a**) Axial section of the posterior fossa showing an increased amount of fluid in the posterior fossa (arrow) with a normal cerebellum; (**b**) Midsagittal section in which an increased amount of fluid in the posterior fossa is visible (arrow) but with a normal vermis and a brainstem-to-vermis angle close to 0°. *P* pons, *M* medulla oblongata, *V* vermis, *MCM* megacisterna magna. (Modified from Paladini D, Volpe P. Ultrasound of congenital fetal anomalies: differential diagnosis and prognostic indicators. CRC press; 2018 Mar 29)

Table 1 Comparison of US parameters in cystic posterior fossa malformations

Malformation	Vermis		4th V/BP	Torcula	Posterior fossa	Tegmento-vermian angle[a]	4th V-CP
	Size	Position					
DWM	Hypoplasia/ partial agenesis	Upward rotation	Enlarged	Elevated	Enlarged	Increased (usually >45°)	Located infero-laterally, distant from the vermian margin and outside the cyst
VH	Hypoplasia	Upward rotation	Normal	Normal	Normal	Increased (usually <45°)	Located inferior to the vermis
BPC	Normal	Upward rotation	Enlarged	Normal	Normal	Increased (usually <35°)	Located superolaterally, close to the vermis and inside the cyst
MCM	Normal	Normal	Normal	Normal	Partially enlarged	Normal	Normal
AC	Normal	Normal	Normal or reduced	Normal	Normal	Normal	Normal

4th V-CP fourth ventricle-choroid plexus, *DWM* Dandy–Walker Malformation, *BPC* Blake's pouch cyst, *VH* vermian hypoplasia, *MCM* megacisterna magna, *AC* arachnoid cyst

[a]A normal TVA is considered between 0° and 15–18° (from *Volpe P.* et al. *Ultrasound Obstet Gynecol. 2012 Jun;39* (6)*:632–5*)

has proven to be a valuable sign for differential diagnosis, especially in the coronal view. In Blake's pouch cyst (BPC), the 4th V-CP is ectopically positioned, but inside the cyst, whereas in DWM, it is displaced infero-laterally [12, 16] (Fig. 8). The location of the choroid plexus reflects the embryologic defect and aids in distinguishing DWM (down and out) from Blake's pouch cyst (up and in, stretched along the inferior vermis). Noteworthy, the visualization of the 4th V-CP and its position may be more difficult in the second trimester in both DWM and BPC cases due to the decreasing size of the 4th V-CP during gestation. The complexity of a prenatal differential diagnosis of cystic posterior fossa malformation is also evidenced by the fact that recently, some authors, have reported that the choroid plexus location, but not the location of the torcula, can be used to distinguish antenatally fetuses with DWM from those without DWM [19]. Conversely, the authors found that the location of the torcula can be useful in the postnatal period. However, the authors did not clearly define the control group (non-DWM), in the prenatal period, as well as the number of cases for each group in the comparison and the diagnostic gold standard for DWM, which could have impacted on the results. This might be the reason why the torcula location resulted to be a sign useful in the distinction of DWM from not-DWM in the postnatal period.

2.4 Association with Other Anomalies

The risk of aneuploidy, syndromic conditions, and other cerebral malformations, ventriculomegaly in particular, is high. The presence of associated malformations serves as a key prognostic indicator, significantly amplifying the risk of aneuploidies such as trisomy 18 and 13, as well as that of syndromic conditions such as *Walker-Warburg syndrome, Meckel-Gruber syndrome, Aicardi syndrome,* and *Neu-Laxova syndrome.*

2.5 Prenatal Management

Given the high risk of genetic anomalies, when DWM is suspected antenatally, genetic testing is indicated. In addition, a thorough anatomical scan conducted by an expert is imperative, considering the heightened risk of associations with other CNS and extra-CNS malformations. Serial US monitoring is warranted to monitor the possible onset of severe hydrocephalus. Delivery is recommended to occur in a tertiary referral center to ensure a conclusive diagnosis and adequate neonatal management.

2.6 Postnatal Treatment

The only possible postnatal intervention involves the placement of a cysto-peritoneal shunt to treat the secondary obstructive hydrocephalus, which is the most common complication in DWM. The approach to primary vermian lesions is supportive and depends on the degree and type of neurological impairment.

2.7 Prognosis

DWM is associated with late-onset hydrocephalus in over 50% of cases. In instances where hydrocephalus occurs, either in utero or in the neonatal period, there is an overall mortality rate exceeding 60%, and the majority of survivors exhibit a low IQ. In cases where hydrocephaly is not present, it has been suggested that the neurological outcome is primarily influenced by the configuration of the cerebellar vermis. When the small vermis displays a normal structure, normal development has been reported in more than 50% of cases. On the contrary, if the vermis is abnormally lobulated, and/or if there are associated cerebral anomalies, the prognosis is unfavorable [1, 18].

3 Blake's Pouch Cyst

3.1 Etiology and Pathogenesis

The Blake's pouch cyst (BPC) arises from the non-perforation of the Blake's pouch (BP), a transient structure typically present in the early stages of fetal brain development. BP originates from the evagination of the PMA, one of the two components of the rhombencephalic roof, the other being the AMA [12, 16, 20]. Initially, the 4th-V at the level of the BP does not communicate with the surrounding subarachnoid space. Subsequently, a spontaneous perforation of the pouch forms the foramen of Magendie (median). The term "BP cyst" was originally introduced in pediatric neuroradiology [20] to describe a form of obstructive hydrocephalus resulting from the failure to form of the foramina of Magendie and Luschka. This failure leads in a compressive cyst of the posterior fossa displacing the cerebellar vermis superiorly. More recently, the term has been employed in fetal imaging studies to denote cases where a posterior fossa cyst displaces an intact cerebellar vermis superiorly. This displacement typically occurs in association with a normal ventricular system and a normal size of the posterior fossa [1, 4, 21, 22]. This finding has been interpreted as an unsuccessful or delayed regression of the BP. The entity described in the original neonatal studies appears to differ from the one later characterized in fetal studies, as the latter typically results in normal outcome and seems to be rarely associated with ventriculomegaly (VM) [1, 4, 22]. For this reason, several authors expressed concerns that the term used might be inaccurate and proposed using the term "upward rotation of the cerebellar vermis (URCV)" instead [23, 24].

3.2 Ultrasound Findings

BPC is characterized, on the axial transcerebellar view, by the presence of an hourglass opening (buttock sign) on the central part of the cerebellum apparently communicating with the cisterna magna (Fig. 10). In the midsagittal view, a normal but moderately upward-rotated vermis is typically observed [4] (Fig. 10). A recent study has shown that the BV angle has good accuracy in distinguishing cases of BPC associated with a spontaneous intrauterine regression of sonographic findings from those persisting after birth. Indeed, in a series of cases of BPC, most of those who experienced de-rotation of the vermis before birth had a BV angle of ≤25°. Conversely, none of the cases with a BV angle >30° experienced a regression [23]. This is in line with the results of a previous neuroradiologic series [24] that suggested a high probability of regression with a BV angle ≤23°.

In BPC, the tentorium and torcular herophili are normally positioned. Additionally, the BPC roof may be visible within the cisterna magna as the content of the latter displays a less translucent echogenicity compared to that of the BPC.

3.3 Differential Diagnosis

Obtaining a midsagittal section of the fetal head is mandatory for accurately assessing the position and characteristics of the vermis, which is crucial for diagnosis. The demonstration of a normal vermis rules out the possibility of a DWM and vermian hypoplasia. In addition, in case of BPC, the rotation of vermis is usually less pronounced compared to DWM [4] (Fig. 10). In addition, choroid plexus location has been proven to be a valuable sign for differential diagnosis. Specifically, in BPC, the choroid plexus is upwardly displaced toward the inferior margin of the vermis, while in DMW, it is displaced inferolaterally (Fig. 8). The location of the choroid plexus reflects the embryologic defect and can help distinguish DWM (down and out) from BPC (up and in, stretched along the inferior vermis) [2, 12, 13, 15–17]. In cases of MCM, the cisterna magna is enlarged, and the fourth ventricle is closed.

3.4 Association with Other Anomalies

About one-third of the antenatally detected BPCs are associated with other anomalies, including chromosomal aberrations (in most cases trisomy 21) [1, 22].

3.5 Prenatal Management

The presence of associated anomalies is the major prognostic indicator, significantly increasing the risk of aneuploidies and syndromic conditions. Therefore, particularly in instances with additional anomalies, genetic testing is mandatory. A detailed anatomical scan performed by an expert is also required to prompt identification of possible other CNS and extra-CNS malformations.

3.6 Postnatal Treatment

In the rare cases of BPC associated with VM, the secondary obstructive hydrocephalus may be treated with a cysto-peritoneal shunt.

3.7 Prognosis

In cases with isolated BPC and normal karyotype, the outcome is typically favorable. Intrauterine regression of sonographic signs is observed in a significant number of cases, with nearly 100% of these cases showing a normal developmental outcome.

4 Vermian Hypoplasia

Vermian hypoplasia (VH), formerly referred to as DWM variant, is characterized by the presence of an isolated and upwardly rotated small vermis. There has been ongoing debate concerning the precise definition of VH. Some experts proposed restricting the term "hypoplasia" to cases where the vermis is small but has a normal morphology. On the other hand, the term "partial agenesis" is suggested, for instances, where a part of the vermis is absent [1, 18]. Not surprisingly, the distinction of these two entities poses important challenges. Moreover, recent studies have demonstrated that over the last decades, the vermis has been incorrectly measured as the 4th V-CP was regularly considered in the measurement, thus overestimating the global vermian size on the midsagittal view. Although never reported before, we have demonstrated that a small 4th V-CP, when properly identified as a separate structure from the vermis, can itself be the cause of an open 4th V [17]. The importance of recognizing the presence of a small 4th V-CP with a normal-sized cerebellar vermis is crucial as it can lead to incorrect conclusions regarding the presumed cause of the open 4th V. Indeed, when a URCV with intact vermis is detected, the most frequent cause is BPC, which is typically associated with a normal postnatal outcome. However, evidence in the literature shows that about 5% of BPC cases, reported as having—by definition—an intact vermis, were associated with adverse neurologic outcome after birth. In the majority of these cases, the 4th V-CP might have been erroneously interpreted as the most caudal part of the vermis, concealing the diagnosis of VH, which is instead associated with a higher rate of adverse postnatal neurological outcome. Conversely, if the vermis is normal and the cause of URCV is the presence of a small 4th V-CP, the postnatal outcome seems favourable [17].

Therefore, it is crucial to distinguish between the cerebellar vermis and the 4th V-CP in order to accurately diagnose the etiology of an 'open' 4th V. This differentiation holds significant implications for both prenatal counseling and postnatal prognosis.

4.1 Etiology and Pathogenesis

It is believed that isolated vermian hypoplasia, such as DWM, derives from an abnormal development of AMA.

4.2 Ultrasound Findings

In axial transcerebellar view, the 4th V communicates with the cisterna magna, which is usually of normal size (Fig. 11). In the midsagittal view, the vermis appears small and upwardly rotated with a BV angle usually not exceeding 45° [4]. Tentorium and torcular herophili are normally positioned.

4.3 Differential Diagnosis

The hypoplastic vermis should be differentiated from other posterior fossa anomalies characterized by an open 4th V. The presence of a communication between the 4th V (open 4th V) and cisterna magna along with the evidence of a normal vermis is indicative of BPC (Fig. 10). In such cases, the rotation of the vermis is typically mild. On the other hand, the presence of a communication between the 4th V (open 4th V) and cisterna magna coupled with a hypoplastic vermis, a superiorly displaced tentorium/torcular herophili and an expanded posterior fossa is indicative of DWM. In these instances, the vermis rotation usually exceeds 45° [4] (Fig. 9). The correct identification of the 4th V-CP as a distinct entity from the vermis helps in the differential diagnosis of the causes of an "open" 4th V. This distinction allows a better definition of the postnatal outcomes.

4.4 Association with Other Anomalies

The most commonly associated anomalies are other CNS anomalies, including supratentorial anomalies. Among syndromic conditions, Joubert syndrome is a very severe albeit rare condition characterized by vermian hypoplasia in association with dysgenesis of the isthmic portion of the brain stem at the pontomesencephalic junction. It presents with a deep posterior interpeduncular fossa and thick, elongated superior cerebellar peduncles. The US diagnosis is difficult and should be confirmed by MRI. The typical aspect of the abnormal superior cerebellar peduncles is commonly referred to as the "molar tooth sign," visible on axial US planes and MRI slices of the brain. Symptoms range from general hypotonia with a frog-like posturing to hyperpnea/apnea, and ataxia. Additionally, associated colobomas, nystagmus, and strabismus might be encountered.

4.5 Prenatal Management

The diagnosis of VH necessitates a thorough assessment of fetal anatomy as it is linked to numerous reported malformations. The presence of associated anomalies is the major prognostic indicator, as it increases the risk of genetic abnormalities and syndromic conditions. Genetic testing is therefore mandatory if VH is suspected.

4.6 Postnatal Therapy

There is no treatment of the primary vermian lesion.

4.7 Prognosis

VH is often a finding associated with multiple anomalies and genetic syndromes [12, 20]. When isolated, asymptomatic cases have been reported. However, the paucity of evidence does not allow to drive any conclusion in this regard [12, 20].

5 Megacisterna Magna

The megacisterna magna (MCM) is defined by the observation of a cisterna magna with an antero-posterior diameter $\geq$10 mm on the axial view of the fetal head. It is characterized by an intact vermis and a normal-sized 4th V.

5.1 Etiology and Pathogenesis

It has been suggested that the enlargement of the cisterna magna may be secondary to a distension of the BP, which, however, does not cause an upward displacement of the cerebellar vermis [1, 4].

5.2 Ultrasound Findings

On the axial transcerebellar view, a CSF collection is observed in the posterior fossa. The vermis is normal, and the fourth ventricle is closed [4] (Figs. 4 and 12). In most cases, the torcula herophili and the tentorium are in normal position.

5.3 Differential Diagnosis

The evaluation of vermis morphology is essential for establishing a differential diagnosis from other cystic anomalies of the posterior fossa. Specifically, the presence of a normal vermis, as observed in cases of MCM, eliminates the possibility of DWM and isolated VH. Likewise, the presence of a closed 4th V and normally positioned vermis excludes the possibility of a BPC. Another cause of cisterna magna enlargement is the presence of arachnoid cysts (AC). However, even in such instances, assessing vermian morphology proves valuable for the differential diagnosis between MCM and AC. Indeed, the mass effect and asymmetric distortion of the cerebellum are typical features of arachnoid cysts.

5.4 Prenatal Management

After MCM diagnosis, a detailed anomaly scan is recommended to exclude the presence of other associated CNS and extra-CNS malformations, as they can worsen the prognosis. Numerous associated anomalies have been documented, with supratentorial anomalies such as periventricular heterotopia and lissencephaly being the most commonly reported. Fetal karyotyping is mandatory, especially in cases where other anomalies are present, because of the risk of chromosomal anomalies.

5.5 Postnatal Therapy

No treatment is required.

6 Aracnoid Cyst

A retrocerebellar arachnoid cyst (AC) is a CSF collection that does not either communicate with the surrounding subarachnoid spaces or with the ventricular system and is not usually associated with brain malformations.

6.1 Ultrasound Findings

Retrocerebellar arachnoid cyst appears as a sonolucent cystic mass at ultrasound evaluation (Fig. 13). Depending on the size, the cyst may compress and displace the cerebellum. In addition, large arachnoid cysts may obstruct the circulation of CSF, leading to a secondary obstructive hydrocephalus.

6.2 Differential Diagnosis

The AC should be distinguished from other cystic anomalies of the posterior fossa, especially the MCM. Notably, posterior fossa AC can mimic MCM, but the former typically presents with mass effect, causing asymmetric distortion of the cerebellum. In addition, and contrary to MCM, AC may cause hydrocephalus.

6.3 Prenatal Management

AC is usually isolated and carries a low risk of associated anomalies, of aneuploidy, and of syndromic conditions. Management should be con-

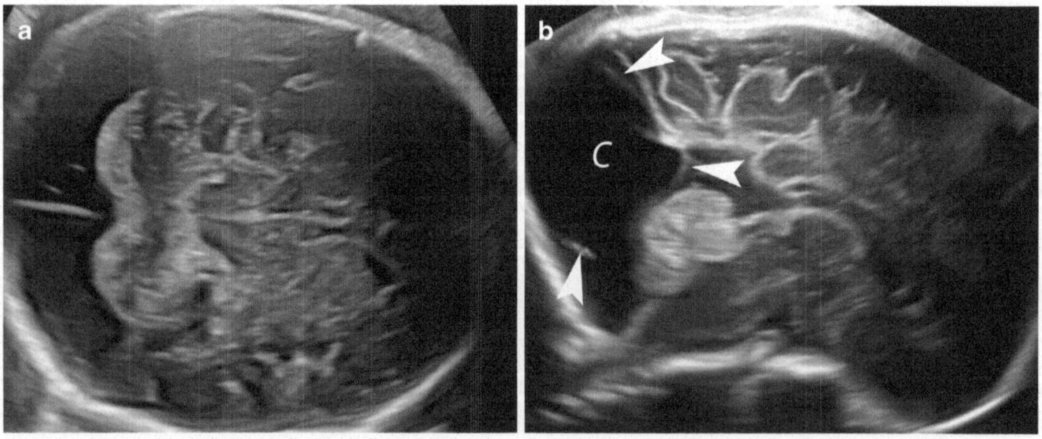

Fig. 13 (**a**) Axial view of the fetal head showing the presence of a fluid collection in the posterior fossa with a normal cerebellum. (**b**) Midsagittal view showing an enlarge cisterna magna because of the presence of the cysts (arrowhead). Of note, the compression of the cerebellar vermis. *C* cyst

servative with serial ultrasound scan to monitor the size of the cyst as it is the most important prognostic factor. Standard obstetric care is advised unless hydrocephalus/macrocrania occurs. In this case, a cesarean section should be performed.

6.4 Postnatal Therapy

In case of symptomatic cysts, cysto-peritoneal shunt may be indicated, although there is controversy surrounding the treatment of AC [20].

6.5 Prognosis

The overall prognosis is good, and shunting is not necessary if compression on the cerebellum is absent or asymptomatic. In contrast, if the cyst is large and symptomatic, it may require surgery [20].

7 Assessment of Cystic Anomalies of the Posterior Fossa: Shifting from the Second to the First Trimester

As previously mentioned, the evaluation of the posterior fossa cystic anomalies has been traditionally performed in the second trimester as the diagnosis of these conditions has been consistently proved to be achievable only at this stage [9]. However, the role of the first-trimester scan has expanded from aneuploidy screening to the diagnosis of fetal malformations, and the assessment of the posterior fossa at 11–14 weeks' gestation is becoming feasible and includes the possibility to identify several ultrasound features that are associated with cystic posterior fossa anomalies. This shift has been made possible for two main reasons: firstly, the introduction of high-frequency probes, both transvaginal and transabdominal, that provide images with higher resolution; secondly, the understanding that the diagnostic signs used for the diagnosis of CPF anomalies in the midtrimester cannot be applied across all gestational ages. Only an in-depth knowledge of the embryologic development of the posterior fossa anatomical structures in normality and pathology allows to infer which signs can be suspicious of CPF anomalies even at earlier gestational ages.

A shift from mid-trimester to first-trimester diagnosis of CNS anomalies has already been reported for the open spina bifida with the introduction of the intracranial translucency (IT) sign observed in the midsagittal view at 11–13 weeks. In fetuses with open spina bifida, the IT is generally absent. This is due to the caudal displacement of the brain observed in Chiari II malformation (which is present in almost all cases of open spina bifida) and loss of the normal appearance of the three hindbrain spaces [25, 26].

Recently, advances have been reported also regarding the first trimester diagnosis of CPF anomalies. However, given that the hypoplasia of the vermis (a diagnostic marker of DWM) cannot be identified in the first trimester, other sonographic markers have been proposed to help in the differential diagnosis of these conditions. To achieve this, a multiplanar approach must be implemented and the following planes must be obtained: a midsagittal plane through the anterior fontanel/fetal face, a midsagittal plane through the posterior fontanel, and a coronal plane of the posterior fossa. These planes allow the assessment of the following aspects: the number of posterior fossa spaces, the brainstem-occipital bone (BSOB) distance, the brainstem-tentorium (BST) angle, the presence and position of the 4th V-CP.

On the same midsagittal view used for nuchal translucency assessment, it is possible to recognize three anechoic spaces which are, from anterior to posterior, the brainstem (BS), the 4th V or intracranial translucency (IT), and the cisterna magna (CM) (Fig. 14). In this section, the parallel line dividing the 4th V and the CM represents the 4th V-CP. The 4th V and the CM can be measured together (in millimeters) by drawing a line from the anterior border of the fourth ventricle to the occipital bone, a measurement called brainstem to occipital bone (BSOB) diameter, and which represents the 4th V-CM complex. It has been shown

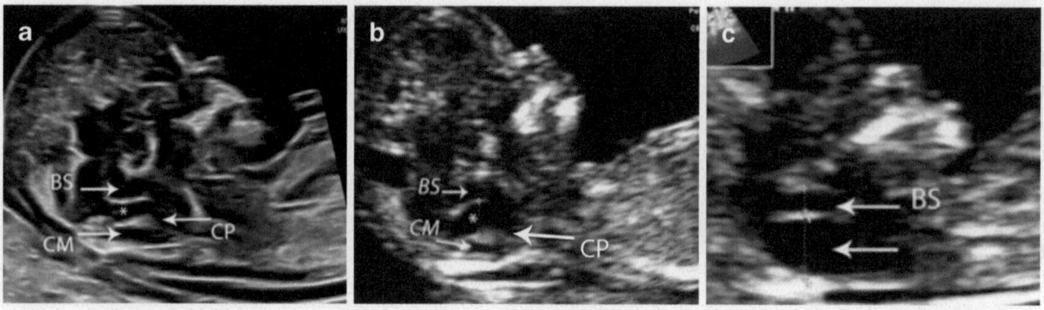

Fig. 14 Midsagittal view of the face and brain at 12 weeks showing the spaces of the posterior fossa. (**a**) The three anechoic spaces are normal, and the choroid plexus is visible (CP). (**b**) Three spaces and the choroid plexus (CP) are still visible but the space corresponding to the fourth ventricle appears enlarged (*). (**c**) Only two brain spaces are visible, the fourth ventricle appears enlarged (lower arrow) and the choroid plexus is not visible. *BS* brainstem, *CM* cisterna magna, * fourth ventricle, *CP* choroid plexus

in a prospective study that fetuses with a BSOB measurement >95th percentile have a high probability to experience a BPC or a DWM in later gestation and that, in these cases, the presence of only two brain spaces (because of the failure to visualize the 4th V-CP) is correlated significantly with DWM especially [10] (Fig. 14). On the same midsagittal section, it is also possible to visualize the tentorium and to measure the brainstem-tentorium angle (BST), previously described as a tool for the assessment of the posterior fossa in the second trimester [4]. The tentorium appears as an echogenic line bridging between the posterior area of the third ventricle and the occipital bone. The BST angle is defined as the angle between a line drawn through to the inferior margin of the brain stem and a line passing through the tentorium. However, the visualization of the tentorium prenatally is technically challenging. Tentorium identification can be aided by the use of high-definition power Doppler or color Doppler imaging with a pulse repetition frequency of 0.3–0.4 MHz to visualize the straight sinus, which runs with the tentorium, and the torcula, which is identified as the confluence of the straight sinus into the superior sagittal sinus (Fig. 15). In this way, once the torcula has been identified by color Doppler, the tentorium can be indirectly visualized allowing the measurement of the BST angle [10]. It has been shown that, after 12 weeks, the superior displacement of the midline ridge of the tentorium and the torcula, secondary to an increased amount of fluid in the posterior fossa, straighten the BST angle by different degree depending on the underlying pathology and can be used in the differential diagnosis of the cystic malformation of the posterior fossa. In particular, in DWM, the tentorium appears upward inserted, and the BST is close to zero (Fig. 16), while in BPC, the BST appears only slightly decreased or similar to normal cases [10]. These signs, which are easily obtained in the same midsagittal view used for the assessment of NT, might be introduced to screen for the various cystic anomalies of the posterior fossa as early as in the first trimester. Moreover, the detection of these signs, which might not be visible in the second trimester, might help in the differential diagnosis of these anomalies.

In instances where a cystic anomaly of the posterior fossa is suspected, a more advanced evaluation of the posterior fossa may provide further signs which can guide toward the correct diagnosis. This can be achieved by obtaining two extra scanning views: a midsagittal view of the posterior fossa through the posterior fontanel, as this allows a better identification of the PCF structure and a coronal view of the PCF (Fig. 7). These views, indeed, enables the visualization of the 4th V-CP as well its position. A recently published study has shown that 4th V-CP is always visible in the midsagittal view in cases of BPC, while it is necessary to obtain a coronal view of the PCF to identify the same structure in DMW. Additionally, in coronal view, the 4th V-CP is observed to be infero-laterally displaced and outside the cyst in DMW cases, while is near the lower extremity of the vermis and inside the cyst in BPC cases (Fig. 8). This

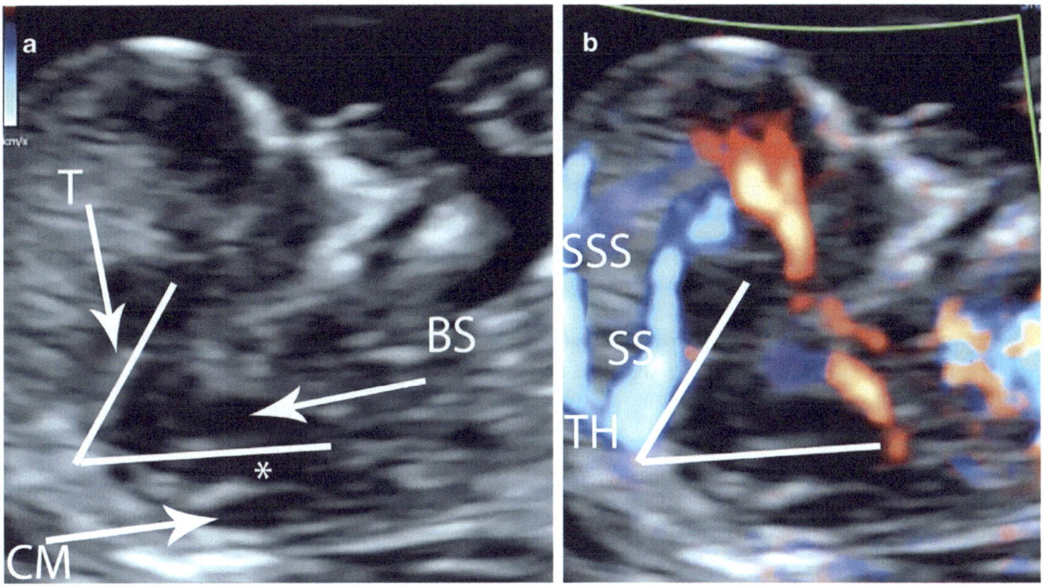

Fig. 15 Midsagittal view of the fetal face and brain in the first trimester with identification of the tentorium with the use of high-definition power Doppler imaging to visualize the straight sinus and the torcula (TH) that was identified as the confluence of the straight sinus into the superior sagittal sinus. (**a** and **b**) The brainstem-tentorium angle was defined as the angle between a line drawn through the inferior margin of the brainstem and a line passing by the tentorium. *T* tentorium, *CM* cisterna magna, * fourth ventricle, *BS* brainstemm, *SSS* superior sagittal sinus, *SS* straight sinus, *TH* torcula herophili

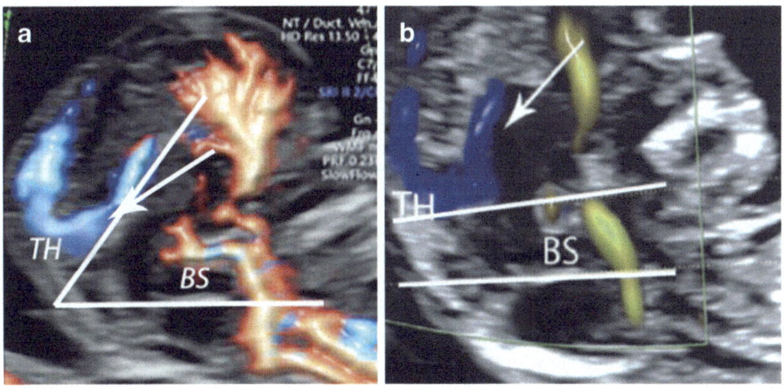

Fig. 16 Measurement of the brainstem-tentorium angle in the midsagittal view of the fetal face and brain with identification of the tentorium with the use of high-definition power Doppler imaging in a fetus with Blake pouch's cyst (**a**) and in a fetus with Dandy–Walker malformation (**b**). In the Dandy–Walker malformation, the tentorium appears upward inserted, and the brainstem-tentorium angle is close to zero; in the Blake pouch's cyst, the brainstem-tentorium angle appears slightly decreased. The upward dislocation of the torcula is clearly seen in DWM. The arrows points to the straight sinus visible at high-definition power Doppler. *TH* torcula herophili, *BS* brainstem

reflects the embryologic pathogenesis of these two conditions: the former due to an abnormal persistence of the AMA and the latter due to abnormal development of PMA. Of note, the visualization of the 4th V-CP as a distinctive structure from the vermis, and consequently, the correct assessment of its position becomes increasingly more difficult as gestation advances and the vermis grows [17]. Indeed, the identification of these signs has been proven to be feasible in the first trimester with a better level of accuracy at 12–13 weeks compared to

15–16 weeks and 20–21 weeks [12]. Given the different prognosis of CPF anomalies, an early identification at first trimester scan might be of great importance in planning diagnostic steps and in guiding the counseling and pregnancy management.

References

1. Gandolfi Colleoni G, Contro E, Carletti A, Ghi T, Campobasso G, Rembouskos G, et al. Prenatal diagnosis and outcome of fetal posterior fossa fluid collections. Ultrasound Obstet Gynecol. 2012;39(6):625–31.
2. Kollias SS, Ball WS, Prenger EC. Cystic malformations of the posterior fossa: differential diagnosis clarified through embryologic analysis. Radiographics. 1993;13(6):1211–31.
3. Robinson AJ, Goldstein R. The cisterna magna septa: vestigial remnants of Blake's pouch and a potential new marker for normal development of the rhombencephalon. J Ultrasound Med. 2007;26(1):83–95.
4. Volpe P, Contro E, De Musso F, Ghi T, Farina A, Tempesta A, et al. Brainstem-vermis and brainstem-tentorium angles allow accurate categorization of fetal upward rotation of cerebellar vermis. Ultrasound Obstet Gynecol. 2012;39(6):632–5.
5. Contro E, Volpe P, De Musso F, Muto B, Ghi T, De Robertis V, et al. Open fourth ventricle prior to 20 weeks' gestation: a benign finding? Ultrasound Obstet Gynecol. 2014;43(2):154–8.
6. Paladini D, Volpe P. Posterior fossa and vermian morphometry in the characterization of fetal cerebellar abnormalities: a prospective three-dimensional ultrasound study. Ultrasound Obstet Gynecol. 2006;27(5):482–9.
7. Barkovich AJ. Developmental disorders of the midbrain and hindbrain. Front Neuroanat. 2012;6:7.
8. Barkovich AJ, Millen KJ, Dobyns WB. A developmental and genetic classification for midbrain-hindbrain malformations. Brain J Neurol. 2009;132(Pt 12):3199–230.
9. Syngelaki A, Hammami A, Bower S, Zidere V, Akolekar R, Nicolaides KH. Diagnosis of fetal non-chromosomal abnormalities on routine ultrasound examination at 11–13 weeks' gestation. Ultrasound Obstet Gynecol. 2019;54(4):468–76.
10. Volpe P, Persico N, Fanelli T, De Robertis V, D'Alessandro J, Boito S, et al. Prospective detection and differential diagnosis of cystic posterior fossa anomalies by assessing posterior brain at 11-14 weeks. Am J Obstet Gynecol MFM. 2019;1(2):173–81.
11. Volpe P, Contro E, Fanelli T, Muto B, Pilu G, Gentile M. Appearance of fetal posterior fossa at 11-14 weeks in fetuses with Dandy-Walker malformation or chromosomal anomalies. Ultrasound Obstet Gynecol. 2016;47(6):720–5.
12. Volpe P, De Robertis V, Volpe G, Boito S, Fanelli T, Olivieri C, et al. Position of the choroid plexus of the fourth ventricle in first- and second-trimester fetuses: a novel approach to early diagnosis of cystic posterior fossa anomalies. Ultrasound Obstet Gynecol. 2021;58(4):568–75.
13. Nelson MD, Maher K, Gilles FH. A different approach to cysts of the posterior fossa. Pediatr Radiol. 2004;34(9):720–32.
14. O'Rahilly: The embryonic human brain: an atlas of... - Google Scholar [Internet]. [cited 2024 Feb 6]. https://scholar.google.com/scholar_lookup?title=The+Embryonic+Human+Brain:+An+Atlas+of+Developmental+Stages&author=R.+R.+O%27Rahilly&author=F.+M%C3%BCller&publication_year=2006&
15. Volpe P, De Robertis V, Volpe G, Olivieri C, Fanelli T, Boito S, et al. Evaluation of cerebellar vermis at 12-22 weeks of gestation: why is traditional assessment incorrect? Ultrasound Obstet Gynecol. 2023;61(3):415–6.
16. Paladini D, Donarini G, Parodi S, Volpe G, Sglavo G, Fulcheri E. Hindbrain morphometry and choroid plexus position in differential diagnosis of posterior fossa cystic malformations. Ultrasound Obstet Gynecol. 2019;54(2):207–14.
17. Volpe P, De Robertis V, Fanelli T, Volpe G, Olivieri C, Boito S, et al. Impact of choroid plexus size in prenatal diagnosis of normal and abnormal closure of fourth ventricle. Ultrasound Obstet Gynecol. 2023;62(6):875–81.
18. Malinger G, Lev D, Lerman-Sagie T. The fetal cerebellum. Pitfalls in diagnosis and management. Prenat Diagn. 2009;29(4):372–80.
19. Whitehead MT, Barkovich MJ, Sidpra J, Alves CA, Mirsky DM, Öztekin Ö, et al. Refining the neuroimaging definition of the Dandy-Walker phenotype. AJNR Am J Neuroradiol. 2022;43(10):1488–93.
20. Tortori-Donati P, Fondelli MP, Rossi A, Carini S. Cystic malformations of the posterior cranial fossa originating from a defect of the posterior membranous area. Mega cisterna magna and persisting Blake's pouch: two separate entities. Childs Nerv Syst ChNS. 1996;12(6):303–8.
21. Guibaud L. Fetal cerebral ventricular measurement and ventriculomegaly: time for procedure standardization. Ultrasound Obstet Gynecol. 2009;34(2):127–30.
22. Paladini D, Quarantelli M, Pastore G, Sorrentino M, Sglavo G, Nappi C. Abnormal or delayed development of the posterior membranous area of the brain: anatomy, ultrasound diagnosis, natural history and outcome of Blake's pouch cyst in the fetus. Ultrasound Obstet Gynecol. 2012;39(3):279–87.
23. Salsi G, Volpe G, Montaguti E, Fanelli T, Toni F, Maffei M, et al. Isolated upward rotation of the fetal cerebellar vermis (Blake's pouch cyst) is a normal variant: an analysis of 111 cases. Fetal Diagn Ther. 2021;48(6):485–92.

24. Conte G, Caschera L, Parazzini C, Cinnante C, Izzo G, Talenti G, et al. Prenatal magnetic resonance imaging within the 26th week of gestation may predict the fate of isolated upward rotation of the cerebellar vermis: insights from a multicentre study. Eur Radiol. 2020;30(4):2161–70.
25. Chaoui R, Nicolaides KH. From nuchal translucency to intracranial translucency: towards the early detection of spina bifida. Ultrasound Obstet Gynecol. 2010;35(2):133–8.
26. Chaoui R, Benoit B, Mitkowska-Wozniak H, Heling KS, Nicolaides KH. Assessment of intracranial translucency (IT) in the detection of spina bifida at the 11-13-week scan. Ultrasound Obstet Gynecol. 2009;34(3):249–52.

Non-cystic Anomalies of the Posterior Fossa

Pierre Mace and Edwin Quarello

Abstract

Non-cystic posterior fossa abnormalities constitute a heterogeneous group of cerebral lesions of diverse primary or secondary etiologies. The incidental finding suspicious for these groups of conditions is usually the late discovery of a transverse cerebellar diameter below the fifth centile. Investigation of the personal and family medical history combined with detailed morphological evaluation of fetal supra- and infratentorial cerebral structures may help in the diagnosis as the presence of specific signs is suggestive of certain specific pathophysiological mechanisms. Fetal MRI, possibly repeated, and genetic analysis according to updated indications, is also mandatory for a better understanding of these complex situations.

Non-cystic anomalies of the posterior fossa (PF) encompass a wide spectrum of abnormalities that may involve one or more of the constituent elements of this region of interest, delimited in its upper part by the tentorium cerebelli and in its lower part by the superior edges of the petrous pyramids. These anomalies may be attributed to numerous causes and pathophysiological mechanisms and may also occur at various stages of cerebral development, from early embryogenesis to later phases of neuronal maturation and migration. Etiologies can thus be generally considered as either primary (genetic) or secondary (disruptive).

As proposed by national and international recommendations regarding the practice of obstetrical ultrasonography screening [1–4], fetal PF should be systematically evaluated in every trimester of pregnancy. Screening examination of the fetal PF in the second and third trimesters of pregnancy, particularly of the cerebellum, depends on the correct insonation of an axial section of the fetal head which allows the visualization, from front to back, of the interhemispheric fissure, the septal cavity, the thalami, the cerebellar peduncles, the fourth ventricle, the vermis, the cerebellar hemispheres, and the retrocerebellar fluid space (Fig. 1). On this view, also known as "transcerebellar" view, the measure of the cerebellar transverse diameter is obtained. It has been demonstrated that this measurement is feasible and reproducible regardless of the operators' expertise [5]. Although this measurement has not been integrated among the recommended measurements by the international scientific societies [2, 4], it is widely obtained in routine clinical practice. In instances where anomaly(ies) are observed on this section, a targeted neurosonography is indicated, ideally by

P. Mace
Image 2 Center, Marseille, France

Prenatal Screening and Diagnostic Unit, Beauregard Hospital, Marseille, France

E. Quarello (✉)
Image 2 Center, Marseille, France

Department of Obstetrics—Gynecology and ART, St Joseph Hospital, Marseille, France

P. Volpe, T. Ghi (eds.), *Fetal Neurosonography*, Ultrasound in Obstetrics and Gynecology,
https://doi.org/10.1007/978-3-031-70192-4_7

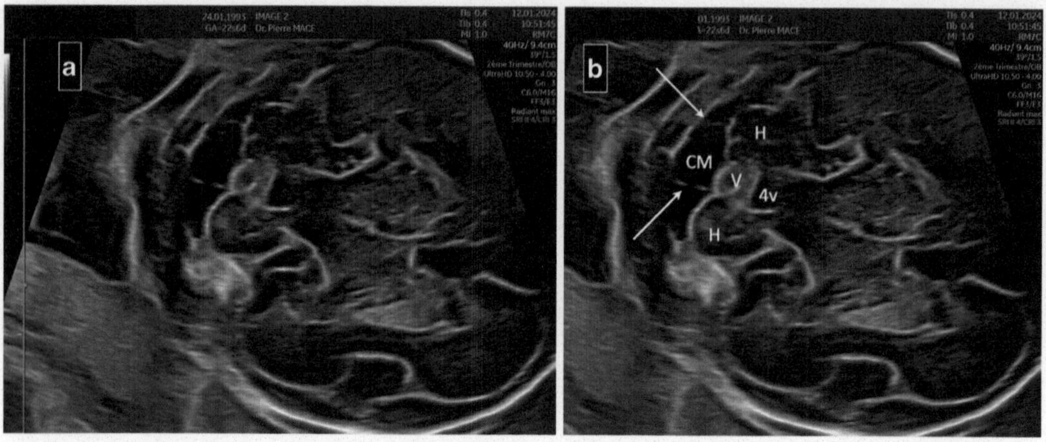

Fig. 1 Transcerebellar axial view of the fetal brain at 22 + 6 weeks displaying a normal posterior fossa with the fourth ventricle (4 V), the cerebellum with its hemispheres (H) and the vermis (V), the cisterna magna (CM), and remnant of Blake's pouch lateral walls (arrows)

using a transvaginal probe, to evaluate the PF in all the three spatial planes: axial, coronal, and sagittal [6]. This can be optimized by exploiting the acoustic window provided by the anterior, and when possible, the posterior, fontanelle. Diagnostic workup will then be based on the evaluation of the PF fluid spaces, the cerebellar biometry and morphology (hemispheres and vermis), the appearance of the fourth ventricle, the orientation of the tentorium cerebelli, and the biometric and morphological analysis of the brainstem [7].

The suspect of possible PF anomalies arises from the observation of measurement(s) outside the normal ranges and/or from the presence of one or more associated image(s) exhibiting an unusual characteristic. The aim of this chapter is to address PF anomalies without associated cystic anomalies.

1 Abnormal Cerebellar Biometry

1.1 Cerebellar Biometry Below Normal Ranges

The observation of a transcerebellar transverse diameter (TCD) equal or below the fifth centile for gestational age during the second and third trimester of pregnancy should be questioned by the clinician regarding the possible etiology. Indeed, a reduced TCD may a be a late finding in the third trimester, with previously normal TCD measurements, and it has been demonstrated that it is significantly associated with major malformations, chromosomal and genetic abnormalities, and unfavorable outcomes [8]. The reduction in TCD may result from a global shortening of the cerebellum or a focal shortening of one or more of its components (i.e., the cerebellar hemispheres and/or the vermis). Therefore, a detailed analysis of each element is mandatory:

Cerebellar Hemispheres: They usually present with regular contours and foliation characterized by the presence of hyperechoic lines parallel to the occipital bone, especially in the third trimester of pregnancy. Generally, the two hemispheres should be separated by the vermis. Measurements of the anteroposterior, lateral diameters, and heights of the two hemispheres should be compared to reference curves [9].

Vermis: It usually has a hyperechoic appearance compared to the lateral cerebellar hemispheres, and it should separate the fourth ventricle from the retrocerebellar space. The following details of the cerebellar vermis should be carefully evaluated: the contours should be regular, the presence of foliation should be detected by identifying the primary fissure, the ratio between the heights of the anterior and posterior vermian lobes should be calculated (the normal anterior-posterior ratio is 1:2), and the vermian axis relative to the brainstem should be assessed with particular attention to the position of the ventral aspect of the anterior and posterior vermian lobes almost in contact to the dorsal aspect of the brainstem, especially the pons. The primary fissure appears embryologically around 14 weeks' gestation, but it becomes visible at prenatal ultrasound around 22 weeks. Measurements of vermis height, anteroposterior diameter, and surface area should also be compared to reference curves [10]. The assessment of vermian structure is facilitated by the use of volumetric probes with thick sections (Fig. 2).

Fourth Ventricle: It is a single and median ependymal cavity at the level of the bulbo-pontine area. Adjacent structures are anteriorly, the pons and the upper half of the medulla oblongata, posteriorly the cerebellum, and laterally, the superior and inferior cerebellar peduncles. The vermis and cerebellum are fully formed by the end of the 15th to 16th week, but the complete closure of the fourth ventricle by these structures is achieved only at 18 weeks' gestation when the communication between the fourth ventricle and the cisterna magna is no longer present [11]. The mature normal fourth ventricle can be assessed from 18 weeks of gestation onward. On the axial plane, the fourth ventricle appears as a trapezoidal anechoic space with the anteroposterior diameter being smaller than the maximum transverse diameter. The short base of the trapezoid structure coincides with the fourth ventricle floor, while the large base coincides with the fourth ventricle roof (Fig. 3). In a sagittal view, the

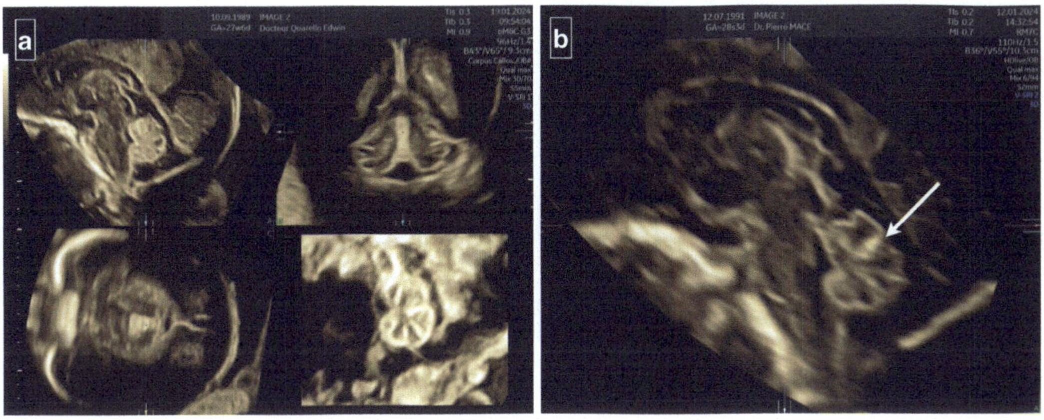

Fig. 2 3D rendering mode of the fetal posterior fossa in the third trimester of pregnancy. Slices of 5 mm (**a**) and 2 mm (**b**) of thickness are used for a better visualization of the vermis. The primary fissure is visible using this rendering technique (arrow)

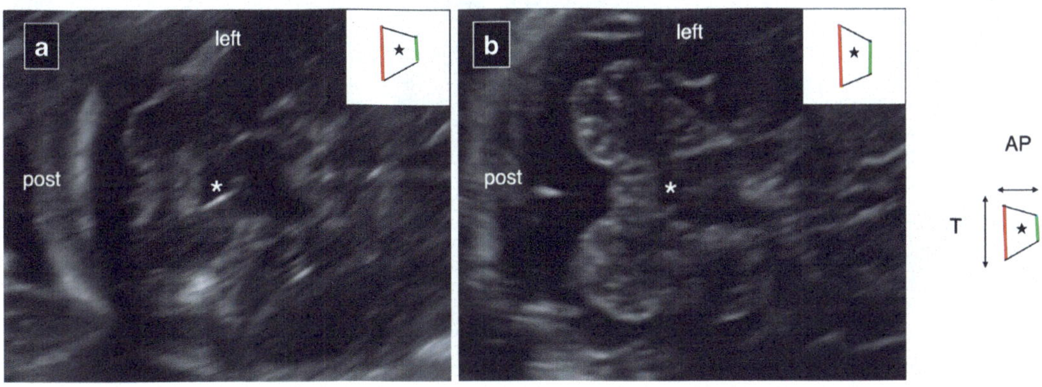

Fig. 3 Axial views of the normal posterior fossa at 22 weeks' gestation (**a**) and 30 weeks' gestation (**b**). In an axial plane, the fourth ventricle appears grossly as a quadrangular anechoic space where the anteroposterior diameter is smaller than the maximum transverse diameter. *Red line* roof of the fourth ventricle, *Green line* floor of the fourth ventricle, *Star* fourth ventricle, *T* transverse diameter, *AP* anteroposterior diameter, *Post* posterior

fourth ventricle looks like a triangular anechoic space where the apex is posterior and is called the fastigium (Fig. 4).

Cerebellar Peduncles: They are two paired median but separated structures that can both be identified on an axial (Fig. 5) or coronal plane. On the transcerebellar axial view, the subjective analysis of the cerebellar peduncles' morphology, symmetry, and size (width and length) is possible.

Brainstem: It can be evaluated by obtaining an axial view of the fetal head although a sagittal section through the anterior fontanelle, and/or preferably the posterior fontanelle, allows a better visualization of this structure (Fig. 6). It consists of three parts: the midbrain, the pons, and the medulla oblongata. The physiological rostro-caudal biometric ratio between these three structures on a median sagittal section is usually about 1:2:1. The pontine protuberance is visible from 18 to 20 weeks onward. The dorsal surface of the brainstem is flat, especially at the level of the pons, and the position of the fastigium is usually identified just below the midpoint of the ventral

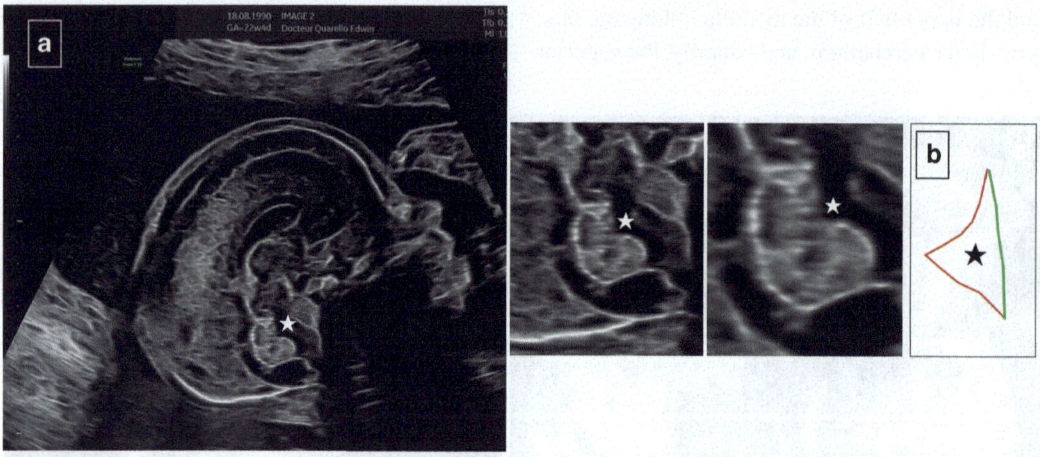

Fig. 4 Sagittal view of the fetal posterior fossa at 22 weeks' gestation (**a**). The fourth ventricle looks like a triangular anechoic space (**b**) where the edge, posterior, is called fastigium. The anterior part, the floor, is straight. *Red line* the roof of the fourth ventricle, *Green line* the floor of the fourth ventricle, *Star*: the fourth ventricle

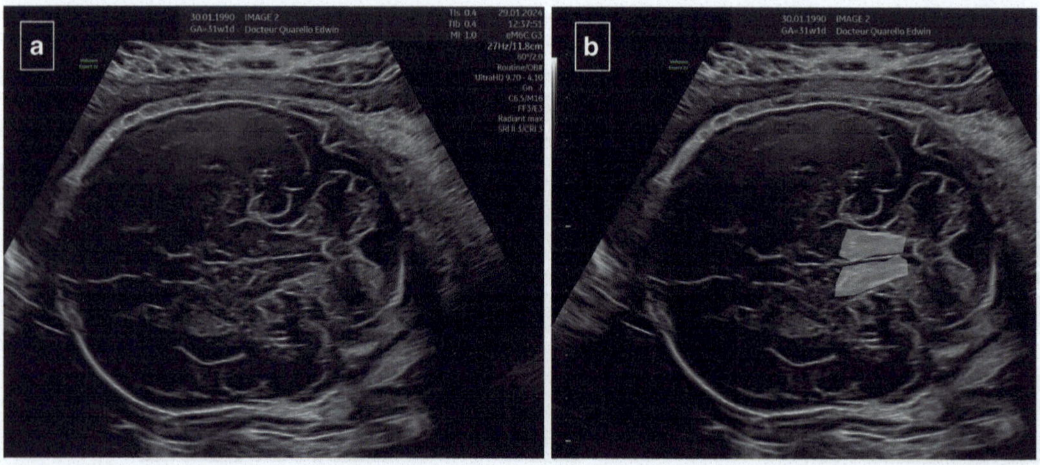

Fig. 5 Axial transcerebellar view of the normal fetal brain displaying the cerebellar peduncles that are paired but separated structures, simultaneously visible (white rectangles)

pons. The prominence of the pons is almost equivalent to the anteroposterior diameter of the brainstem. The brainstem has a typical bichromatic aspect, especially in the third trimester, being the pontine protuberance rather hyperechoic compared to the non-protuberant part (Fig. 7). This aspect can be attributed to the different cellular components of these structures, namely the tegmentum in front and the tectum behind (Fig. 7).

In the case of a shortening in cerebellar transverse diameter, two distinct conditions should be considered:

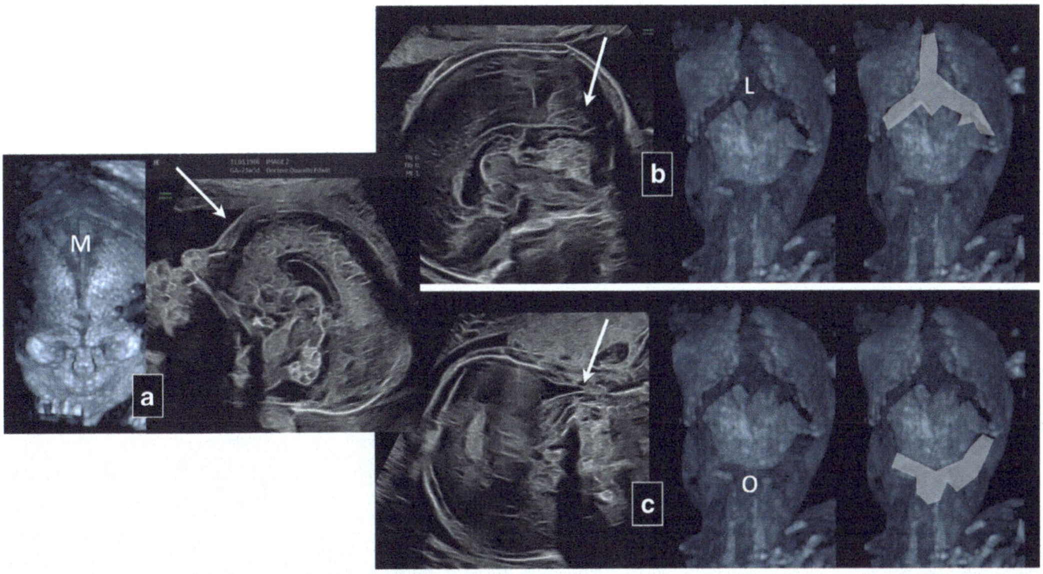

Fig. 6 Different approaches for fetal brainstem assessment using the metopic suture (M) and anterior fontanelle (**a**), the lambdoid suture (L) and posterior fontanelle (**b**), or the window below the occipital bone (O) (**c**)

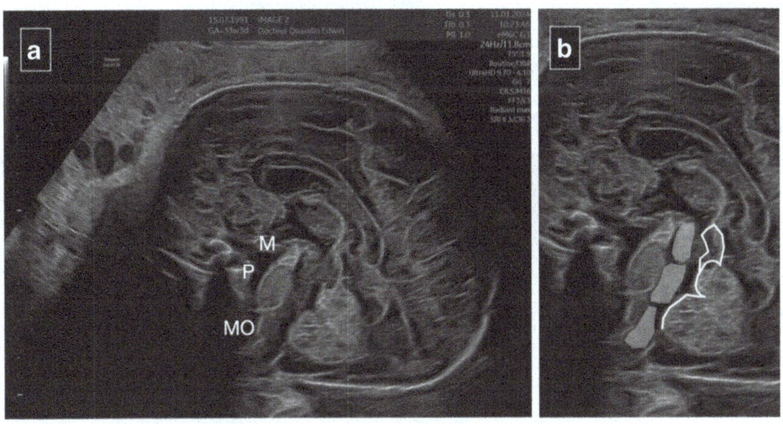

Fig. 7 Visualization of the fetal brainstem at 33 weeks' gestation with its three components: the mesencephalon (M), the pons (P), and the medulla oblongata (MO). The prominence of the pons is almost equivalent in size to the anteroposterior diameter of the brainstem. There is usually a bichromatic aspect of the brainstem—especially in the third trimester—with a pontine protuberance rather hyperechoic compared to the non-protuberant part. This aspect can be attributed to the different cellular components that make up these structures, namely the tegmentum in front (white rectangles) and the tectum (white line) behind

1.1.1 Asymmetric Appearance of a Small Cerebellum

In cases of cerebellar asymmetry, history and imaging findings help in the differential diagnosis. Postnatally, partial cerebellar hypoplasia has been reported to be secondary to prematurity, prenatal hypoxia, hemorrhagic processes, prenatal infections, or exposure to teratogens. Antenatal imaging suggestive of a secondary/disruptive origin of a partial cerebellar hypoplasia includes unilateral or asymmetric involvement of the cerebellum (Fig. 8), the presence of signs of hemorrhage or ischemia, irregular and heterogeneous echogenic appearance evolving over time, irregular borders (Fig. 9), a cerebellar cleft, posterior cerebral nodules, intraparenchymal calcifications, or cysts (Fig. 10). Of note, the prognosis of unilateral ischemic-hemorrhagic cerebellar lesions depends more on the fact that the vermis is involved rather than on the degree of cerebellar parenchymal involvement [12, 13].

Although unilateral cerebellar hypoplasia is most often of disruptive nature, while global cerebellar hypoplasia (with symmetrical cerebellar involvement, regular cerebellar borders, and persistently homogeneous echogenicity over time) has more likely a primary/developmental etiology, the differential diagnosis between the two origins is not straightforward. In fact, some primary genetic etiologies are predisposing factors to disruptive complications, such as the autosomal dominant COL4A1-related disorders which is characterized by small-vessel brain disease with hemorrhage [14]. Additionally, cerebellar asymmetry can also

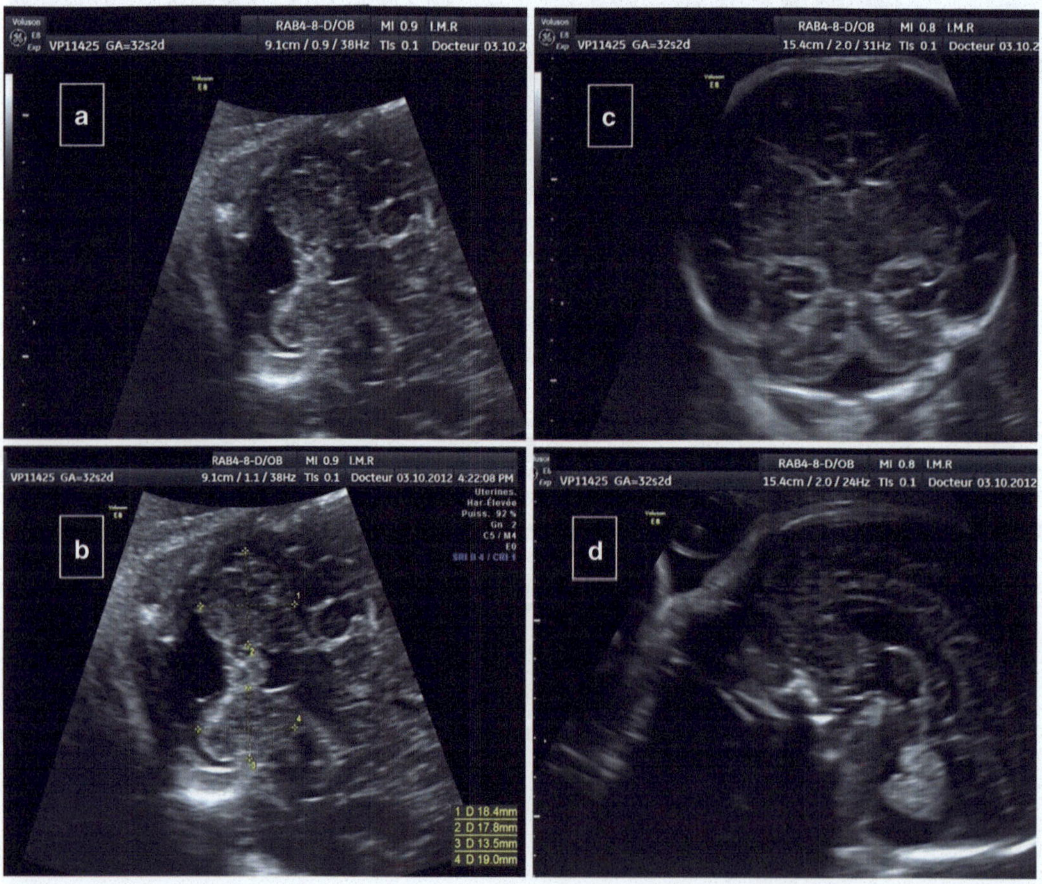

Fig. 8 Fetal cerebellar asymmetry in a possible case of vascular insult (acquired condition). The shape of both cerebellar hemispheres looks grossly normal (**a**–**c**). The vermis looks normal as well. However, the cerebellar borders are of difficult assessment in cases of hypoplastic hemisphere, and MRI is indicated in these cases

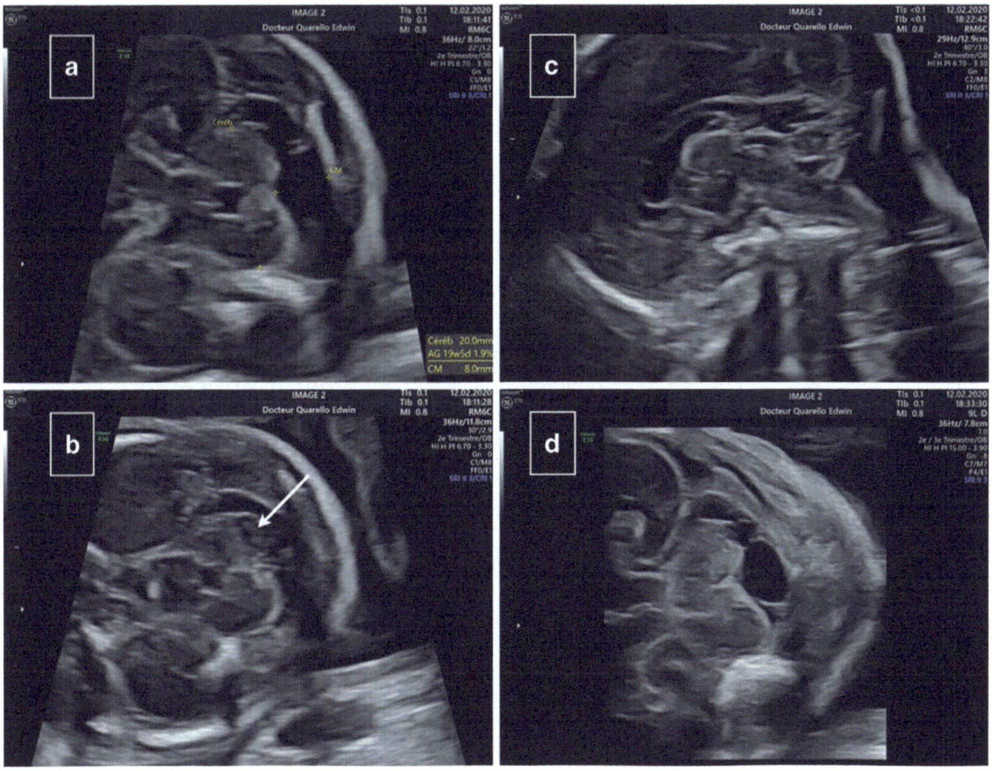

Fig. 9 Fetal cerebellar asymmetry in a case of possible vascular insult. The transverse cerebellar diameter is below the third percentile (**a**), and one of the two hemispheres looks heterogeneous (arrow) with irregular borders (**b**). In sagittal view, the vermis looks dysplastic (**c**), and a remnant of Blake's pouch cyst is visible (**d**)

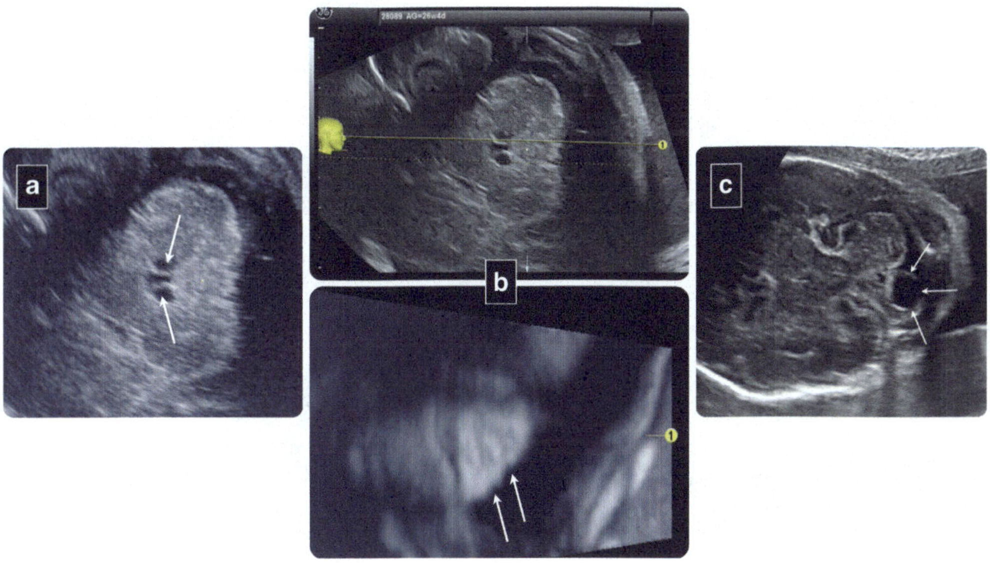

Fig. 10 Fetal cerebellar asymmetry in a fetus with CMV infection. The fourth ventricle looks unusual (**a**) with cystic structures (arrows) inside. It is also possible to observe the irregular borders of one hemisphere in parasagittal view (**b**). A cystic structure is also present at the infero-posterior part of the abnormal hemisphere (white arrows) (**c**)

be found in Moebius syndrome, neurofibromatosis type 1, and PHACE syndrome. The latter corresponds to a rare group of neurocutaneous anomalies of unknown origin, presenting with a large segmental facial, cervical, or high thoracic hemangioma associated with central nervous system (CNS) and cutaneous anomalies in 45% and 35% of cases, respectively [15]. Unilateral cerebellar hypoplasia is the most common CNS anomaly, encountered in 20% of the cases, and it is considered a major diagnostic criterion for this condition. On a coronal view, both at US and MRI imaging, the "tilted telephone receiver" sign can be observed, which is highly suggestive for PHACE syndrome (Fig. 11). This sign reflects the presence of unilateral cerebellar hypoplasia displaced upwards, asymmetric dilation of the fourth ventricle connected to an ipsilateral retrocerebellar cyst, and a deviated vermis fused with the contralateral cerebellar peduncle, forming an oblique connection between the two hemispheres [15]. In addition to this sign, the presence of smooth contours of the posterior part of the affected hemisphere is also highly suggestive, as well as the presence of ipsilateral vascular malformations (absence of the posterior communicating artery or the inferior cerebellar artery, persistence of the trigeminal artery, etc.). Conversely, the absence of suggestive signs of typical clastic lesions such as transient hyperechoic cerebellar parenchyma, presence of calcifications and/or cysts, and irregular contours should be kept in mind for etiological purposes.

1.1.2 Symmetric Appearance of a Small Cerebellum

In instances when the TCD is reduced without obvious morphological anomalies of its intrinsic components (the vermis and the cerebellar hemispheres), it is key to perform a thorough evaluation (morphology and biometry) also of the aforementioned-related structures: the cerebellar peduncles, the fourth ventricle, the brainstem—the pons in particular—as well as the supratentorial structures.

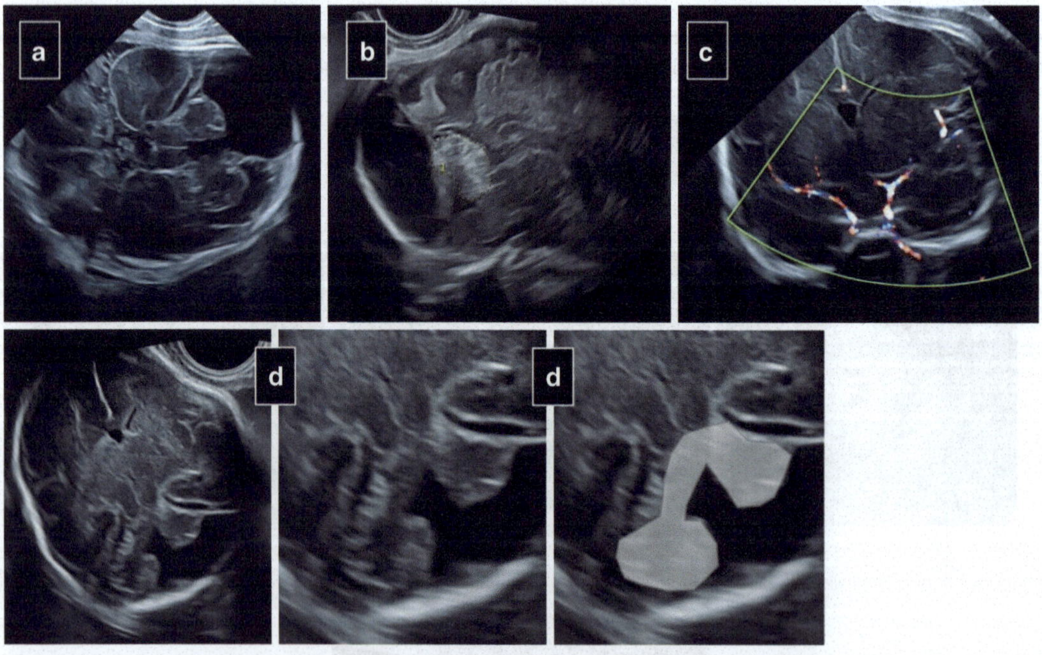

Fig. 11 Fetal cerebellar asymmetry in PHACE syndrome. A large posterior and lateral cyst is visible on the axial view, communicating with the fourth ventricle (**a**, **d**). On the sagittal view, the vermis looks hypoplastic (**b**). It is also possible to visualize an asymmetry in the size of the cerebral vessels (**c**). On the coronal view (**d**), the "tilted telephone receiver" sign is observed and indicative of PHACE syndrome (**e**)

The term "cerebellar hypoplasia" refers to a subjectively defined total or partial reduction in the cerebellar volume although a clear biometric definition for postnatal diagnosis of this condition is not available. In cases where a global cerebellar size reduction is present (hemispheres + vermis), a differential diagnosis between cerebellar hypoplasia and atrophy should be attempted. In cerebellar hypoplasia, the cerebellar volume is reduced but the morphology is preserved, specifically cerebellar foliation can be appreciated. Conversely, a widening of spaces between fissures might be observed in cerebellar atrophy. Cerebellar or vermian hypoplasia may be either syndromic (Fig. 12) or non-syndromic. Therefore, the clinician should carefully look for other associated signs suggestive of CHARGE syndrome or even other conditions possibly confirmed by genetic analyses using high-resolution sequencing techniques (WES or WGS). Cerebellar and pontocerebellar hypoplasia will be discussed later in this chapter.

1.2 Cerebellar Biometry Above Normal Ranges

Situations where the cerebellum appears larger than normal, with a TCD above the normal range, are exceptional. On the axial plane, the TCD might appear falsely increased in cases of total vermian agenesis or severe vermian hypoplasia associated with abnormal separation of the two cerebellar hemispheres (Fig. 13). As it will be reviewed later in this chapter, some cases of cerebellar cortical dysplasia may be associated with

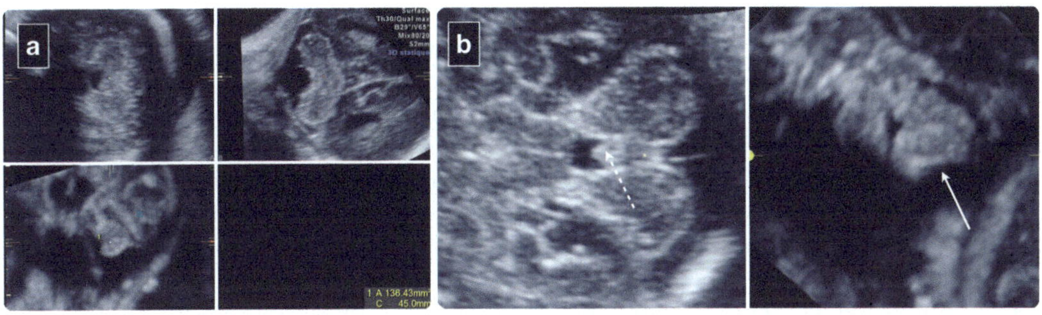

Fig. 12 Slightly asymmetric (**a**) or symmetric (**b**) cerebellar hypoplasia in trisomy 13 and CHARGE syndrome, respectively. The shape of fourth ventricle has an abnormal appearance (dotted arrow), and the inferior part of the vermis is hypoplastic (full arrow)

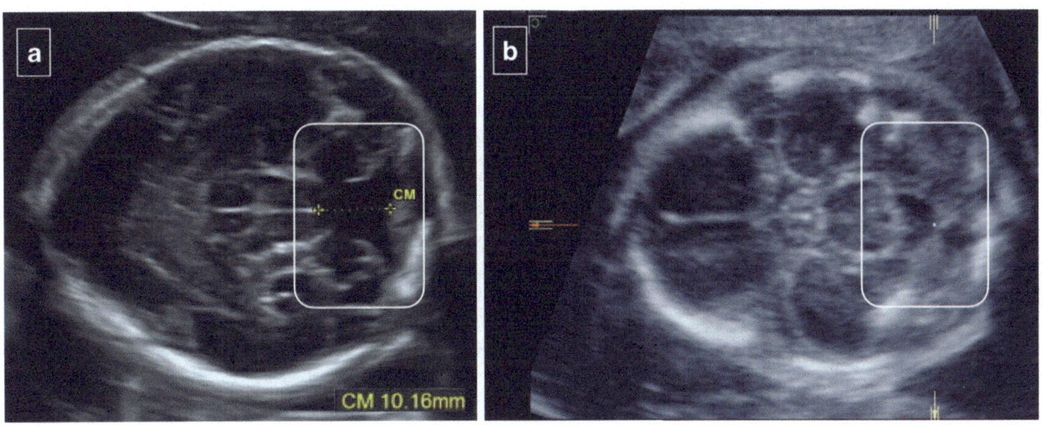

Fig. 13 Severe hypoplastic vermis (**a**) and cerebellar agenesis (**b**) are characterized by an abnormal appearance of the cerebellum on the axial view

focal hypertrophy leading to an increased size of one or both cerebellar hemispheres. Another cause of increased cerebellar size might be the presence of an acute intra-cerebellar hemorrhage with mass effect. The involved area usually appears hyperechoic and poorly defined. Macrocerebellum, characterized by an abnormally large cerebellum with normal morphology [16], is characterized by a hypertrophy of the cerebellar hemispheres with a usually normal vermis. This entity can be observed in isolation (non-syndromic) or associated (syndromic) with other anomalies in Costello syndrome, Sotos syndrome, or neurometabolic abnormalities. In this case, cerebellar hypertrophy is often due to gray matter hypertrophy and a mass effect of adjacent structures, such as the brainstem. Indeed, the hypertrophic cerebellar hemispheres expand toward adjacent anatomical regions wrapping around the brainstem and herniating upward or downward.

2 Abnormal Morphology of the Posterior Fossa

2.1 Abnormal Cerebellar Aspect

2.1.1 Abnormal Aspect of Cerebellar Hemispheres

Unusual Echogenicity: In the presence of unusual echogenicity in one or both cerebellar hemispheres, the following elements need to be evaluated:

- Size of the hemisphere(s): larger or smaller than the reference values for gestational age.
- Borders: regular or irregular.
- Aspect of the lesion: homogeneous or heterogeneous.
- Evolution over time: progression, stability, involution, or disappearance.
- Normality or abnormality of the vermis.
- Coexistence of supratentorial anomalies.

Of note, the abnormal aspect of the PF should be carefully evaluated through the different spatial planes.

In the presence of a hyperechogenic, irregular area, possibly associated with evolving changes over time such as irregular borders, reduction in size, or relative/total disappearance, an ischemic-hemorrhagic lesion is likely (Figs. 9 and 14). MRI will confirm the hemorrhagic nature of the lesion (MRI signals indicative of bleeding). It is key that MRI imaging should be performed shortly after ultrasound diagnosis given the evolutive nature of the lesion with possible disappearance over time.

In instances when a hyperechogenic lesion is observed with no associated changes in dimension and borders that is visible in all three spatial planes, stable over time, and possibly present in the vermis, cerebellar capillary telangiectasia should be considered, with diagnosis confirmed by MRI, especially postnatally after Gadolinium injection [17].

In the presence of hyperechogenicity not visible in all three spatial planes, loss of normal

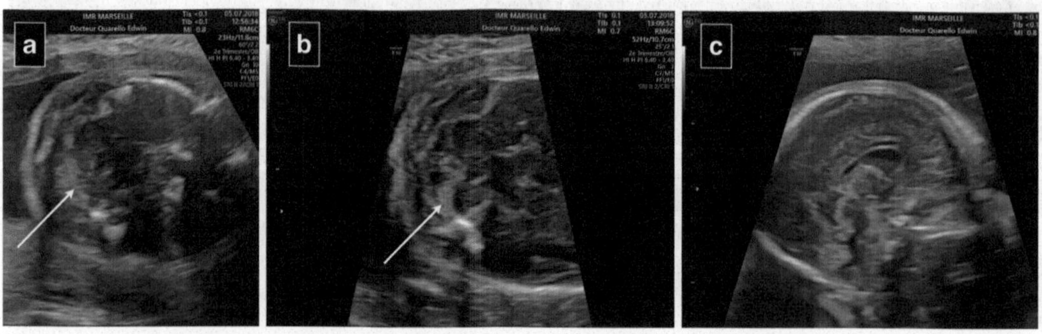

Fig. 14 Abnormal aspect of one cerebellar hemisphere in a case of cerebellar hemorrhage. The vermis is normal. (**c**) The hemisphere appears hyperechogenic with irregular borders (**a**, **b**)

transverse foliation, presence of vertical foliation, increased volume indicative of focal hypertrophy, and irregular borders, focal anomalies such as cerebellar cortical dysplasia should be considered. This lesion remains stable over time and is confirmed by MRI data [18].

Irregular borders of one or both cerebellar hemispheres: As described earlier, the presence of irregular borders on one or both cerebellar hemispheres should be analyzed along with other parameters such as echogenicity, evolution over time, biometries, etc. Thus, a disruptive origin or cerebellar cortical dysplasia may be considered in most of the time.

2.1.2 Abnormal Aspect of the Vermis

An abnormal vermis appearance is almost always a secondary finding identified in the context of anomalies of the pericerebellar fluid spaces, transverse cerebellar diameter, or fourth ventricle. The abnormal vermian morphology, both in its contours and foliation, is generally associated with abnormal measurements. The loss of the 1:2 ratio between the anterior and posterior lobes (Fig. 15) and the presence of irregular contours at the vermis' lower border is suggestive of vermian hypoplasia, often of ischemic origin. The detailed characterization of vermian dysgenesis includes the analysis of supra- and infratentorial anatomical structures and the search for associated extracerebral anomalies. Indeed, the complementary analysis of the cerebellar peduncles, fourth ventricle, vermis axis, and supratentorial structures could shed light on this condition. Different types of vermis anomalies may be associated with conditions described in the following sections. The primary fissure, usually visible around 22 weeks, may not be present in some dysgenesis. In rare cases of complete cerebellar agenesis, pericerebellar fluid spaces may be increased or decreased due to medial ptosis of the occipital lobes [19].

2.2 Abnormal Pericerebellar Fluid Spaces

Pericerebellar fluid spaces are subjectively assessed by visualizing hypoechoic areas located behind the vermis and laterally to the cerebellar hemispheres. As mentioned, from 18 weeks' gestation onwards, the retrocerebellar fluid space or retrocerebellar cistern does not physiologically communicate with the fourth ventricle. Retrocerebellar space measurement

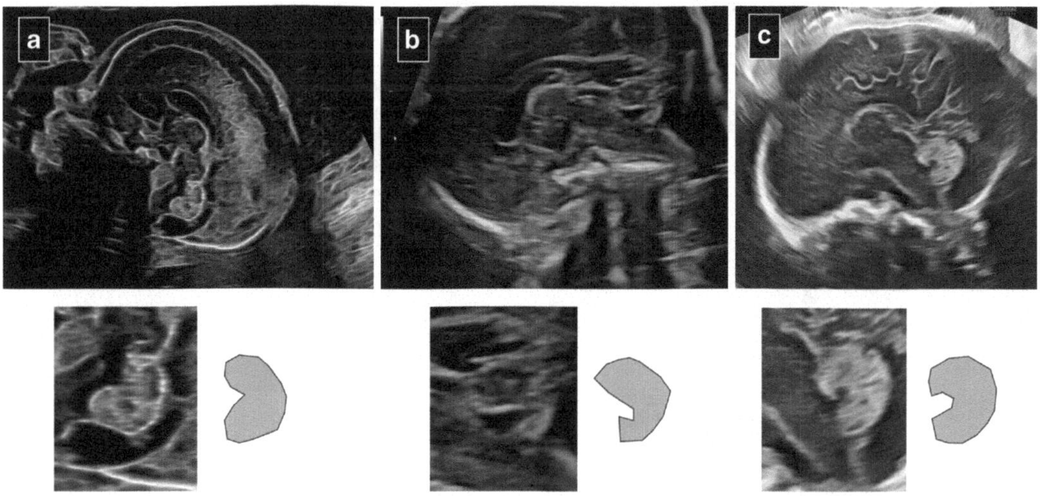

Fig. 15 Normal (**a**) and abnormal (**b**, **c**) appearance of the vermis. In (**b**) the shape of the vermis is abnormal with a hypoplasia of its inferior part. In (**c**), the anterior and posterior parts appear grossly equal in size instead of displaying the usual 1:2 ratio; in addition, the position of the fourth ventricle is also atypical as it is localized in the middle

can be usually performed on the axial plane, although not recommended by expert societies, and these measurements are referenced. Cystic anomalies of the posterior fossa will not be addressed in this chapter. However, the presence of a poorly defined hyperechogenic collection at the edge of one of the cerebellar hemispheres (Fig. 16) may indicate a subdural hemorrhage, especially if changes in echogenicity, dimensions (potentially leading to disappearance), and visualization of transverse/sigmoid sinuses adjacent to the hemorrhagic collection are observed over time (Fig. 16). A detailed analysis of the hemispheres and vermis should be complemented by MRI imaging in order to identify any ischemic/hemorrhagic or clastic injuries, which significantly alter the associated prognosis. Other vascular lesions such as thrombosis of the torcular and/or transverse sinuses will be described in another chapter. The presence of a non-vascularized echogenic tissue behind the vermis should raise suspicion of rare conditions such as extra-cerebellar ectopia of cerebral tissue or intracranial extracerebral glioneuronal heterotopia (IEGH) which are confirmed by MRI. Supporting findings to the diagnosis are

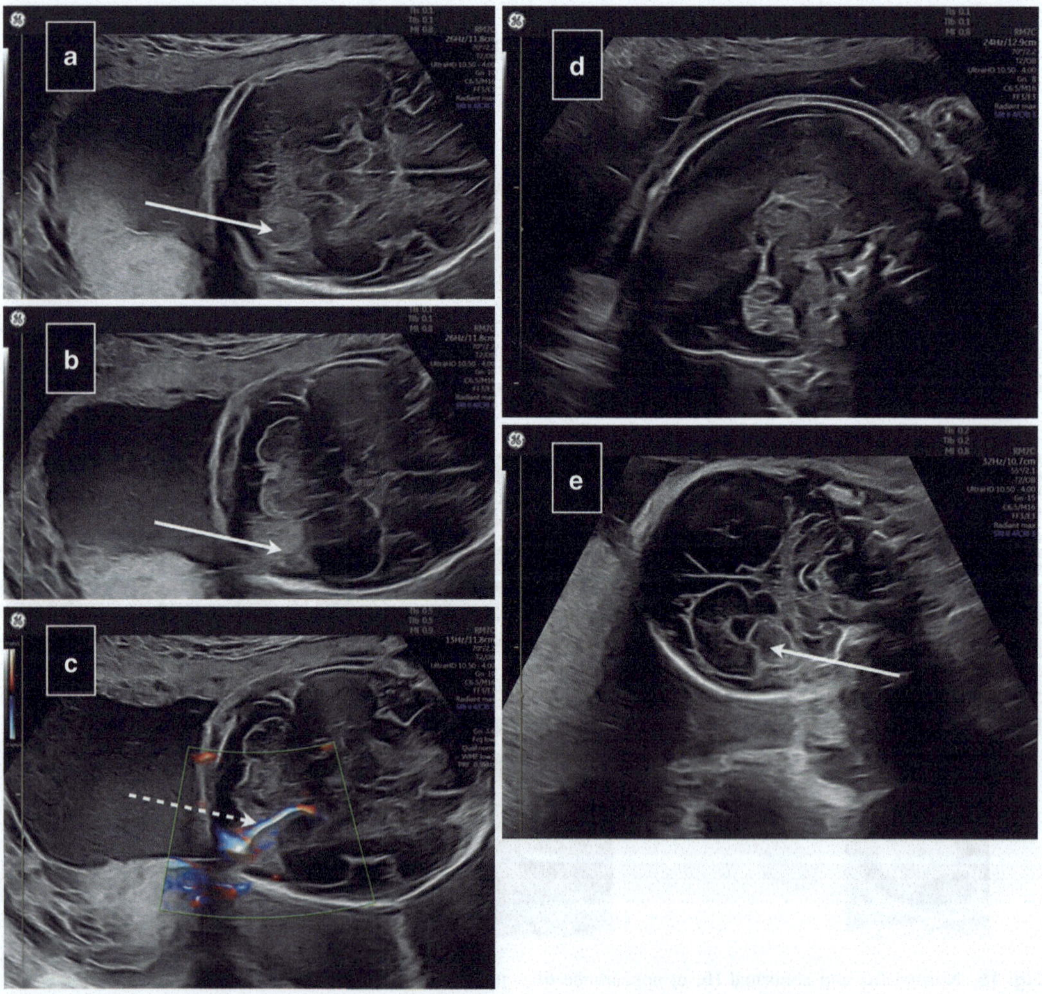

Fig. 16 Abnormal pericerebellar space in a case of possible subdural hemorrhage (**a**, **b**, **e**) (full arrows). A hyperechogenic collection is visible on the edge of one of the cerebellar hemispheres, and it might indicate a subdural hemorrhage with visualization of transverse/sigmoid sinuses adjacent to it (dotted arrow) (**c**)

the isolated nature of the latter and the integrity of adjacent cerebellar and supratentorial cerebral structures [20].

3 Non-cystic Anomalies of the Posterior Fossa

3.1 Cerebellar/Pontocerebellar Hypoplasia

Definition: Cerebellar hypoplasia (CH), or pontocerebellar hypoplasia (PCH) when associated pontine involvement is present, is a nonspecific generic term used to describe a wide spectrum of heterogeneous abnormalities. They can be associated with various imaging findings, clinical characteristics, and neurodevelopmental impairments that can be attributed to multiple primary (genetic) or secondary (acquired/disruptive) causes. CH- or PCH-related disorders are characterized by a reduction in the volume of the cerebellum, or even of the cerebellum and pons together where the two components might be not equally involved. These disorders might be also associated with supratentorial structures' anomalies. Cerebellar involvement is heterogeneous: it can affect the whole cerebellum (most common), or it can selectively involve the vermis alone or one or both cerebellar hemispheres without vermis involvement. No clear biometric thresholds have been identified to define these anomalies, both in the postnatal and prenatal period. Thus, the term hypoplasia is purely descriptive and often inappropriate because subsequent diagnosis of true cerebellar atrophy is made in cases initially described as PCH [21].

Epidemiology: The prevalence of CH/PCH is unknown. These are extremely rare conditions as evidenced by the available literature which mainly consists of case series. The most recent is a retrospective single-center study of 42 cases of PCH diagnosed prenatally over 13 years (2008–2021) [21]. The exact incidence of CH/PCH is unknown. However, HPC2A caused by homozygous mutation of p.A307S in the TSEN54 gene is the most frequent type with an estimated incidence of 1:200,000 [22].

Etiology: CH/PCH is mostly characterized by a progressive reduction in cerebellar or cerebellar/pontine volumes. Although PCH typically begins prenatally, identification during this period remains anecdotal [23]. Indeed, the term PCH is descriptive and not pathognomonic of any etiology. The term PCH was introduced in 1993 by Peter G. Barth, who initially proposed a classification into two types based on neuropathological and clinical data. The classification of this broad group of anomalies can be based on etiologies, thanks to the growing knowledge on genetic aberrations [13], or based on imaging characteristics [14, 24]. Both primary and secondary causes may be implicated. As mentioned earlier, in the postnatal period, secondary causes of CH/PCH are associated with situations of hypoxia, hemorrhage, infections (such as CMV), and exposure to certain toxins and teratogens (retinoic acid and valproic acid, alcohol, cocaine). A classification based on neuroimaging findings is proposed by various authors. A recent one, proposed by Accogli et al. in 2021 [14], allows for a more concise description of this broad group of conditions by proposing a diagnostic algorithm for CH-related disorders [14]:

- Isolated CH: isolated hypoplasia of the vermis and/or cerebellar hemispheres.
- CH with abnormalities of cerebrospinal fluid in the posterior fossa.
- CH with brainstem abnormalities (specific or hypoplasia).
- CH with brainstem involvement and cortical abnormality of neuronal migration.
- CH with cerebellar dysplasia.

It is important to note that, in addition to classic forms of PCH, other entities may resemble PCH. Jaillard et al. [21] recently proposed a PCH classification also according to the suspected etiology:

- Classic PCH.
- Non-classic PCH.
- PCH associated with chromosomal anomalies.
- PCH of unknown origin.

The pathogenesis of the different entities of PCH is highly heterogeneous. However, some forms of PCH share the same pathophysiological mechanism, such as the involvement of the exosome complex, which is implicated in mRNA degradation in certain forms of PCH1 (HPC1B, HPC1C, HPC1D), or the involvement of the TSEN complex, which is implicated in the aberrant tRNA splicing in other forms of PCH (e.g., HPC2A, HPC2B, HPC2D, HPC2F, HPC4, and HPC5) [24]. In cases of non-classic forms listed in the OMIM database, the pathogenic mechanisms may involve the CASK pathway as well.

Genetic background: Genetic studies might allow the differentiation between so-called fixed causes (PCH type 3 and 8) and progressive, evolutionary, or neurodegenerative causes (PCH 1, 2, 4, 5, 6, and 7) [13, 21]. To date, there are 13 described types of PCH with 17 subtypes and as many identified involved genes (VRK1, EXOSC3, EXOSC8, TSEN54, RARS2, PCLO, etc.). The number of (sub)types of PCH is constantly growing due to the introduction of the next-generation sequencing techniques, with (sub)type classification for each new gene associated with PCH. Mutate genes in PCH are often associated with an autosomal recessive transmission [13]. Conversely, genes such as CASK, RELN, VLDLR, TUB seem to be implicated in the so-called non-classic forms listed in the OMIM database. Of these, CASK gene is inherited with an X-linked transmission.

Sonographic findings: As previously highlighted, the classical ultrasound characteristic suspicion for CH/PCH, usually identified in the third trimester, is the incidental observation of a reduced TCD, often below the fifth percentile [21], and its possible association with a decreased anteroposterior diameter of the pons [25] (Fig. 17). However, these signs can be also identified in the context of a diagnostic ultrasound performed for a detailed evaluation of supratentorial and/or extracerebral anomalies (Fig. 17). Vermis evaluation may be challenging, particularly in cases of severe hypoplasia, due to the superposition in a sagittal plane of the medial borders of the cerebellar hemispheres. CH/PCH is mostly progressive and late-onset (third trimester of pregnancy or even perinatal period), making early detection usually impossible during the second-trimester ultrasound examination [22].

Differential diagnosis: The diagnosis of CH/PCH is suspected when a TCD below the fifth centile is observed, with or without pontine hypoplasia. Thus, this hypothesis cannot, a priori, be erroneously confused with other malformative entities. The differential diagnosis will be considered more in terms of the isolated or non-isolated nature of this CH/PCH and the presence of a genetic anomaly different from the classic causes of PCH. However, the presence of an enlarged posterior fossa due to the existence of a cystic structure (Dandy– Walker malformation, arachnoid cyst, etc.) or to an abnormally enlarged fluid

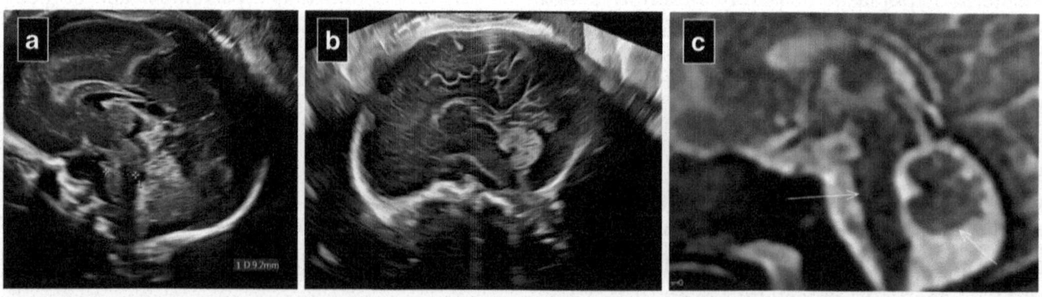

Fig. 17 Pontocerebellar hypoplasia (PCH) in two different conditions (**a**, **b**). The anteroposterior diameter of the pons is below normal ranges, and a flattening or disappearance of the normal pontine protuberance is also visible, especially in the second case which was confirmed at MRI (**c**). In case (**a**), PCH was identified in a patient evaluated for a transverse cerebellar diameter below the third percentile at 33 weeks' gestation and associated with 1p36 deletion. In case (**b**), PCH was diagnosed during a referral scan in a patient with a bilateral club foot in the third trimester of pregnancy with normal chromosomal array

space (mega cisterna magna), which might displace the vermis, will point toward cystic anomalies associated with cerebellar dysgenesis.

MRI imaging: The use of MRI, especially in the third trimester of pregnancy, is key in cases of suspected CH/PCH, particularly for a detailed analysis of the brainstem and its adjacent structures (anterior and posterior part of the pons, diencephalic/mesencephalic junction, etc.) as well as of the cerebral cortex. In coronal sections, MRI may, in some cases, identify the typical "dragonfly" pattern, indicative of predominant involvement of the cerebellar hemispheres compared to the vermis. However, this sign, similarly to other signs at MRI/US, is not pathognomonic. Accurate evaluation of the mesencephalon and brainstem might lead to a specific diagnostic entity in this group of conditions.

Prognosis: In cases of CH/PCH, it has been demonstrated that pontine biometry, particularly its anteroposterior diameter, is significantly correlated with clinical outcomes, with smaller measurements associated with less favorable outcomes in the series published by Jaillard et al. [21].

Treatment options: No curative treatment is available to date for any of these conditions. Treatment is only symptomatic.

Obstetric management: Not applicable.

3.2 Joubert Syndrome and Related Disorders (JSRD)

Definition: The diagnosis of Joubert syndrome (JS) is based on the identification of three key elements: (1) the "molar tooth sign" associated with cerebellar vermis hypoplasia in PF imaging; (2) the presence of hypotonia or low muscle tone; (3) the presence of developmental delay or intellectual disability. In addition to these three cardinal features, other anomalies are often described in infants and children with JS.

Epidemiology: The prevalence of JS has been estimated to range between 1:80,000 and 1:100,000. However, given the growing number genes found to be implicated and the broad range of phenotypic findings, the prevalence might be underestimated.

Etiology: JS is classified in the heterogenous group of the ciliopathies. The term "ciliopathies" refers to an emerging class of genetic multisystemic human disorders caused by the mutation of several—mainly unrelated—genes involved in the ciliary structure/function. These conditions, including the Joubert syndromes and related disorders (JSRD), are characterized by a wide range of multisystemic features resulting from the impaired cilia function and affecting often the brain, eyes, kidney, liver, and skeleton. Most of the proteins codified by the genes mutated in JSRD are either components of the primary cilium, the basal body, and/or the mother centriole from which it arises, or they are regulatory proteins and transcription factors involved in the primary cilium development and function.

Genetic Background: Thirty-five genes have been recognized to be implicated in the pathogenesis of JSRD. The inheritance is autosomal recessive for most of them although OFD1 (Oral Facial Syndrome 1) has an X-linked recessive inheritance. A few genes have been suggested to have autosomal dominant inheritance, but this is highly speculative [26]. Some of the causative genes in JSRD have been also observed to be involved in other ciliopathies such as Meckel-Gruber syndrome, Bardet–Biedl syndrome, and nephronophthisis, which share some features with JSRD.

Sonographic Findings: Few authors have reported the antenatal detection of the "Molar Tooth Sign" (MTS) at ultrasound or MRI [27]. This pathognomonic sign corresponds to a complex midbrain–hindbrain malformation—the dysgenesis of the brainstem isthmus—which is characterized by the elongation and thinning of the ponto-mesencephalic junction. These changes lead to an increase in the depth of the interpeduncular anterior fossa with an associated thickening, elongation, and horizontalization of the superior cerebellar peduncles which results in the pathognomonic MTS observed on the axial views (Fig. 18). The shape of the fourth ventricle (4th V) is also abnormal in cases of JSRD [28]. Indeed, on axial view, the fourth ventricle appears enlarged with its floor pointing anteriorly due to the lack of normal decussation of the cerebellar peduncles in the tegmentum. The visualization of this specific feature depends on the level of insonation of the fourth ventricle on the axial view. Indeed, it is visible only if the axial view is obtained at the upper level of the pons. We also observed a change in the normal antero/posterior—lateral ratio, with antero/posterior diameter being larger than the lateral diameter (Fig. 19). In sagittal view, the fourth ventricle in JSRD appears to be abnormally enlarged and rounded, lacking the characteristic posterior "fastigial point" and with a convex roof (Fig. 20). Antenatal diagnosis of JSRD relies on a positive family history and/or on the ultrasound finding of abnormal posterior fossa anatomy and/or the presence of associated suggestive features, such as kidney anomalies or polydactyly.

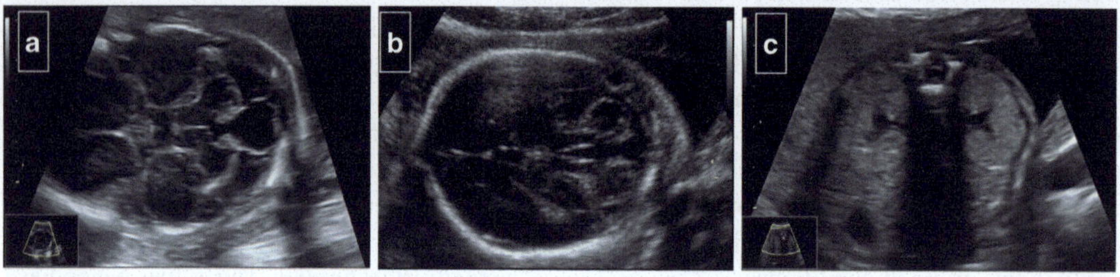

Fig. 18 Joubert syndrome and related disorder (JSRD) are suspected at midtrimester anomaly scan in the presence of an abnormal posterior fossa where the fourth ventricle and the cisterna magna are in communication (**a**), the molar tooth sign with abnormal cerebellar peduncles is observed (**b**), and abnormal kidneys (enlarged and hyperechogenic) are evidenced (**c**)

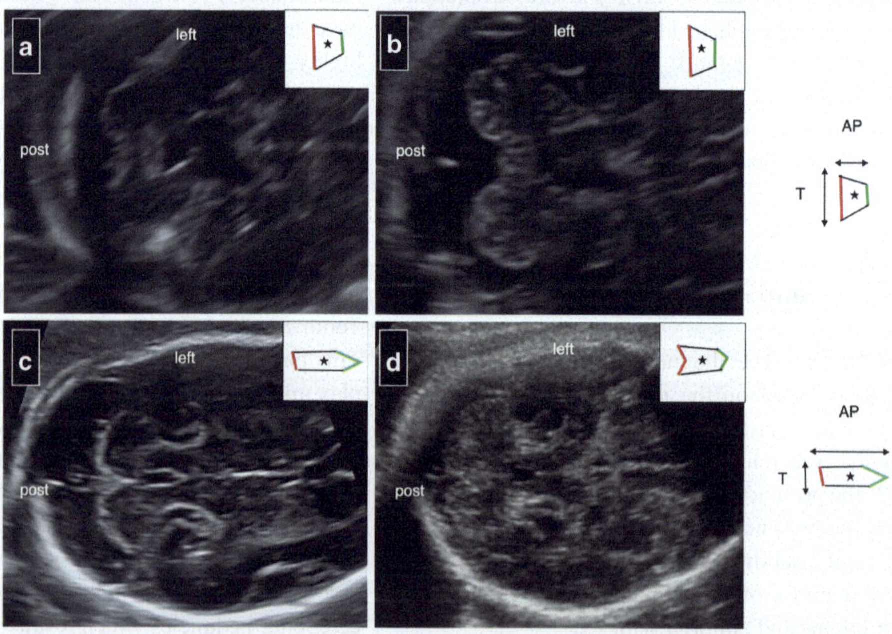

Fig. 19 Axial views of the posterior fossa in a normal fetus at 22 weeks (**a**) and 30 weeks (**b**) and in a fetus diagnosed with JSRD (**c**, **d**). In **c** and **d**, the fourth ventricle is enlarged. The ventricular floor is abnormal, pointing anteriorly (**c**, **d**) due to the lack of normal decussation of the cerebellar peduncles in the tegmentum. In JSRD, the anteroposterior diameter of the superior aspect of the fourth ventricle is longer than its transverse diameter. A pictorial representation of the fourth ventricle in normal (**a**, **b**) and JSRD cases (**c**, **d**) is displayed on the right of the figure. *Red line* the roof of the fourth ventricle, *Green line* the floor of the fourth ventricle, *Star* fourth ventricle, *AP* antero–posterior, *T* transverse, *Post* posterior

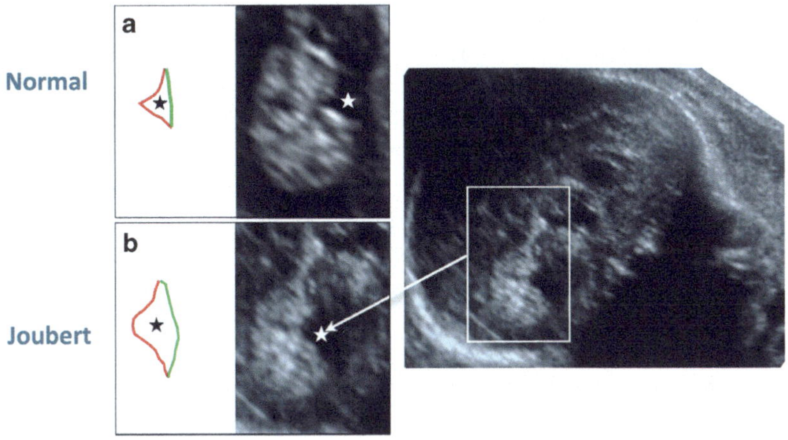

Fig. 20 The sagittal view of the posterior fossa at 27 weeks' gestation in a normal fetus (**a**). In JSRD (**b**), the fourth ventricle appears to be enlarged, rounded and it lacks the characteristic posterior pointed triangular shape with the so-called "fastigial point" (white arrow). *Red line* the roof of the fourth ventricle, *Green line* the floor of the fourth ventricle, *Star* fourth ventricle

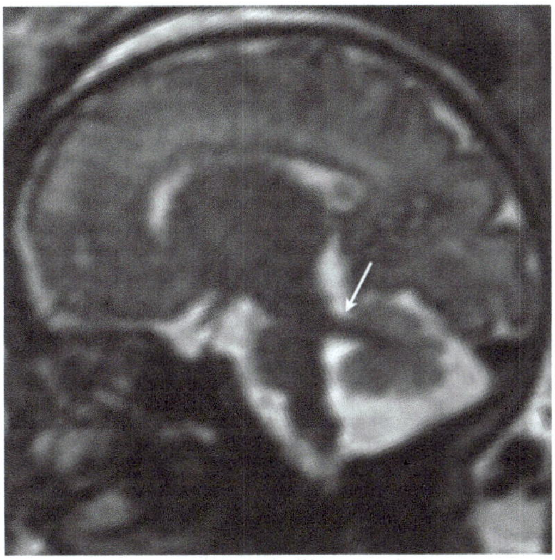

Fig. 21 Parasagittal views at MRI allow the visualization of thick superior cerebellar peduncles perpendicular to the posterior surface of the brainstem (white arrow). Note that the cisterna magna looks subjectively mildly dilated as a consequence of the hypoplasia of the posterior part of the vermis

Differential Diagnosis: Open fourth ventricle is a sonographic sign frequently observed in the second trimester, where the fourth ventricle funnels into the cisterna magna. It is the most common indicator of midbrain–hindbrain malformations and suggests dysgenesis, agenesis, or upward displacement and rotation of the cerebellar vermis. Of note, this finding may be transient in up to 10% of normal fetuses between 15 and 18 weeks and present in all conditions where a vermian dysgenesis is observed JSRD might be suspected. The presence of associated cerebral and/or extracerebral anomalies will support the diagnosis, conversely, will point toward other specific entities.

MRI imaging: MRI imaging of the parasagittal views may allow visualization of other subtle features typical of JSRD, such as thick superior cerebellar peduncles perpendicular to the posterior surface of the brainstem (Fig. 21). MRI also helps to exclude other fetal cerebral malformations, especially those involving the cortex.

Prognosis: Global prognosis varies considerably among JSRD subgroups, depending on the extent and severity of organ involvement.

Options of Treatment: Treatment is only supportive.

Obstetric Management: not relevant.

3.3 Rhombencephalosynapsis

Definition: Rhombencephalosynapsis (RES) is a rare developmental midbrain–hindbrain malformation, generally associated with a poor outcome, characterized by partial (hypoplasia) or complete absence (aplasia) of the vermis and midline fusion of the cerebellar hemispheres [29] and of dentate nuclei [30]. The cerebellar tonsils and deep cerebellar nuclei can also be fused. This variety of findings suggests that RES should be described as a malformative spectrum of cerebellar fusion with variable vermian involvement. Evidence in the literature shows that the posterior vermis is the most commonly and severely affected, followed by the anterior vermis and then the nodulus [29, 31].

The classification of RES is based on the pattern of vermis agenesis and hence the region and degree of hemispheric fusion:

- *Complete* RES: total absence of the vermis.
- *Partial* RES: classified according to the missing part of the vermis.
  - Partial severe RES: absence of the posterior and anterior vermis, with nodulus remnants.
  - Posterior RES: absence of the posterior vermis and variable remnants of the anterior vermis and nodulus.
  - Anterior RES: absence of the anterior vermis and variable remnants of vermian tissue caudal to the primary fissure.
  - Mixed RES: fusion of the central part of the vermis—mostly involving the posterior vermis—with some remnants of the anterior and posterior vermis above and below the fusion level.

The prenatal diagnosis of RES remains challenging and usually is made in the late second or third trimester of pregnancy. Suspicion is most often raised by major ventriculomegaly, associated with a small and abnormally shaped cerebellum, in which the vermis is not identified. The cerebellar hemispheres seem to be fused with the cerebellum displaying a posterior convexity (Fig. 22).

Epidemiology: RES is a rare congenital defect, first described by Obersteiner in 1914. Despite the growing use and advances in neurosonography and fetal imaging, RES can be missed even in cases of aqueduct stenosis and congenital hydrocephalus. In a postnatal series of 3000 pediatric brain magnetic resonance imaging (MRI), the estimated prevalence was 0,13% [32] but since the pediatric series do not include cases of termination of pregnancies and neonatal demise, the exact incidence remains unknown.

Etiology/ Pathogenesis: Our understanding of the pathogenetic mechanisms of RES is limited by the absence of known genetic causes or animal models. It has been postulated that this cerebellar anomaly results from a regulation disorder in the developmental pathway involving the cerebellar primordium, an unpaired structure located at the junction of the metencephalon and the mesencephalon. The cerebellar primordium normally divides into a median part, the vermis, and a pair of hemispheres that grow from the rhombic lips. It is still debated whether the failure of vermis differentiation—between post conception days 28 and 42—is the cause or the consequence of the fusion (or undivided pattern) of the cerebellar hemisphere [30, 33, 34]. Associated midline malformations (impaired mesencephalic, pontine, and diencephalic cleavage and holoprosencephaly) point to a still unknown but shared developmental mechanism along the cranio-caudal axis. The theory of a dorsal–ventral patterning defects resulting in loss of midline and fusion of lateral structures can explain some of these malformative associations [29, 35]. Severe ventriculomegaly is most often due to an associated aqueductal stenosis [30, 36], and it should also be kept in mind that many supratentorial anomalies are often consequences of hydrocephalus and not primary defects of these structures.

Genetic background: To date, no genetic nor molecular causes have been identified, and no animal models exist for RES. The most extensive exome sequencing analysis of a cohort of patients with RES failed to identify a single gene with variants meeting the criteria for de novo dominant and recessive modes of inheritance in more than one family. However, a genetic cause for RES seems to be plausible [37]. RES is a malformation similar to other stereotyped brain malformations with a known genetic causes (e.g., holoprosencephaly, Joubert syndrome) and which seems to present in line with the "developmental field defect" concept [38].

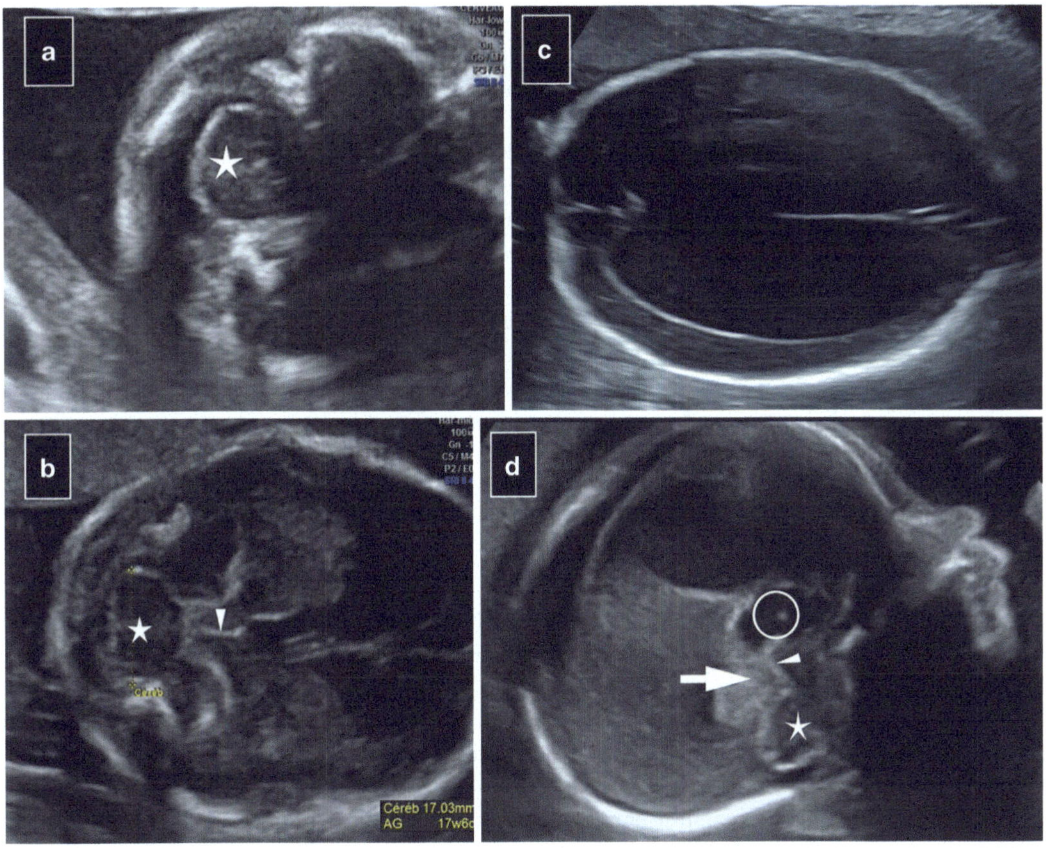

Fig. 22 Complete rhombencephalosynapsis at 22 weeks' gestation. The axial views of the fetal brain at the level of the posterior fossa (**a**) and mesencephalon (**b**). Figure (**a**) displays a small and round-shaped cerebellum (TCD < 3rd centile) with the absence of the vallecula (star). Neither the vermis nor the fourth ventricle is identified. The cisterna magna is not enlarged. (**b**) The hyperechoic line (arrowhead), without identification of aqueductal of Sylvius lumen at level of mesencephalon, is suggestive of aqueductal stenosis with dilated third ventricle. (**c**) On the axial view, a severe ventriculomegaly with septal rupture is evidenced. (**d**) On the midsagittal view of the brain, the vermis is not identified; instead, a "midline" cerebellum is observed which can be misinterpreted as the vermis (star). Note the hyperechoic atretic aqueduct (arrow head), the thickened tectum (arrow), and stretched interthalamic adhesion (circle). The pons has a normal appearance

Most RES cases are sporadic and possibly due to a de novo mutation with dominant inheritance pattern. Thus, the lack of recurrence, especially in consanguineous families does not suggest recessive inheritance [29, 37]. In a series of 115 RES [37], RES was diagnosed as an isolated brain malformation in 24% of patients. The first syndrome to be associated with RES was described by Gómez and Lopez who defined a congenital anomaly syndrome in a series of patients characterized by RES, parietal-occipital scalp alopecia, and trigeminal anesthesia (Gómez-López-Hernández syndrome). Craniosynostosis and distinctive dysmorphic facial features had also been described [39]. RES has also been confirmed to be associated with VACTERL features (vertebral anomalies, anal atresia, cardiac defect, tracheoesophageal fistula, renal anomalies, radial dysplasia, or other limb defects) and hydrocephalus (VACTERL-H) [30, 38], and some authors suggest that this association should be referred to the term of VACTERL-R.

Notably, a recent study [40], which employed a "genotype-first" approach on a cohort of individuals with recognizable neurodevelopmental disorders and distinctive craniofacial features, identified "de novo" C-terminal truncating mutations in MN1 in eight patients with partial RES. This finding provides new insights into the developmental mechanisms of RES.

Sonographic findings: The prenatal diagnosis of RES remains challenging and usually occurs in the late second or third trimester of pregnancy, although early signs of RES have been reported as early as in the first trimester [41]. Suspicion is most often raised by the presence of severe ventriculomegaly associated with a small (the shortening of the TCD is more marked that that of the anterior-posterior diameter) and abnormally shaped cerebellum. The vermis is not well identified, and the cerebellar hemispheres look fused with posterior convexity and loss of the classic posterior cerebellar notch (vallecula) (Fig. 22). On the coronal or axial view of the cerebellum, the characteristic transverse-oriented folia crossing the midline can be appreciated, especially from the second trimester onwards (Fig. 22). The posterior fossa is usually small with no cystic malformations. Of note, on the midsagittal view, the "midline cerebellum" might be erroneously interpreted as the vermis (although it presents a hypochogenic appearance with shallow folia and no deep fissure) (Fig. 22). Additionally, the "midline cerebellum" height is usually >2 SD compared to that of a normal vermis; this might help to differentiate RES from other causes of reduced transverse cerebellar diameter with small vermis. Lastly, less severe forms of the RES spectrum might present with a more defined cerebellar shape and with a small vermis remnant.

In a recent series of 62 cases (48 complete RES and 14 partial RES) [31], the primary fissure of the vermis was not identified on sagittal views in all cases. The transverse cerebellar diameter was below the third centile in 87.1% of the cases (complete RES 91.7%, partial RES 71.4%), and an abnormal fourth ventricle was observed in 72.6% and 87.1% of complete RES and partial RES cases, respectively, and absent or shallow vallecula in 95.2% of all cases. Ventriculomegaly was present in 80% of cases with subsequent anomalies like ventricular septal or brain parenchyma and rupture in the severe cases. The association between RES and ventriculomegaly is explained by the frequent underlying aqueductal stenosis due to an obstructive mechanism at the mesencephalic level [29, 36].

The evidence of an abnormal aqueduct of Sylvius (AoS) in RES is well established. Indeed, a large neuropathological study of 40 fetal cases found isolated stenosis, atresia, complex forking, and dysmorphism of the AoS in 13%, 39%, 31%, and 12% of cases, respectively [30] (Fig. 23). In another series of RES cases [31], a developmental anomaly of the midbrain was present in 92% cases. Aqueductal stenosis was the most frequent abnormality (77.4%), anteroposterior midbrain diameter was below the fifth centile in 54.8% of cases, and associated mesencephalosynapsis was present in 54.8% of the cases. Pontine anomalies were seen in 77% of cases, with different degrees of hypoplasia. The severity of midbrain abnormalities seems to strongly be correlated with the severity of RES [31]. Associated abnormal cleavage at the diencephalic level (diencephalosynapsis) [42] has also been described. Other intracranial supratentorial anomalies possibly associated are corpus callosum agenesis/dysgenesis, septo-optic dysplasia, holoprosencephaly, and cortical anomalies.

Differential diagnosis: Possible differential diagnosis includes other causes of cerebellar hypoplasia described in this chapter, where the cerebellum is small but anatomically complete with intact vermis and cerebellar lobes not fused. Cases of unilateral cerebellar hypoplasia show small but asymmetric cerebellum, cerebellar lobes are not fused, and the vermis can be intact or also affected. Pathologies with reduced or absent vermis like Dandy–Walker malformation spectrum or vermian agenesis usually present with enlarged posterior fossa, and an open fourth ventricle in communication with the cisterna magna, which is not present in RES.

MRI imaging: The ultrasound anomalies described above can be confirmed at MRI imaging.

On the axial view, the rounded appearance of the posterior border of the cerebellum with fused lobes, characteristic fusion or joining of the dentate nuclei, and absent midline notch are observed. On coronal or axial view, the highly

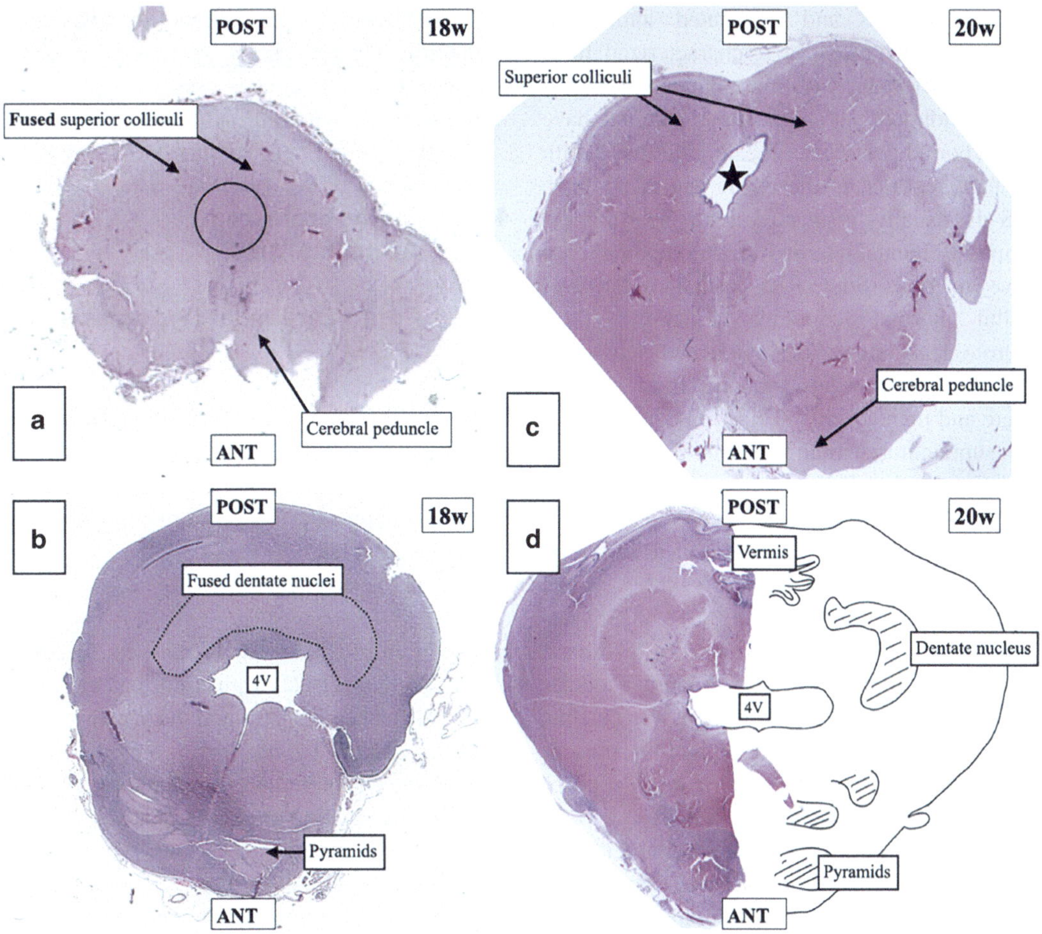

Fig. 23 Histological findings of rhombencephalosynapsis in a fetus at 18 weeks (**a**, **b**) and in a normal fetus at 20 weeks' gestation (**c**, **d**). (**a**) Transverse section through the upper part of midbrain, showing atresia of aqueduct of Sylvius (circle), replaced by few small tubules lined with ependymal cells. (**b**) Transverse section through brainstem and cerebellum, showing rhombencephalosynapsis with fused dentate nuclei and narrowed fourth ventricle (4 V) with "diamond shape." (**c**) Transverse section through the upper part of midbrain, showing a normal aqueduct of Sylvius (star) and non-fused colliculi. (**d**) Transverse section through the brainstem and cerebellum showing normal 4 V, normal vermis, and two distinct dentate nuclei

characteristic transverse folding can be of difficult evaluation at MRI [43, 44]. The fourth ventricle might appear with normal size or with a small round shape. However, it can also be enlarged presenting an oval or diamond-shaped configuration [31].

On sagittal view, the characteristic signs of a normal vermis are absent, as neither the primary fissure nor the fastigial point can be identified. Also at MRI imaging, the "midline cerebellum" can falsely mimic the vermis [43, 44]. In partial RES, the presence of the nodulus can also appears as a "thumb-like" projection into the floor of the fourth ventricle, simulating a fastigial point [31]. MRI imaging can also be useful to characterize above-described associated anomalies of the pons, midbrain, and diencephalon. Similarly, MRI can also help in the diagnosis of agenesis of the corpus callosum, holoprosencephaly, severe ventriculomegaly, and cortical abnormalities [29, 31, 42].

Prognosis: RES presents with a wide spectrum of clinical findings, and the clinical presentation seems to correlate with the severity of the imaging features and associated anomalies. Generally, the prognosis is characterized by a shortened lifespan, with most patients dying in early childhood, although some patients have been reported to survive till early adulthood with one case reported to die at the age of 55 [45]. RES is usually associated with neurological symptoms, mental retardation, and impaired cognitive functions. Some RES cases may however exhibit normal cognitive functions [46]. Neurological defects and associated symptoms with RES vary widely, ranging from mild to severe and their severity seems linked to concurrent supratentorial malformations [29, 31] and reduction of cerebellar volume [47]. Prenatal hydrocephalus is considered an unfavorable prognostic feature. Ataxia, both truncal and limb, involuntary head movements with typical "Figure-of-eight" head shaking [38, 48], dysarthria, swallowing difficulties, seizure disorders, hypothalamic pituitary axis dysfunction, ocular abnormalities such as abnormal eye movements, strabismus, and optic nerve atrophy [49], muscular hypotonia, and spastic quadriparesis contribute to the clinical presentation [50].

Options of treatment: No specific curative treatment exists. A careful postnatal examination (also provided by an endocrinologist) during neonatal period is mandatory. Medical management is supportive with palliation of associated symptoms. Hydrocephalus may require shunt placement.

Obstetric management: Not relevant.

4 Major Brainstem Abnormalities

4.1 Ponto Cerebellar Hypoplasia (PCH)

PCHs have been previously described (III.A/ cerebellar and pontocerebellar hypoplasia), and they can be associated with various anomalies affecting the structures developed from the midbrain–hindbrain complex.

PCH is suspected:

- *On the axial plane*: a short transverse cerebellar diameter (TCD) with a normal morphology of the hemispheres and the vermis.
- *On the sagittal plane*:
  - Reduced anteroposterior diameter of brainstem at pontine level, with possible flattening or disappearance of the pontine protuberance (Fig. 24).
  - Reduced height, surface, and anteroposterior diameter of the vermis.

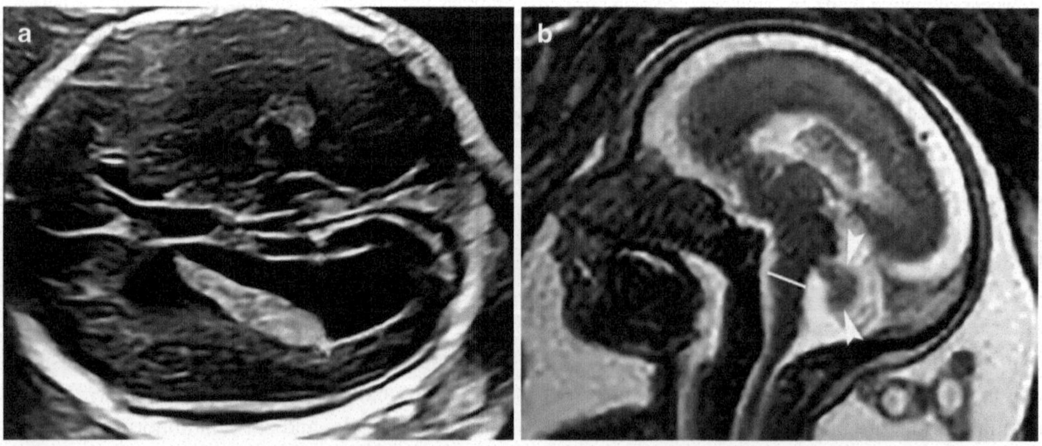

Fig. 24 Pontocerebellar hypoplasia at 24 weeks' gestation. (**a**) On the axial transventricular plane, a moderate ventriculomegaly (12.6 mm) is observed. (**b**) T2-weighted MR image. On a midsagittal section of the posterior fossa ponto-vermian hypoplasia is evidenced. A flattened pons lacking the typical protuberance is observed. The anteroposterior diameter of the pons (white line) is below the fifth centile. The arrowheads indicate the hypoplastic vermis

4.2 Cobblestone Malformations (COB)

Cobblestone cortical malformations correspond to a group of syndromes attributed to abnormal glycosylation of alpha-dystroglycan. This is associated with neuroglial overmigration into the arachnoid space resulting in the formation of an extracortical neuroglial layer responsible for agyria and/or irregular, "cobblestone," surface of the brain and ventriculomegaly. Diagnosis can be suspected antenatally when a thick hyperechogenic band is observed supratentorially. Ultrasound findings are the following:

- *On the axial plane*:
  - Supratentorially, the presence of the cortical hyperechogenic.
  - Filling of peri-cerebral spaces.
  - Tri-ventricular dilatation of the ventricular system with Sylvian aqueduct stenosis.
- *On the sagittal plane*:
  - Infratentorially, a folded appearance of the brainstem (Kinking brainstem) strongly suggestive of cobblestone lissencephaly in association with ventriculomegaly and agyria (Fig. 25).

4.3 Joubert Syndrome and Related Disorders (JSRD)

Joubert syndrome and related disorders are associated with primary cilia function abnormalities affecting the brainstem and other organs. In the brainstem, dysgenesis of the mesencephalic isthmus is observed, including:

- *On the axial plane*:
  - Elongated and thickened superior cerebellar peduncles at the mesencephalon, leading to the characteristic "molar tooth" appearance.
  - Dysmorphic fourth ventricle with elongated appearance and anteroposterior diameter greater than lateral diameter, reversing typical proportions.
- *On the sagittal plane* (Fig. 26):
  - Dysgenesis of the mesencephalic isthmus (isthmus narrowing).
  - Thickened and horizontal superior cerebellar peduncles.
  - Enlarged and quadrangular fourth ventricle.
  - Flattened fastigium.
  - Absent or aplastic vermis and/or dysplastic with absence of primary and secondary fissures.

4.4 Cap Tegmentum Pontine Dysplasia

Cap tegmentum pontine dysplasia is a rare hindbrain malformation possibly resulting from abnormal neuronal migration or axonal guidance which leads to a distinctive hindbrain malformation, cranial nerve dysfunction, and developmental delay. At brainstem level, the following findings can be detected [52, 53]:

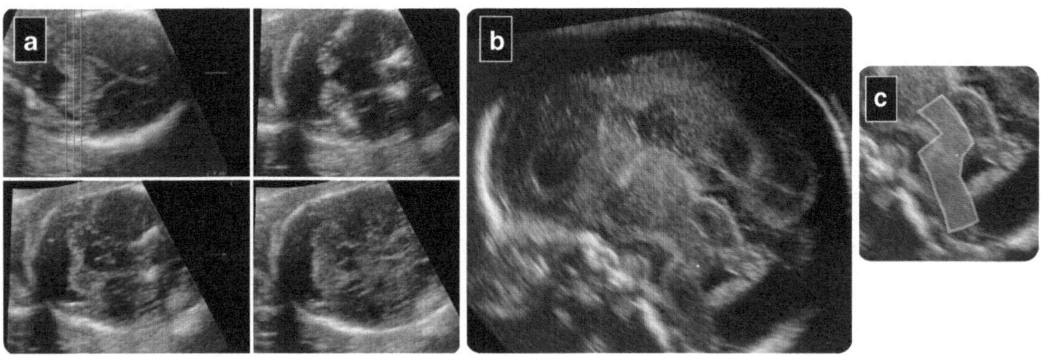

Fig. 25 Kinked fetal brainstem (**b**, **c**) in the setting of Walker–Walburg syndrome with dysplastic vermis (**a**)

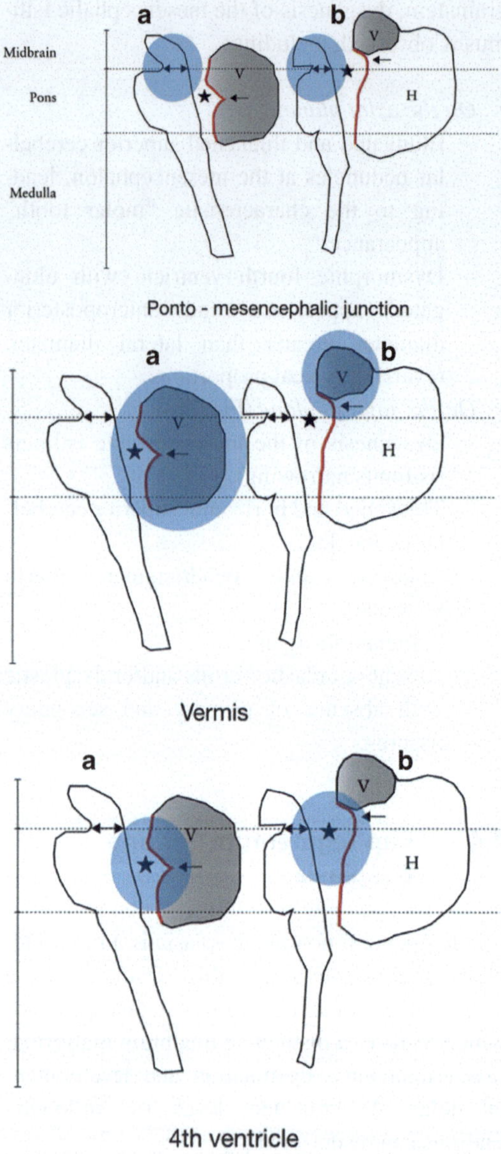

Fig. 26 Different drawings of the brainstem in normal (**a**) and JSRD (**b**) fetuses. Three main features are usually seen: the narrowing of the pontomesencephalic junction, a dysplastic vermis, and an abnormal fourth ventricle. star: fourth ventricle; V: vermis; H: cerebellar hemisphere; red line: roof of the fourth ventricle

- *On the axial plane*:
  - Near disappearance of middle cerebellar peduncles.
  - Thinning of superior and inferior cerebellar peduncles.
- *On the sagittal plane*:
  - Shortening of the mesencephalic isthmus (ponto-mesencephalic junction).
  - Ventral hypoplasia of the pontine ventral part, with loss of pontine protuberance.
  - Presence of a dorsal tissue projection (cap) covering the middle third of the pontine tegmentum, extending into the fourth ventricle.
  - A kinked appearance of the brainstem.
  - Vermian hypoplasia/dysplasia often associated with cerebellar hypoplasia.

4.5 Diencephalic-Mesencephalic Junction Dysplasia

Diencephalic-mesencephalic junction dysplasia is a rare malformation spectrum characterized by a poorly defined junction between the two entities. It is associated with a wide range of anomalies, including callosal anomalies and/or supratentorial ventricular dilatations. Ultrasound findings at the brainstem level are the following [54, 55]:

- *On the axial plane* (for DM dysplasia type A):
  - No separation between the mesencephalon and thalami resulting in ventro-dorsal axis enlargement and abnormal contours of the mesencephalon.
  - Often, a ventral fissure in the DM resulting in the characteristic "butterfly sign."
- *On the sagittal plane*:
  - Poor delineation of the diencephalic-mesencephalic junction.
  - Abnormal ventral position of thalami.
  - Enlargement of the interthalamic adhesion.
  - Pontine hypoplasia.
  - Poorly-identified or stenosed Sylvian aqueduct.
  - A kinked appearance of the brainstem, particularly at the ponto-medullary junction.

4.6 Tubulinopathies

Tubulinopathies are characterized by mutations in tubulin genes that affect the tubulin heterodimerization process and/or their stability, leading to disruption in neuronal division and migration, resulting in brain malformations. During the prenatal period, two main types, severe and intermediate forms, have been described, both affecting the brainstem [56].

In cases of severe involvement, there is an enlargement of the germinal matrices, indicative of precursor cell entrapment, with a significant reduction in cortical parenchymal thickness, presenting as an agyric cortical surface (referred to as micro lissencephaly), microcephaly, and severe brainstem dysgenesis characterized by a thin and folded brainstem.

In cases of intermediate involvement, there is no microcephaly, but various presentations within the spectrum of tubulinopathies, including:

- *On the axial plane*:
  - Supratentorial:
    - Distortion of the interhemispheric fissure, with frontal lobe asymmetry.
    - Dysmorphic/asymmetric and dilated frontal horn ventricles.
    - Anomaly in the operculation of the Sylvian fissure.
    - Callosal dysplasias.
  - Infratentorial:
    - Asymmetry of the brainstem and/or cerebellum.
    - Cerebellar dysplasia.
- *On the sagittal plane*:
  - Supratentorial:
    - Callosal dysplasias.
  - Infratentorial:
    - Cerebellar dysplasia.
    - Dysplastic, folded brainstem of varying thickness.

5 Conclusion

Non-cystic posterior fossa abnormalities constitute a heterogeneous group of cerebral lesions of diverse primary or secondary etiologies. The incidental finding suspicious for these groups of conditions is usually the late discovery of a transverse cerebellar diameter below the fifth centile. Investigation of the personal and family medical history combined with detailed morphological evaluation of fetal supra- and infratentorial cerebral structures may help in the diagnosis as the presence of specific signs is suggestive of certain specific pathophysiological mechanisms. Fetal MRI, possibly repeated, and genetic analysis according to updated indications, is also mandatory for a better understanding of these complex situations.

Special thanks to: Dr. JP Bault, Dr. C.Colmant, Dr. D.Grevent, Dr. P.Volpe for providing some figures and cases to illustrate our chapter.

References

1. International Society of Ultrasound in Obstetrics and Gynecology, Bilardo CM, Chaoui R, Hyett JA, Kagan KO, Karim JN, et al. ISUOG practice guidelines (updated): performance of 11-14-week ultrasound scan. Ultrasound Obstet Gynecol. 2023;61(1):127–43.
2. Salomon LJ, Alfirevic Z, Berghella V, Bilardo CM, Chalouhi GE, Da Silva CF, et al. ISUOG practice guidelines (updated): performance of the routine mid-trimester fetal ultrasound scan. Ultrasound Obstet Gynecol. 2022;59(6):840–56.
3. Khalil A, Sotiriadis A, D'Antonio F, Da Silva CF, Odibo A, Prefumo F, et al. ISUOG practice guidelines: performance of third-trimester obstetric ultrasound scan. Ultrasound Obstet Gynecol. 2024;63(1):131–47.
4. Malinger G, Paladini D, Haratz KK, Monteagudo A, Pilu GL, Timor-Tritsch IE. ISUOG practice guidelines (updated): sonographic examination of the fetal central nervous system. Part 1: performance of screening examination and indications for targeted neurosonography. Ultrasound Obstet Gynecol. 2020;56(3):476–84.

5. Sciard C, Lacalme A, Combourieu D, Gaucherand P, Lajeunesse C, Massardier J, et al. Fetal transcerebellar diameter measured in screening ultrasound: feasibility and reproducibility. J Gynecol Obstet Biol Reprod (Paris). 2016;45(5):516–20.
6. Paladini D, Malinger G, Birnbaum R, Monteagudo A, Pilu G, Salomon LJ, et al. ISUOG practice guidelines (updated): sonographic examination of the fetal central nervous system. Part 2: performance of targeted neurosonography. Ultrasound Obstet Gynecol. Apr 2021;57(4):661–71.
7. Guibaud L, des Portes V. Plea for an anatomical approach to abnormalities of the posterior fossa in prenatal diagnosis. Ultrasound Obstet Gynecol. 2006;27(5):477–81.
8. Atallah A, Guibaud L, Gaucherand P, Massardier J, des Portes V, Massoud M. Fetal and perinatal outcome associated with small cerebellar diameter based on second- or third-trimester ultrasonography. Prenat Diagn. 2019;39(7):536–43.
9. Takano M, Nakata M, Oji A, Nagasaki S, Umemura N, Maemura T, et al. Utility of fetal anteroposterior to transverse cerebellar diameter ratio to exclude cerebellar hypoplasia in trisomy 18. J Obstet Gynaecol Res. 2018;44(6):1031–5.
10. Katorza E, Bertucci E, Perlman S, Taschini S, Ber R, Gilboa Y, et al. Development of the fetal vermis: new biometry reference data and comparison of 3 diagnostic modalities-3D ultrasound, 2D ultrasound, and MR imaging. AJNR Am J Neuroradiol. 2016 Jul;37(7):1359–66.
11. Zalel Y, Yagel S, Achiron R, Kivilevich Z, Gindes L. Three-dimensional ultrasonography of the fetal vermis at 18 to 26 weeks' gestation: time of appearance of the primary fissure. J Ultrasound Med. 2009;28(1):1–8.
12. Massoud M, Cagneaux M, Garel C, Varene N, Moutard ML, Billette T, et al. Prenatal unilateral cerebellar hypoplasia in a series of 26 cases: significance and implications for prenatal diagnosis. Ultrasound Obstet Gynecol. 2014;44(4):447–54.
13. Poretti A, Boltshauser E, Doherty D. Cerebellar hypoplasia: differential diagnosis and diagnostic approach. Am J Med Genet C Semin Med Genet. 2014;166C(2):211–26.
14. Accogli A, Addour-Boudrahem N, Srour M. Diagnostic approach to cerebellar hypoplasia. Cerebellum. 2021;20(4):631–58.
15. Leibovitz Z, Guibaud L, Garel C, Massoud M, Karl K, Malinger G, et al. The cerebellar "tilted telephone receiver sign" enables prenatal diagnosis of PHACES syndrome. Eur J Paediatr Neurol. 2018;22(6):900–9.
16. Moosavi A, Kanekar S. Congenital malformations of cerebellum. Clin Perinatol. 2022;49(3):603–21.
17. Guibaud L, Garel C, Annie B, Pascal G, François V, Vavasseur C, et al. Prenatal diagnosis of capillary telangiectasia of the cerebellum--ultrasound and MRI features. Prenat Diagn. 2003;23(10):791–6.
18. Massoud M, Clerc J, Cagneux M, Vasiljevic A, Massardier J, Doret M, et al. Prenatal diagnosis of cerebellar cortical dysplasia associated with abnormalities of foliation. Ultrasound Obstet Gynecol. 2012;40(2):243–4.
19. Huissoud C, Rudigoz RC, Bisch C, Brahimi P, Alias F, Tixier H, et al. Complete cerebellar agenesis: a very rare abnormality of the posterior fossa. Ultrasound Obstet Gynecol. 2009;33(6):730–1.
20. Guibaud L, Devonec S, Des Portes V, Roth P, Gaucherand P, Pracros JP. Extracerebellar ectopic brain tissue in the posterior fossa. Ultrasound Obstet Gynecol. 2005;26(6):687–9.
21. Jaillard A, Valence S, Vande Perre S, Dhombres F, Héron D, Billette de Villemeur T, et al. Prenatal diagnosis of pontocerebellar hypoplasia with postnatal follow-up. Prenat Diagn. 2024;44(1):35–48.
22. van Dijk T, Baas F, Barth PG, Poll-The BT. What's new in pontocerebellar hypoplasia? An update on genes and subtypes. Orphanet J Rare Dis. 2018;13(1):92.
23. Desai S, Desai T. Prenatal diagnosis of pontocerebellar hypoplasia associated with rare syndromes: expanding the genetic and phenotypic spectrum. Ultrasound Obstet Gynecol. 2021;57(3):498–9.
24. Rüsch CT, Bölsterli BK, Kottke R, Steinfeld R, Boltshauser E. Pontocerebellar hypoplasia: a pattern recognition approach. Cerebellum. 2020;19(4):569–82.
25. Leibovitz Z, Shkolnik C, Haratz KK, Malinger G, Shapiro I, Lerman-Sagie T. Assessment of fetal midbrain and hindbrain in mid-sagittal cranial plane by three-dimensional multiplanar sonography. Part 2: application of nomograms to fetuses with posterior fossa malformations. Ultrasound Obstet Gynecol. 2014;44(5):581–7.
26. Parisi MA. The molecular genetics of Joubert syndrome and related ciliopathies: The challenges of genetic and phenotypic heterogeneity. Transl Sci Rare Dis. 2019;4(1–2):25–49.
27. Quarello E, Molho M, Garel C, Couture A, Legac MP, Moutard ML, et al. Prenatal abnormal features of the fourth ventricle in Joubert syndrome and related disorders. Ultrasound Obstet Gynecol. 2014;43(2):227–32.
28. Haratz KK, Shulevitz SL, Leibovitz Z, Lev D, Shalev J, Tomarkin M, et al. Fourth ventricle index: sonographic marker for severe fetal vermian dysgenesis/agenesis. Ultrasound Obstet Gynecol. 2019;53(3):390–5.
29. Ishak GE, Dempsey JC, Shaw DWW, Tully H, Adam MP, Sanchez-Lara PA, et al. Rhombencephalosynapsis: a hindbrain malformation associated with incomplete separation of midbrain and forebrain, hydrocephalus and a broad spectrum of severity. Brain. 2012;135(5):1370–86.
30. Pasquier L, Marcorelles P, Loget P, Pelluard F, Carles D, Perez MJ, et al. Rhombencephalosynapsis and related anomalies: a neuropathological study of 40 fetal cases. Acta Neuropathol. 2009;117(2):185–200.

31. Krajden Haratz K, Oliveira Szejnfeld P, Govindaswamy M, Leibovitz Z, Gindes L, Severino M, et al. Prenatal diagnosis of rhombencephalosynapsis: neuroimaging features and severity of vermian anomaly. Ultrasound Obstet Gynecol. 2021;58(6):864–74.
32. Sener RN. Unusual MRI findings in rhombencephalosynapsis. Comput Med Imaging Graph. 2000;24(4):277–82.
33. Utsunomiya H, Takano K, Ogasawara T, Hashimoto T, Fukushima T, Okazaki M. Rhombencephalosynapsis: cerebellar embryogenesis. AJNR Am J Neuroradiol. 1998;19(3):547–9.
34. Takanashi J, Sugita K, Barkovich AJ, Takano H, Kohno Y. Partial midline fusion of the cerebellar hemispheres with vertical folia: a new cerebellar malformation? AJNR Am J Neuroradiol. 1999;20(6):1151–3.
35. Yachnis AT. Rhombencephalosynapsis with massive hydrocephalus: case report and pathogenetic considerations. Acta Neuropathol. 2002;103(3):301–4.
36. Barkovich AJ, Raybaud C. Pediatric neuroimaging: 5th edition. 2012. 1.
37. Aldinger KA, Dempsey JC, Tully HM, Grout ME, Mehaffey MG, Dobyns WB, et al. Rhombencephalosynapsis: fused cerebellum, confused geneticists. Am J Med Genet C Semin Med Genet. 2018;178(4):432–9.
38. Tully HM, Dempsey JC, Ishak GE, Adam MP, Curry CJ, Sanchez-Lara P, et al. Beyond Gómez-López-Hernández syndrome: recurring phenotypic themes in Rhombencephalosynapsis. Am J Med Genet A. 2012;158A(10):2393–406.
39. Gomez MR. Cerebellotrigeminal and focal dermal dysplasia: a newly recognized neurocutaneous syndrome. Brain and Development. 1979;1(4):253–6.
40. Mak CCY, Doherty D, Lin AE, Vegas N, Cho MT, Viot G, et al. MN1 C-terminal truncation syndrome is a novel neurodevelopmental and craniofacial disorder with partial rhombencephalosynapsis. Brain. 2020;143(1):55–68.
41. Macé P, Ville Y, Bessière B, Quarello E. Early diagnosis of rhombencephalosynapsis: the limits of intracranial translucency at first-trimester screening and a plea for assessment of aqueduct of Sylvius. Ultrasound Obstet Gynecol. 2021;57(5):846–8.
42. Cagneaux M, Vasiljevic A, Massoud M, Allias F, Massardier J, Gaucherand P, et al. Severe second-trimester obstructive ventriculomegaly related to disorders of diencephalic, mesencephalic and rhombencephalic differentiation. Ultrasound Obstet Gynecol. 2013;42(5):596–602.
43. Napolitano M, Righini A, Zirpoli S, Rustico M, Nicolini U, Triulzi F. Prenatal magnetic resonance imaging of rhombencephalosynapsis and associated brain anomalies: report of 3 cases. J Comput Assist Tomogr. 2004;28(6):762–5.
44. McAuliffe F, Chitayat D, Halliday W, Keating S, Shah V, Fink M, et al. Rhombencephalosynapsis: prenatal imaging and autopsy findings. Ultrasound Obstet Gynecol. 2008;31(5):542–8.
45. Bell BD, Stanko HA, Levine RL. Normal IQ in a 55-year-old with newly diagnosed rhombencephalosynapsis. Arch Clin Neuropsychol. 2005;20(5):613–21.
46. Poretti A, Alber FD, Bürki S, Toelle SP, Boltshauser E. Cognitive outcome in children with rhombencephalosynapsis. Eur J Paediatr Neurol. 2009;13(1):28–33.
47. Altman NR, Naidich TP, Braffman BH. Posterior fossa malformations. AJNR Am J Neuroradiol. 1992;13(2):691–724.
48. Pinchefsky EF, Accogli A, Shevell MI, Saint-Martin C, Srour M. Developmental outcomes in children with congenital cerebellar malformations. Dev Med Child Neurol. 2019;61(3):350–8.
49. Phillips PH, Glasier CM, Brodsky MC. Neuro-ophthalmologic findings in patients with rhombencephalosynapsis. J AAPOS. 2008;12(1):97–9.
50. Toelle SP, Yalcinkaya C, Kocer N, Deonna T, Overweg-Plandsoen WCG, Bast T, et al. Rhombencephalosynapsis: clinical findings and neuroimaging in 9 children. Neuropediatrics. 2002;33(4):209–14.
51. Lacalm A, Nadaud B, Massoud M, Putoux A, Gaucherand P, Guibaud L. Prenatal diagnosis of cobblestone lissencephaly associated with Walker-Warburg syndrome based on a specific sonographic pattern. Ultrasound Obstet Gynecol. 2016;47(1):117–22.
52. Blondiaux E, Valence S, Friszer S, Rodriguez D, Burglen L, Ducou le Pointe H, et al. Prenatal imaging findings of pontine tegmental cap dysplasia: report of four cases. Fetal Diagn Ther. 2019;45(3):197–204.
53. Haratz KK, Lerman-Sagie T. Prenatal diagnosis of brainstem anomalies. Eur J Paediatr Neurol. 2018;22(6):1016–26.
54. Severino M, Tortora D, Pistorio A, Ramenghi LA, Napoli F, Mancardi MM, et al. Expanding the spectrum of congenital anomalies of the diencephalic-mesencephalic junction. Neuroradiology. 2016;58(1):33–44.
55. Severino M, Righini A, Tortora D, Pinelli L, Parazzini C, Morana G, et al. MR imaging diagnosis of diencephalic-mesencephalic junction dysplasia in fetuses with developmental ventriculomegaly. AJNR Am J Neuroradiol. 2017;38(8):1643–6.
56. Cabet S, Karl K, Garel C, Delius M, Hartung J, Lesca G, et al. Two different prenatal imaging cerebral patterns of tubulinopathy. Ultrasound Obstet Gynecol. 2021;57(3):493–7.

Malformations of Cortical Development (MCDs)

Ritsuko K. Pooh

Abstract

Malformations of cortical development (MCDs), though individually rare, are collectively a significant health concern. These conditions originate in the womb due to a range of genetic and environmental factors and their intricate interplays. Technological advances, particularly next-generation sequencing (NGS) in molecular genetics, alongside diagnostic efforts, have progressively elucidated the causes of MCD and transformed its classification system. Historically, MCD classification relied on pediatric MRI findings and gene identification, but recent enhancements in fetal neurosonography now allow for early indirect detection of MCD, predicting its presence before the formation of cortical gyri and sulci is evident.

Recent upgrades in ultrasound technology have enhanced our capability to assess both the normal development and the maldevelopment of the cerebral cortex, identifying not just overt cortical anomalies but also subtle indicators. Ongoing discoveries in molecular genetics are yielding new pathogenic genes regularly. Despite having the same genetic mutations, a wide array of phenotypic expressions has been observed, challenging the assumption of a direct phenotype–genotype correlation. This field is expected to benefit from further structuring and categorization with the help of artificial intelligence in upcoming years.

Keywords

Malformations of cortical development · Fetus · Neurosonography

1 Introduction

Malformations of cortical development (MCDs) are of rare occurrence but represent a significant burden of disease; MCD is a disease that forms in utero due to environmental and genetic causes and their complex interplay. Advances in molecular genetics using next-generation sequencing (NGS) and diagnostic efforts have gradually clarified the etiology of MCD and changed the classification of MCD. Originally, MCD was classified based on pediatric MRI and causative genes, but recently, fetal neurosonography has increasingly revealed MCD, making it possible to indirectly predict MCD before the manifestation of cortical gyri and sulci.

R. K. Pooh (✉)
Fetal Brain Center, CRIFM Prenatal Medical Clinic, Osaka, Japan
e-mail: ritsuko.pooh.brain@fetal-medicine-pooh.jp

P. Volpe, T. Ghi (eds.), *Fetal Neurosonography*, Ultrasound in Obstetrics and Gynecology,
https://doi.org/10.1007/978-3-031-70192-4_8

2 Cortical Neurogenesis

The developing brain is segmented into six zones: ventricular zone (VZ), subventricular zone (SVZ), intermediate zone (IZ), subplate (SP), cortical plate (CP), and marginal zone (MZ), progressing from bottom to top. Further, SVZ is divided into inner SVZ (iSVZ) and outer SVZ (oSVZ). Pugash et al. first showed cerebral lamination by neurosonography in 2012 [1], and now it is not difficult to detect lamination with advanced technology as shown in Fig. 1: VZ + iSVZ, oSVZ+IZ, SP, and CP. In the cerebral cortex, neurons are organized in a structured manner, with the neocortex forming a six-layered structure. Cell migration is an important process during embryogenesis that allows different types of cells originating in different brain regions to settle in the cerebral cortex. Initially, migrating cells contribute to the transient preplate (PP). Subsequent migrations then divide the PP into the superficial MZ, destined to become layer I, and the SP, creating a central layer known as the CP. As development proceeds, the CP forms in an inside-out pattern, with successive waves of migrating neurons settling into deeper layers, eventually forming layers II-VI. Over time, the SP regresses postnatally, primarily serving as a scaffold for developing cortical axons. New neurons arise from radial glia, producing post-mitotic daughter neurons. Approximately 70–80% of the neurons in the cerebral cortex are excitatory neurons, which originate during embryonic development in the VZ or the adjacent SVZ. These neurons migrate radially to the surface of the brain. In contrast, inhibitory neurons, also known as cortical interneurons, in the cerebral cortex are not produced in the mantle but rather in the ventral basal ganglionic eminence (GE). Interneurons migrate tangentially into the cortex from GE as shown in Fig. 2.

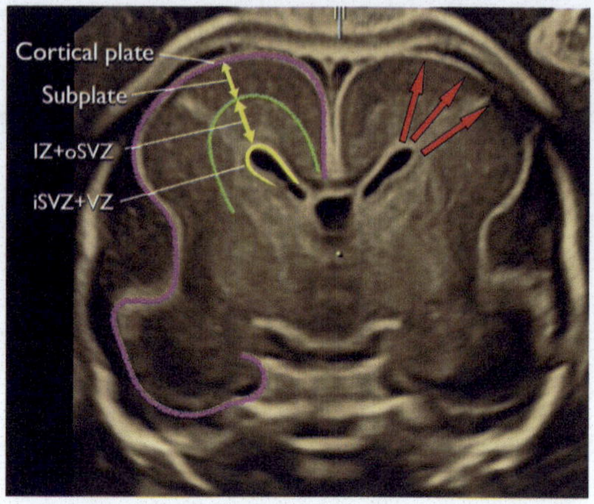

Fig. 1 Lamination of the brain and migration route of excitatory neurons. Transvaginal neurosonography shows brain lamination. Ventricular zone (VZ) + into inner SVZ (iSVZ), outer SVZ (oSVZ) + intermediate zone (IZ), subplate (SP), and cortical plate (CP). Excitatory neurons are born in VZ and SVZ and migrate radially (red arrows) toward CP. The borderline between SP and IZ is visualized in the second trimester

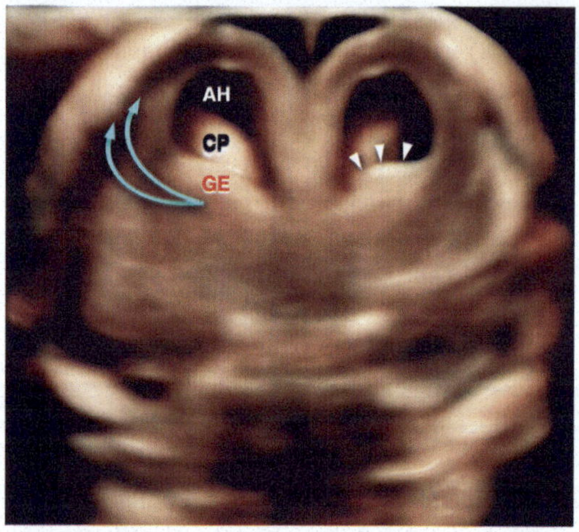

Fig. 2 Ganglionic eminence and migration route of interneurons. Transvaginal 3D thick slice image shows ganglionic eminence (GE) visualized as hyperechoic region. Cortical interneurons (inhibitory neurons) are born in the GE and migrate tangentially (blue arrows). *CP* choroid plexus, *AH* anterior horn of the lateral ventricle

The evolution of the primate cerebral cortex has been marked by expansion and complexification, evident in increased cortical areas, network density, and cortical column diversity [2–4]. A significant contributor to this expansion, particularly in humans, is the oSVZ, an anatomical innovation in cortical development [5]. Differences in cortical connectivity between primates and rodents underscore the importance of understanding the developmental origin of cortical structures [3, 6, 7]. Recently, it was reported that modern human transketolase-like 1 (TKTL1), which differs from Neanderthal TKTL1 by a lysine-to-arginine amino acid substitution, implies greater neurogenesis in frontal neocortex of modern humans [8]. Evolutionary adaptations in the cell cycle regulation, including primate-specific microRNA expression targeting cell cycle genes, likely contribute to cortical expansion and complexity [9, 10]. The complexity of gene networks associated with neurogenesis suggests that the origin and expansion of the oSVZ result from multiple genetic changes rather than from a single master gene [11]. Understanding how these diverse genetic changes collectively shape cortical anatomy remains a challenging question in cortical neurogenesis [12].

3 Definition and Classification of MCD

Malformations of cortical development (MCDs) encompass rare disorders associated with developmental delay, cerebral palsy, and seizures, with diverse causes including genetic, infectious, vascular, and metabolic factors. The classification of MCD has evolved over time, with Barkovich et al. proposing a model in 1996 [13] and subsequent updates in 2001 [14] and 2005 [15]. In 2012, Barkovich et al. introduced the concept that disruptions in three major stages of cortical development contribute to MCD: cell proliferation and apoptosis, cell migration, and postmigration development [16]. This concept emphasizes the role of temporal patterning in achieving cortical diversity, with different neuronal populations migrating to distinct layers [17]. Microcephaly and macrocephaly can result from disruptions in proliferation and apoptosis, leading to dysmorphic neurons and focal cortical dysplasia [18]. Migration defects, regulated by genes and molecular processes, can cause conditions like periventricular nodal ectopia [19]. Mutations in genes controlling migration contribute to MCD spectrum disorders, including microcephaly and heterotopia [20]. Disruptions in postmigration development, such as axon and dendrite formation, are associated with secondary microcephaly and specific types of focal cortical dysplasia [16, 21]. Cortical development extends beyond birth, leading to developmental disorders affecting gray and white matter [22]. Classifications of MCD are dynamic models that evolve with advancements in understanding pathological mechanisms [12]. Identifying genes and pathways involved in cortical development has complicated classification schemes, as mutations in the same gene can result in different MCD types, and mutations in different genes within the same pathway may produce similar cortical malformations [12, 23]. Recent research has highlighted significant implications regarding genetic MCDs, revealing that many MCDs of genetic origin cut across multiple classification categories based on morphology and primary mechanisms such as proliferation, differentiation, and migration. For instance, polymicrogyria, a type of MCD, spans several categories due to the involvement of genes like tubulins in diverse processes ranging from cell division to axon growth. This indicates the complex interplay of genetic factors in cortical development and underscores the need for a comprehension of the genetic basis underlying the interconnectivity of signaling pathways and the multifaceted nature of genetic influences on MCD [12, 24, 25]. Table 1 shows the relations between main MCD and causative genes.

Table 1 Main MCD and causative genes

MCD	Causative genes
Microcephaly, microencephaly	*MFSD2A, STIL, SASS6, ASPM, KIF14, NCAPH, BUB1, PDCD6IP, COPB2, CEP135, WDFY3, CENPE, LMNB1,CDK6, MAP11, MCPH1, CDK5RAP2, NCAPD3, NCAPD2, PHC1, NUP37, CIT, ANKLE2, CENPJ, KNL1(CASC5), CEP152, LMNB2, WDR62, ZNF335, RRP7A*
Macrocephaly and brain overgrowth	*CHD8, EXT2, HERC1, MITF, NFIB, PAK1, PTEN, RIN2, RNF135, SPOP, TBC1D7, TRIO, ZBTB7A, AKT1,GCDH, GFAP, HEXB, NDUFS4, PIK3CA, Other genes in PI3K/AKT/mTOR pathway*
Lissencephaly	*MACF1, CEP85L, RELN, LAMB1, CDK5, TUBA1A, TMTC3, NDE1, KATNB1, MDLS, PAFAH1B1, ARX, DCX,ADGRG1 (GPR56)*
Microlissencephaly	*CIT, KATNB1, KIF14, NDE1, RELN, RNU4ATAC, PAFAH1B1, TUBA4A (TUBA1), TUBB2B, TUBB3, TUBG1*
Polymicrogyria	*AKT3, CCND2, PIK3R2, RTTN, PIK3CA, OCLN , ADGRG1, TUBB2B, PI4KA, COL3A1, ATP1A2, WDR62,FKTN, KIFBP, FIG4, TUBA1A, SNAP29, NEDD4L, ATP1A3, HSD17B4, POMT2, LAMC3, GRIN1, MAN2C1,COL18A1, GPSM2, CCDC88A, ATN1, TMX2, MN1, DEPDC5, DYNC1H1, COL4A1, COL4A2, TUBB3, ARX*
Focal cortical dysplasia	*AKT3, CNTNAP2, COL4A1, COPB2, DEPDC5, DYNC1H1, MTOR, NPRL2, NPRL3, NUP133, PIK3CA, POMT1,SCO2, TSC1, TSC2, FGFR3, Other genes in PI3K/AKT/mTOR pathway*
Dysgyria	*ACTA2, LAMB1, MED11, PAFAH1B1, TUBA1A, TUBB2B, TUBB3*
Heterotopia	*ARF1, PVNH3, MAP1B, PVNH5, ERMARD, NEDD4L, ARFGEF2, FLNA, DCX, PAFAH1B1, EML1, ACTB,MEF2C, FAT4, WDR62, APC2, GPSM2, CEP85L, TUBA1A, DCHS1, MMRCS1, LAMB1, MPDZ, MYMK*
Schizencephaly	*COL4A1, COL4A2, EMX2, EPG5, KIF26A, SHH, SIX3, TUBB2B, WDR62, WNT1*

This list is based on the genes known to be causative of MCD as of May 2024 from OMIM, Human Phenotype Ontology (HPO), and other genome databases

4 Indirect Neurosonographic Signs of MCD

4.1 Sylvian Fissure

In the fetal brain, the upper part of the Sylvian fissures gets deeper from the second to the third trimester as shown in Fig. 3. There has been much sonographic research on Sylvian fissures' development. Toi et al. found that in 50 normal fetuses, the Sylvian fissure starts as a smooth dent early in pregnancy and develops sharp edges around the circular sulcus after 17 weeks. Initially wide, the insula/operculum angle sharpens, noticeably by 24.5 weeks [26]. Mittal et al. used the distance from the Sylvian fissure to the parietal bone, measured by 3D ultrasound, as a reliable indicator of the fissure's development from 12 to 41 weeks of gestation, noting that the fissure widens linearly with pregnancy [27]. Quarello et al. proposed a score for Sylvian fissure operculization (SFO) based on the temporal lobe's coverage over the insula, evaluated through ultrasound at 22 to 32 weeks [28]. Similar findings came from a study using ultrasound to score fetal cortical development, including the Sylvian fissure from 20 to 40 weeks [28], linking the SFO score positively with gestational age. However, those methods work only on the distal hemisphere on the transabdominal axial plane due to shadow cast from the skull on the proximal one. Pooh noted in 2008 that delayed sulcation of the Sylvian fissure in cases of migration disorders could be detected in the anterior coronal plane using transvaginal 3D ultrasound [29]. Later on, Poon et al. introduced the Sylvian fissure angle in 2019, measured bilaterally on the coronal section and based on specific landmarks as a method for quantitative assessment of the Sylvian fissure [30]. Pooh et al. also found that most MCD cases exhibit delayed Sylvian fissure angles on both sides [31]. Figure 4 shows abnormal Sylvian fis-

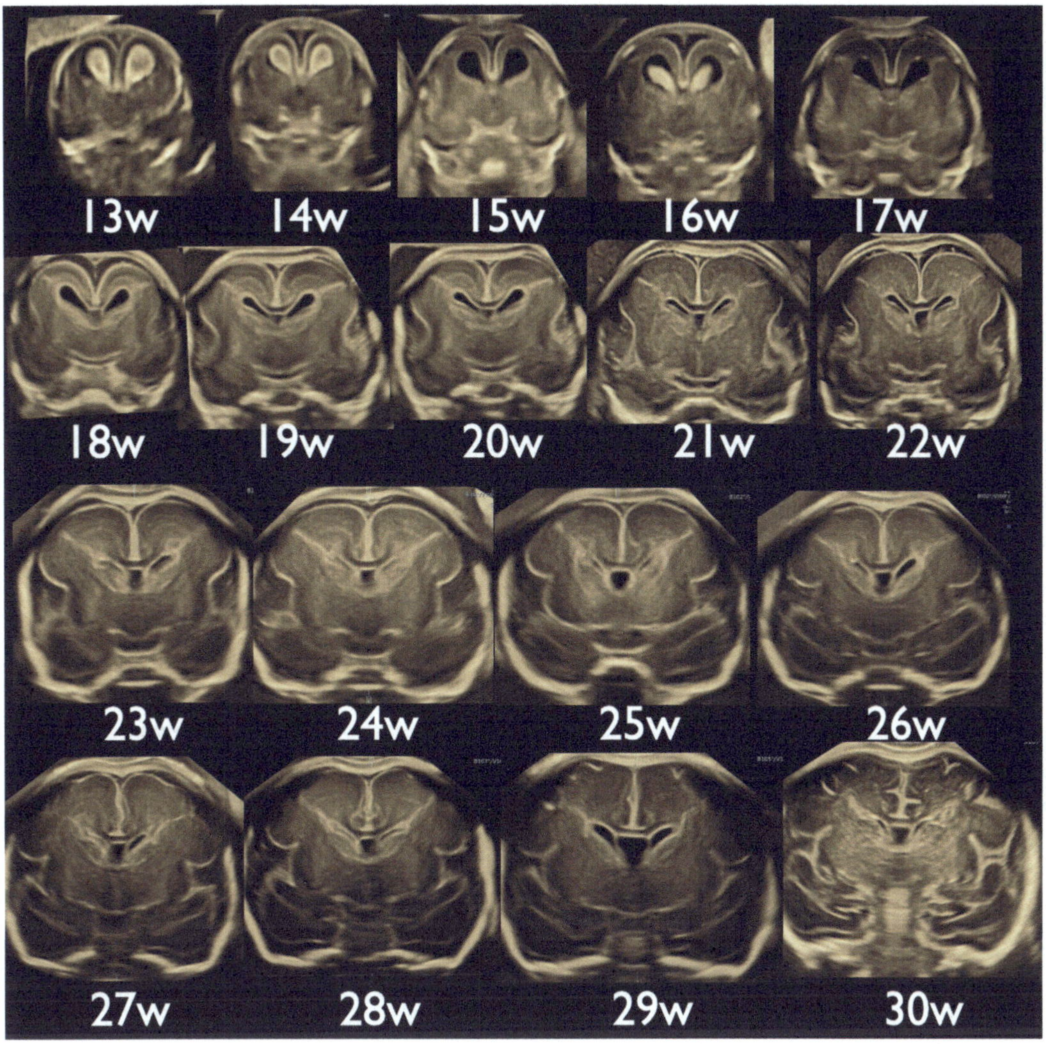

Fig. 3 Normal brain images in the anterior coronal plane between 13 and 30 weeks of gestation. Dramatically changing appearance of fetal brain between 13 and 30 weeks. Note that the upper part of the Sylvian fissures rotates inward from the second to the third trimester, and gyrification is gradually visualized by neurosonography at around 28–30 weeks

sures in cases of MCD compared to normal at the same gestation. Monitoring the Sylvian fissures during the second trimester is crucial for identifying fetuses at risk of developing MCD later.

4.2 Ganglionic Eminence

As mentioned above, cortical interneurons, which are both inhibitory and connecting neurons, are born in Ganglionic Eminence (GE) and from there tangentially migrate toward the cortical mantle. Del Bigio found histopathologically in 2011 that the GE reduced progressively in the fetal period [32], and Stuempflen et al. did MRI volumetry in 2023 and found objectively that GE reduced its volume with advancing gestational age [33]. It is easy to imagine that impaired interneuron migration can cause MCD with a variety of neurological disorders. Some reports of abnormalities in the GE, such as GE cavitation during pregnancy, detected by MRI or sonography have

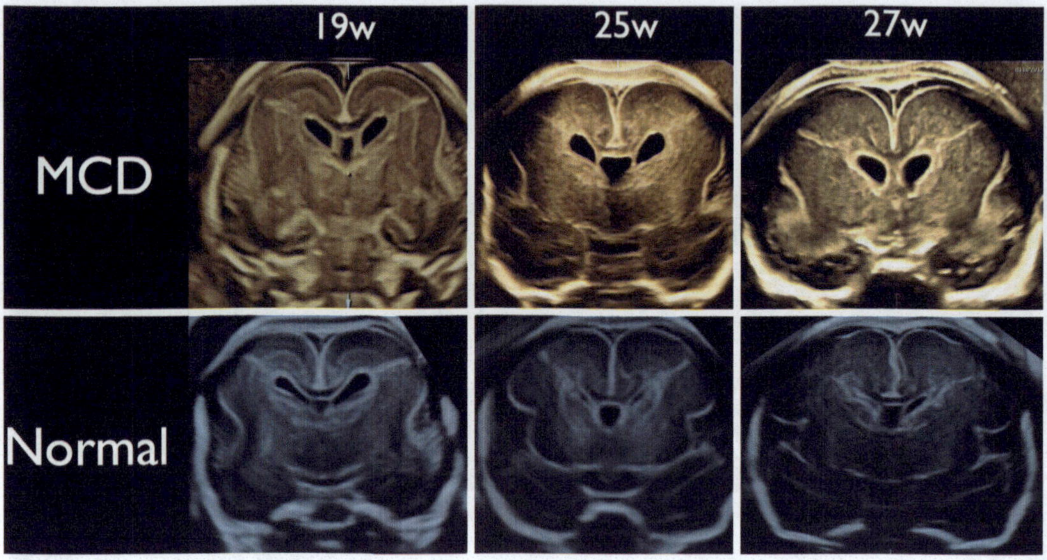

Fig. 4 Abnormal Sylvian fissures in MCD cases compared to normal cases. Abnormal Sylvian fissures in three cases of MCD at 19, 25, and 27 weeks of gestation, compared to normal at the same gestation. All cases are different monogenic disorders

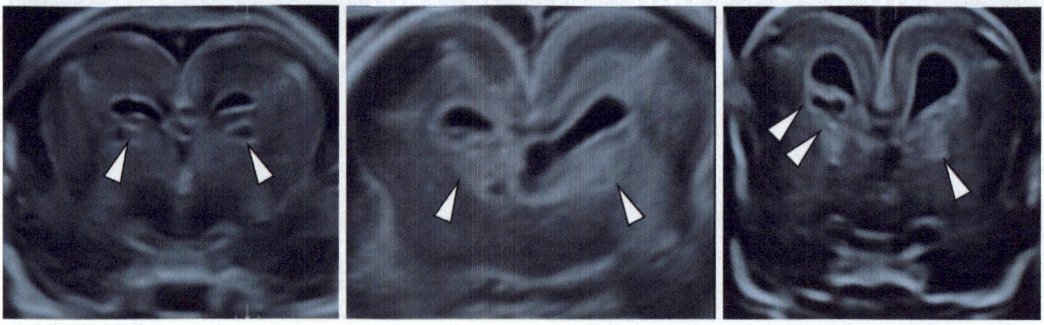

Fig. 5 Persistent GE with intra-GE cavitation. GE reduces its size and volume. However, in those three cases show abnormal GE in the anterior coronal section of transvaginal 3D neurosonography. From left, *TUBA1A* variant case at 19 weeks, Jacobsen syndrome (microdeletion of 11q) at 18 weeks, and *SCN3A* variant at 19 weeks

been reported in cases of developmental delay of the brain [34–37]. Figure 5 shows a persistent GE with internal cysts by transvaginal 3D neurosonography in cases with MCD caused by chromosomal microdeletion or monogenic disorders.

4.3 Microcephaly, Microencephaly

Microcephaly is characterized by a small head with a head circumference (HC) significantly below −2 standard deviations (SD) compared to age- and gender-matched controls [38, 39]. Mild microcephaly is defined by a HC below −2 and severe below −3 SD [38]. While microcephaly indicates a small head circumference, microencephaly suggests a reduced brain volume. In practice, both terms are often used interchangeably, as brain growth arrest typically results in a small head circumference [40].

Microcephaly is categorized into primary and secondary forms based on the time of occurrence [39, 41, 42]. Primary microcephaly, previously

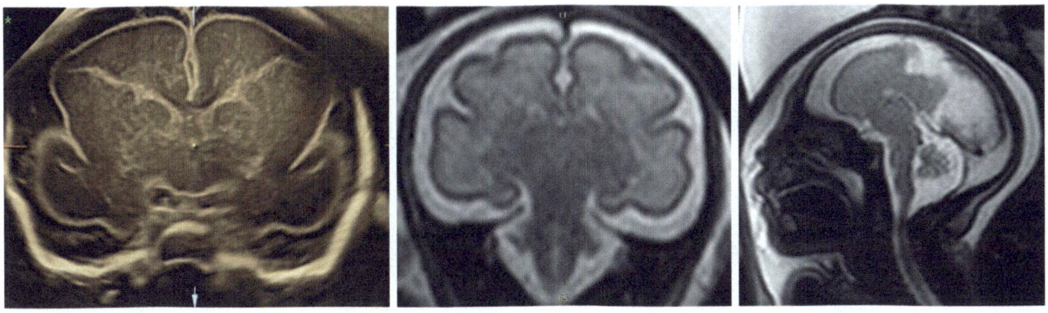

Fig. 6 Microcephaly (MCPH5) at 30 weeks of gestation. At 30 weeks, BPD was −3.1sd, and HC was −3.7sd. Genetic test resulted in *ASPM* variant, responsible for MCPH5. Left image; transvaginal neurosonography shows less gyri/sulci with abnormal Sylvian fissure. Middle and right images; MR images at 31 weeks in the posterior coronal section(middle) and mid-sagittal (right) cutting section

known as "microcephalia vera," is congenital and is usually associated with a simplified gyral pattern, presenting at birth or even before birth. It is believed to result from abnormalities in neurogenesis, but the underlying genetic defect is identified in only 59% of cases [43]. To date, 18 primary microcephaly (MCPH) loci (MCPH1–MCPH18) from diverse global populations have been identified, encompassing genes such as Microcephalin, *WDR62, CDK5RAP2, CASC5, ASPM* [44], *CENPJ, STIL, CEP135, CEP152, ZNF335, PHC1, CDK6, CENPE, SASS6, MFSD2A, ANKLE2, CIT*, and *WDFY3*. This has enhanced our knowledge of the genetic underpinnings of microcephaly [45]. Figure 6 shows the MCPH5 case due to the *ASPM* variant. Primary microcephalic heads also tend to grow more slowly than average. Secondary microcephaly develops postnatally, often with a HC in the lower normal range at birth, and is typically a consequence of disruptions occurring after neurogenesis [41].

Both primary and secondary microcephalies can further be classified as acquired/environmental or genetic (syndromic and non-syndromic) forms [38]. Microcephaly can also be associated with various cortical anomalies, including simplified gyral patterns, lissencephaly, gray matter heterotopia, and polymicrogyria [46, 47]. The case shown in Fig. 7 has extremely severe microcephaly, and its intracranial anatomy shows the most severe developmental defect that does not fit into any of the above classifications.

The degree of gyral pattern simplification correlates with the severity of microcephaly, and cases of microcephaly with lissencephaly may involve a simplified gyral pattern with a thickened cortex. However, microcephaly with lissencephaly encompasses a heterogeneous group of disorders with diverse underlying mechanisms. Additionally, microcephaly may be associated with other brain malformations, white matter signal alterations, calcifications, and basal ganglia or callosal anomalies, which can aid in determining specific etiological diagnoses [40, 48].

4.4 Macrocephaly and Brain Overgrowth

Macrocephaly, or macrocrania, denotes a generalized head enlargement, with a HC exceeding the mean for age and gender by at least two standard deviations (SD), corresponding to the 97th percentile. Mild macrocephaly falls within a HC range of 3 SD above the mean, corresponding to the 99.7th percentile [49, 50]. On the other hand, megalencephaly refers to the enlargement of the brain itself, distinct from macrocephaly. Unlike microcephaly and microencephaly, macrocephaly can result from various causes other than megalencephaly, including hydrocephalus, enlargement of extra-axial spaces, and skeletal dysplasia [51–53].

Megalencephaly does not necessarily simply macrocrania, as brain overgrowth can be unilat-

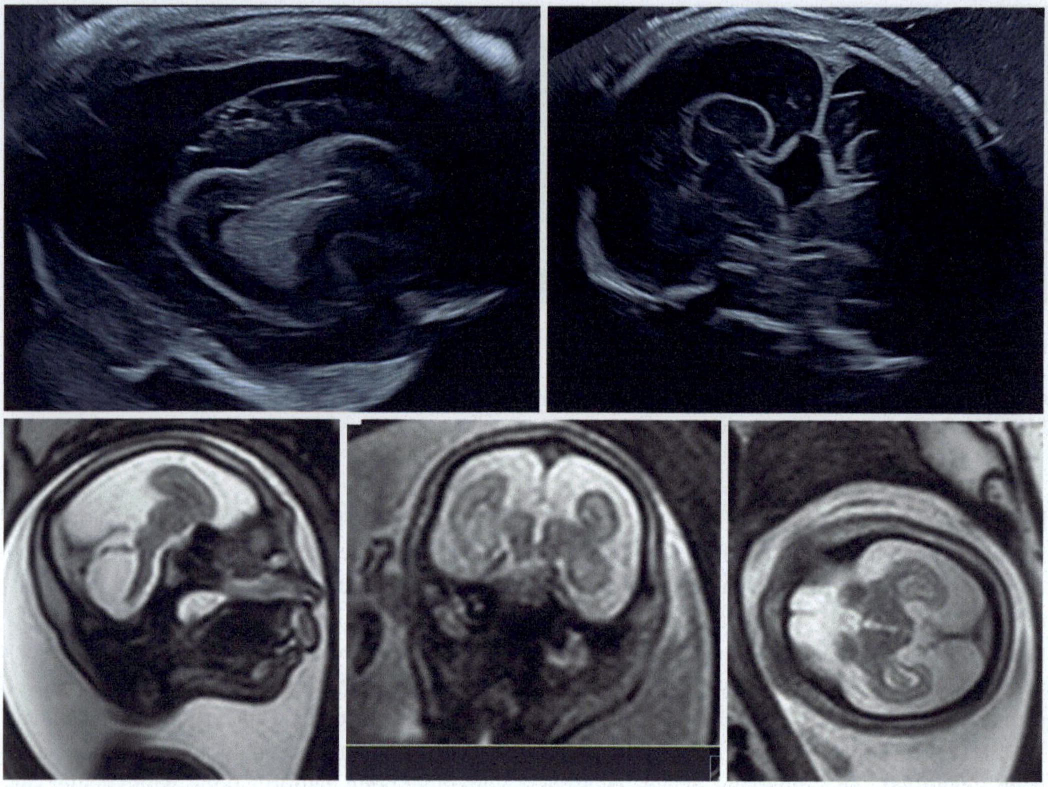

Fig. 7 Severe microcephaly with extremely maldeveloped brain at 29 weeks of gestation. This case shows extreme microcephaly with BPD -6.2sd and HC -6.8sd. Genetic tests revealed no genetic variants responsible for microcephaly. Transvaginal sonography in the parasagittal (upper left) and coronal (upper right) images shows microencephaly with large subarachnoid cysts. The lower figures are fetal MR images in the mid-sagittal, coronal, and axial planes, respectively, from the left. Note the flat face due to microcephaly

eral or focal, not significantly affecting head circumference [54]. It can be due to disruptions in signaling pathways regulating brain cellular processes, leading to developmental megalencephaly, or caused by inborn errors of metabolism and leukodystrophies, resulting in metabolic megalencephaly [51]. Megalencephaly is nowadays recognized as a spectrum of brain overgrowth disorders, which may involve bilateral or unilateral growth, and cause complete or partial hemispheric involvement, or focal megalencephaly affecting up to three cerebral lobes [51, 54]. Figure 8 shows an example of megalencephaly with asymmetrical MCD caused by a *PTEN* variant associated with mosaic uniparental disomy of chromosome 10q, which the author reported in 2021 [55].

Complete unilateral megalencephaly involving one hemisphere is termed hemimegalencephaly (HMEG). In contrast, focal megalencephaly involving up to three cerebral lobes may be referred to as quadrantic dysplasia, lobar HMEG, or hemi-HMEG. HMEG often exhibits thickened or deviated septum pellucidum, fornices, and mid-sagittal band-like structures connecting the frontal lobe with the limbic system, visible in diffusion tensor imaging studies [56]. Megalencephaly and HMEG may be associated with normal-appearing cortex, cortical malformations, and/or white matter signal abnormalities [25]. Some dysplastic HMEG cases have been found to show large areas of focal cortical dysplasia (FCD) type II, depending on the causative mutation's timing and extent [57].

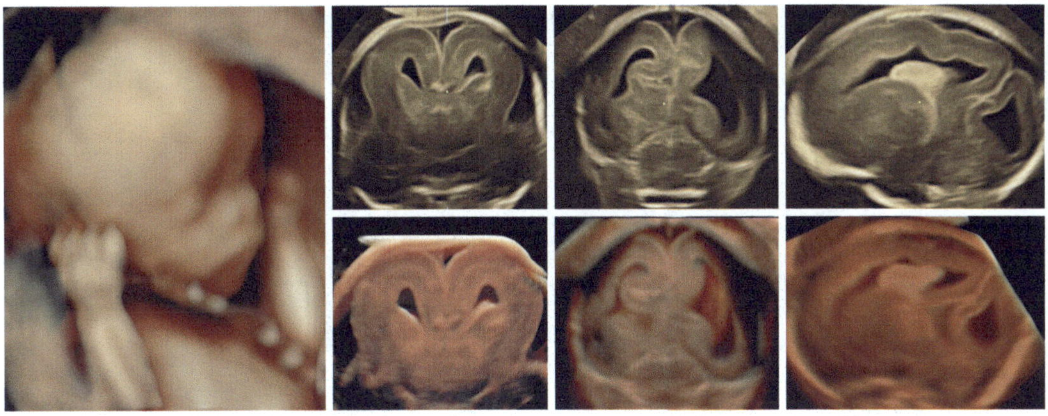

Fig. 8 Megalencephaly with abnormal cortical development at 18 weeks of gestation. At 18 weeks, macrocephaly was obvious with BPD +6.1 SD, and HC +6.2 SD. The causal factor was found in a case of paternal uniparental disomy (UPD) mosaicism of 10q with PTEN (on a chromosome 10q) variation. Left image shows fetal profile by 3D surface rendering. Note the typical macrocephaly face with frontal bossing and low nasal bridge. Neurosonography images (upper row) are in the anterior coronal, posterior coronal, and parasagittal sections, respectively, from the left. Note asymmetrical ventricles with abnormal shapes and abnormal sulci, especially in the middle image; the parasagittal image shows obviously irregular ventricular wall and irregular brain surface. The lower row figures are thick slices of 3D Silhouette images of the three images in the upper row

Posterior cranial fossa structures, such as the cerebellum, can also be involved in megalencephaly, leading to cerebellar overgrowth and potential cerebellar cortical dysplasia, with rapid progression during early life and acquired cerebellar tonsillar ectopia [58]. This condition has been termed "total HMEG" but may not be exclusive to HMEG as it can be observed in other megalencephaly forms due to mosaic mutations [57].

Megalencephaly may also present with varying cortical phenotypes on MRI or neurosonography, including polymicrogyria as shown in Fig. 9. It can be isolated or part of syndromic conditions like megalencephaly-capillary malformation (MCAP) syndrome [58], megalencephaly polymicrogyria-polydactyly hydrocephalus (MPPH) syndrome [58, 59], epidermal nevus syndrome, congenital lipomatous asymmetric overgrowth of the trunk with vascular malformations, epidermal nevi, scoliosis/skeletal/spinal anomalies (CLOVES) syndrome, and mechanistic target of rapamycin (mTOR) related diseases, mTORopathies [60]. The PI3K/AKT/mTOR signaling pathway is critical in mediating signal transduction and influencing biological activities, including cell proliferation, apoptosis, metabolism, and angiogenesis. The components of this pathway are more intricated than those found in other signaling cascades. Understanding the regulatory mechanisms and functions of the PI3K/AKT/mTOR pathway is crucial due to its association with various pathologies, encompassing ischemic brain injury, neurodegenerative disorders, and neoplasms [61–64]. Consequently, abnormal activation of this pathway is linked to developmental abnormalities and the initiation of epilepsy [65]. The syndromes described above are characterized by body overgrowth and cutaneous hallmarks, such as cutaneous nevi, often resulting from post-zygotic somatic mosaicism involving neural crest cells [53, 58].

4.5 Lissencephaly

Lissencephaly, meaning a smooth brain, typically results from impaired neuronal migration [66]. It is characterized by a thickened cortex and abnormal gyral patterns, ranging from agyria (absent gyration) to pachygyria (reduced gyration) [20, 66]. Initially, two distinct types of lissencephaly

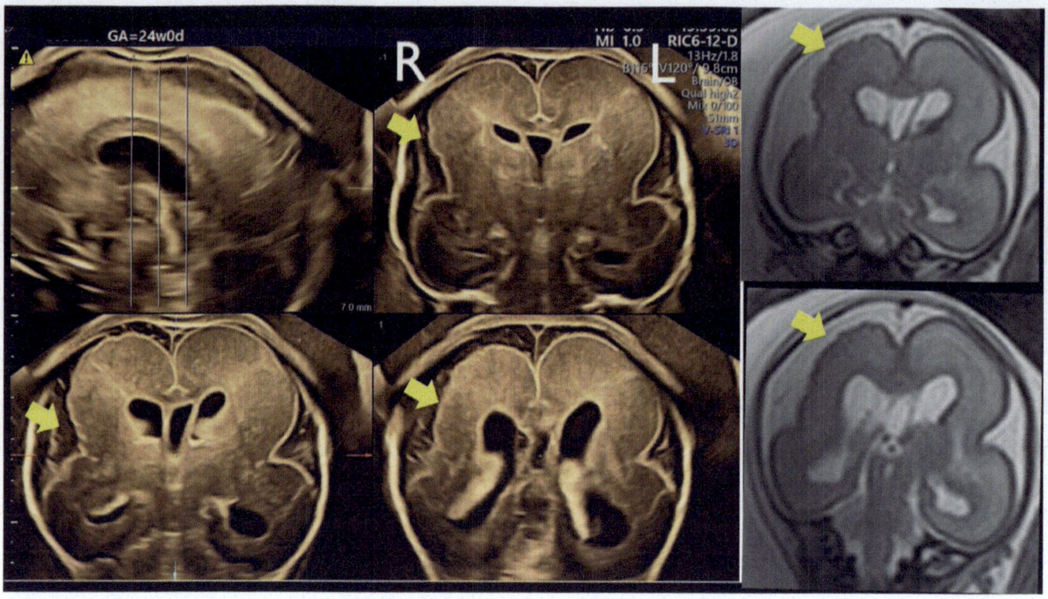

Fig. 9 Hemimegalencephaly with focal polymicrogyria (PMG) at 24 weeks of gestation. Left picture; Tomographic ultrasound images showing consecutive anterior coronal sections of the brain. Note the abnormal Sylvian fissures with focal polymicrogyria (yellow arrows) in the right brain surface. The right two pictures are MR images at the same gestational age. MRI demonstrates polymicrogyria more precisely

were proposed: type 1, the classic agyria syndrome, and type 2, with polymicrogyria and a more severely disorganized cortex. Agyria indicates a complete lack of cortical convolutions, while pachygyria refers to a simplified convolutional pattern with broadened and shallow gyri [20, 66]. Malformations related to improper neuronal cell migration frequently coincide with unusual cell number, duplication, and growth. For instance, in classic lissencephaly type I, there is typically a decrease in brain mass. Thus, malformations from both growth and migration issues are addressed together. Causes of cobblestone malformations and classic type II differ from those of type I. Cobblestone malformations stem from defects in the pial-limiting membrane, leading to an overmigration of neurons beyond the arachnoid membranes and into the subarachnoid space. The spectrum of cobblestone malformations further encompasses localized leptomeningeal glioneuronal heterotopia and more widespread conditions often referred to as polymicrogyria, like the bilateral opercular cobblestone cortex resulting from *GPR56* variants [67, 68]. Figure 10 shows cobblestone malformation detected by neurosonography and MRI at 36 weeks of gestation.

The differentiation between lissencephaly types I and II has been discarded due to advancements in understanding their distinct pathophysiological mechanisms [13]. Current classification emphasizes severity, gradient of gyral malformation, cortical thickness, and associated brain anomalies [69]. Imaging features include a thick cortex with reduced gyration, with agyria presenting the most severe phenotype [66]. Additionally, lissencephaly can be classified as "thin," "variable," or may coexist with subcortical band heterotopia [20]. Associated anomalies may include reduced white matter volume, cerebellar malformations, and abnormalities in basal ganglia and brainstem [20, 40].

4.6 Microlissencephaly

Microlissencephaly is a heterogeneous group of rare diseases [20], characterized by lissencephaly in combination with severe congenital microcephaly [70, 71]. Miller–Dieker syndrome is a

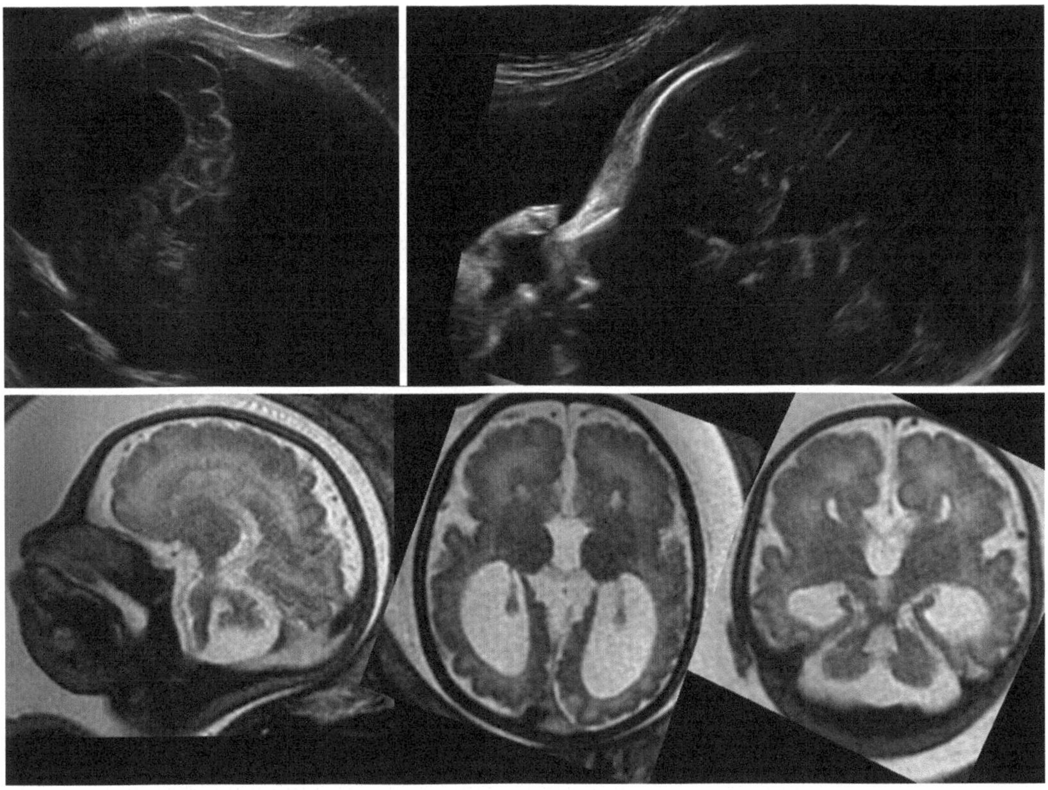

Fig. 10 Cobblestone lissencephaly with agenesis of the corpus callosum and cerebellar hypoplasia at 36 weeks of gestation. (upper) Sonographic pictures of the posterior coronal (left) and mid-sagittal (middle) sections. Abnormal gyral formation is depicted. (lower) Fetal MR images at the same gestation. Cobblestone lissencephaly with hypoplastic cerebellum and agenesis of the corpus callosum are clearly demonstrated

consecutive gene deletion syndrome of chromosome 17p13 including *PAFAH1B1* gene (also known as *LIS1*) to *YWHAE* gene, associated with classical lissencephaly and distinct facial features. Dobyns et al. described in 1984 the differences of Miller–Dieker, Norman–Roberts syndromes caused by *RELN* variants and isolated lissencephaly [72]. Figure 11 shows the microlissencephaly case due to the *PAFAH1B1* variant at 28 weeks of gestation.

Several tubulinopathies or tubulin-related cortical dysgenesis cause microlissencephaly [73], many of which are associated with *TUBA1* variants and rarely with *TUBB2B*, *TUBB3*, or *TUBG1*variant [73–75]. Figure 12 shows neurosonography image and postnatal MRI in the microlissencephaly case due to *TUBA1* variant. Variants in *CIT* (encoding citron kinase, important for mitosis) are also associated with microlissencephaly [76]. Juric-Sekhar et al. reported microcephalic osteodysplastic primordial dwarfism (MOPD-1), which exhibits primarily anterior three-layer, ectopic glioneuronal, microcephaly, corpus callosum hypoplasia, and midbrain and hindbrain abnormalities [77]. In 2013, Abdel-Salam et al. reported that *RNU4ATAC* variants are associated with MOPD-1 [78].

4.7 Polymicrogyria

Polymicrogyria is characterized by an excess of small cerebral gyri, with varied anatomical distribution and etiologies [79]. It can be focal, multifocal, or generalized, and may be unilateral or bilateral, asymmetric or symmetric [79, 80]. Both genetic factors (variants in genes such as *AKT3, PIK3CA, DYNC1H1, COL4A1/COL4A2,*

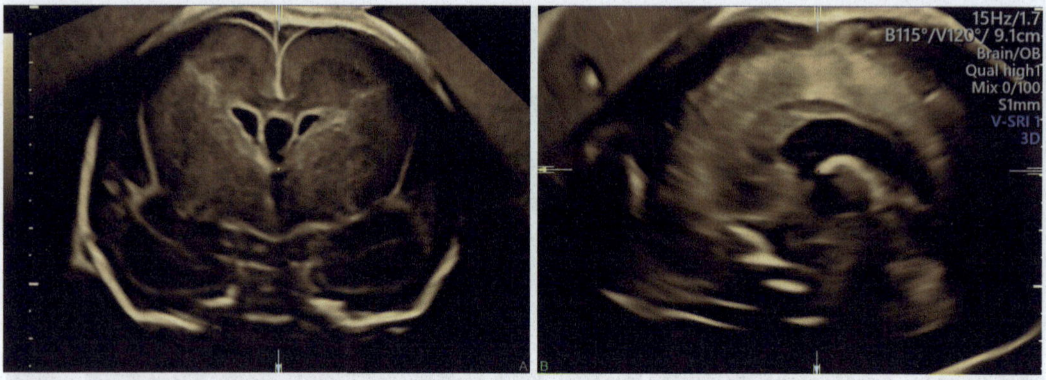

Fig. 11 Microlissencephaly due to *PAFAH1B1(LIS1)* variant. At 28 weeks. Abnormal Sylvian fissure with agyria is obvious in the coronal image (left). Abnormally thick anterior corpus callosum is visualized in the mid-sagittal image (right)

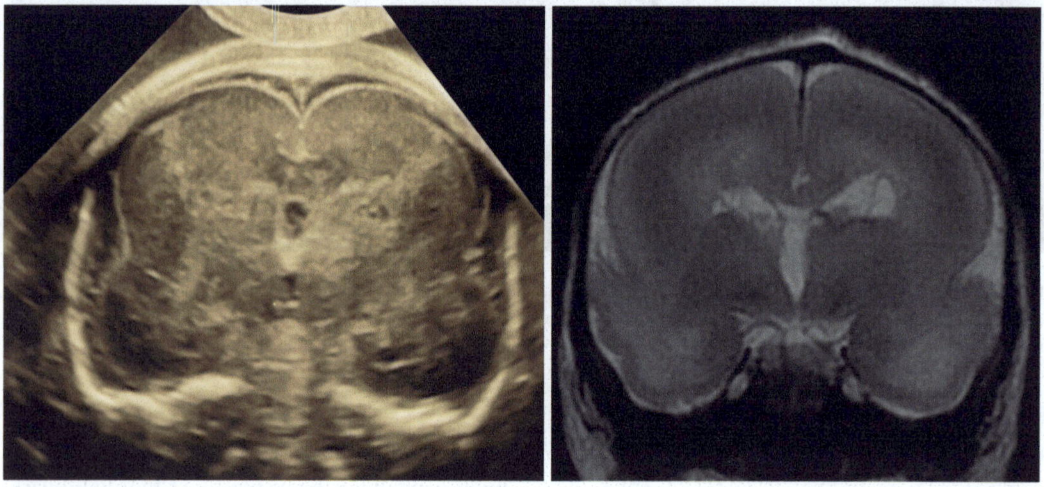

Fig. 12 Microlissencephaly due to *TUBA1A* variant. The left is an anterior coronal image by transvaginal 3D neurosonography at 24 weeks of gestation. Note the extremely primordial Sylvian fissures. The right picture is postnatal MRI showing literally "smooth" brain

TUBA1A, TUBB2B, TUBB3, OCLN, RTTN, WDR62, ARX, and others) [79] and non-genetic causes (infections, trauma, teratogen exposure) contribute to its development [40, 79]. Polymicrogyria often affects the Sylvian fissures as shown in Fig. 9, but can extend into other cerebral lobes, with varied appearances on imaging, including fine delicate gyri, irregularly bumpy surfaces, or paradoxically smooth cortex [80]. The condition's appearance can vary based on MRI technical factors, brain maturity, and myelination stage [81]. It is important to note that occasionally, PMG is diagnosed histologically, although it does not appear to be PMG on neuroimaging or even macroscopic examination, as shown in Fig. 13.

4.8 Focal Cortical Dysplasia

Focal cortical dysplasia (FCD) encompasses a spectrum of brain malformations categorized into three subgroups by the International League Against Epilepsy (ILAE) in 2011 [82, 83]: Type I

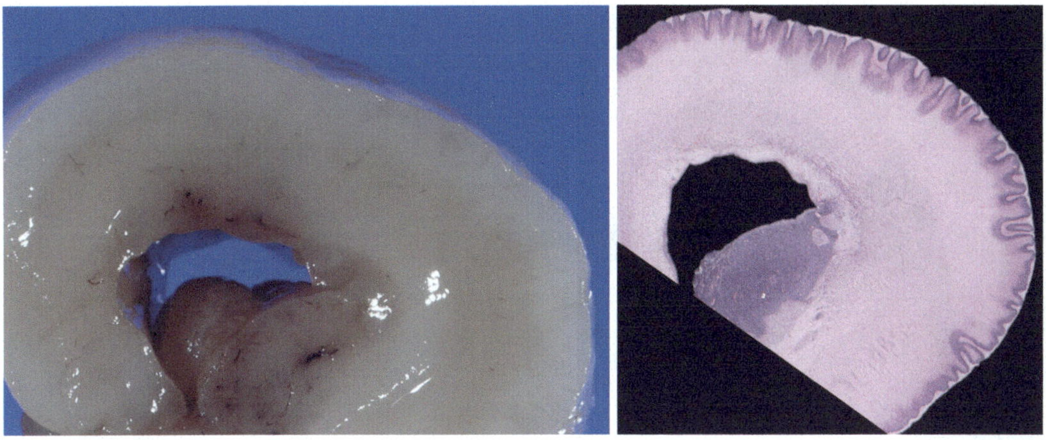

Fig. 13 Histological polymicrogyria (PMG). Occasionally, polymicrogyria is diagnosed histologically (right picture), although it does not appear to be PMG on neuroimaging or even macroscopic examination (left picture)

(a–c), Type II (a, b), and Type III. Type I involves alterations in cortical structure, Type II exhibits marked disruption of cortical lamination with abnormal cell types, and Type III includes additional lesions in the same lobe. A critical update by Najm et al. in 2018 [83] emphasized challenges in classifying FCD, particularly regarding types I and III, advocating for an integrated clinico-pathological and genetic approach. Incidence rates suggest FCD IIa as most common, followed by FCD IIb, Ia, and Ib. Recently, many cortical overgrowth malformations, and some of FCD, especially type II, have been linked to mutations that cause overactivation of the receptor tyrosine kinase (RTK), PI3K-AKT-mTOR signaling pathway [84–86]. Although RTK is a major activator of the PI3K-AKT-mTOR pathway, mutations involving RTK are much less common in brain overgrowth disorders [24]. *FGFR3* is deeply related to the brain size [87]. In severe lethal dwarfism, known as thanatophoric dysplasia, activating mutations in *FGFR3* have been reported to result in brain overgrowth with excessive gyration confined to the occipitotemporal region but without cytoplasmic neurons [88]. Since *FGFR3* activates PI3K-AKT-mTOR signaling [89], this pathway is presumed to contribute to brain overgrowth. Interestingly, occipitotemporal overgrowth reflects a gradient in *FGFR3* expression during development [88]. The brain focal overgrowth in cases of thanatophoric dysplasia has been reported from 2012 [90–92]. It is not clear when the focal brain overgrowth begins in the fetal period, but it is likely to occur very early. Figure 14 shows focal brain hyperplasia in a case of thanatophoric dysplasia at 16 weeks gestation.

Associated imaging features include changes in cortical thickness, abnormal gyral patterns, and the "transmantle sign," highly specific for FCD IIb. Diagnosis may require advanced techniques such as subdural electrodes or hybrid imaging. Additionally, hypointense bands on susceptibility-weighted images and calcifications on CT scans may aid diagnosis. Early detection is crucial, as subtle FCDs may be initially overlooked [83, 93, 94].

4.9 Dysgyria

"Dysgyria is a term recently coined to describe a non-specific cortical malformation characterized by an abnormal gyral pattern [95], not typical for pachygyria or polymicrogyria. Diagnostic imaging reveals that the cortex maintains normal thickness, yet exhibits dysmorphic gyration patterns. This includes deviations in sulcal depth and direction, presenting with a smooth cortical surface and sulci that are oriented radially, or with narrow gyri divided by sulci that are either unusu-

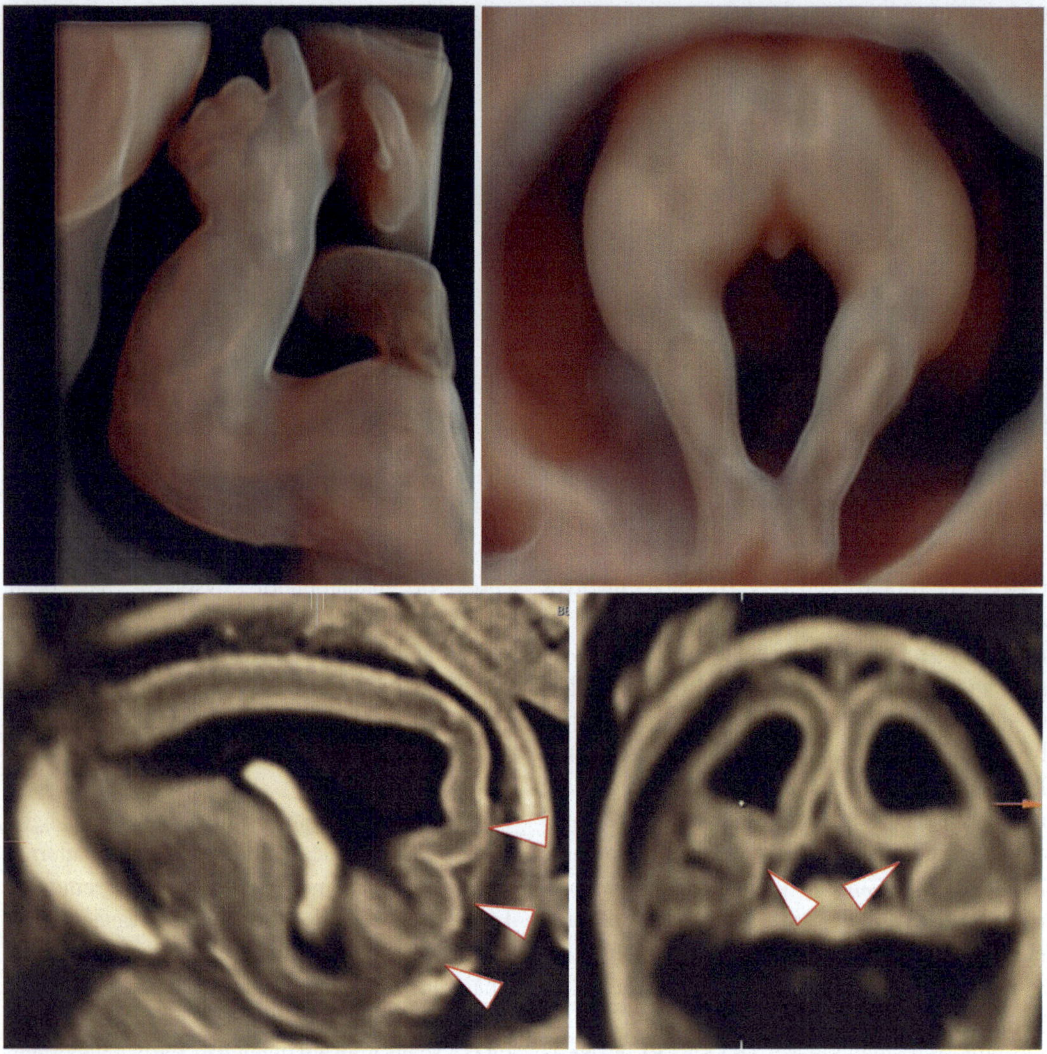

Fig. 14 Focal brain overgrowth in a thanatophoric dysplasia case at 16 weeks. Upper row: 3D surface rendering images of fetal left arm and legs, showing characteristic limb morphology in thanatophoric dysplasia. Lower row: parasagittal (left) and posterior coronal (right) neurosonography images. Arrowheads indicate focal brain overgrowth. A genetic test resulted in an *FGFR3* variant

ally deep or shallow. Such regions display sulci with irregular orientations and produce an imaging profile distinct from those seen in conditions like polymicrogyria, pachygyria, or a simplified gyral pattern. Often seen in cases of tubulinopathies and cobblestone lissencephaly [73, 95–97]. Some of these cases are associated with callosal agenesis [98]. Figure 15 shows the *TUBB3* variant case showing cortical dysgyria and abnormal corpus callosum Sylvian fissures.

4.10 Heterotopia

Heterotopia refers to a large cluster of misplaced neurons which vary greatly in shape and size, from the common periventricular nodular heterotopia (PNH) to a smooth gray matter layer along ventricular walls, to organized columns of neurons spanning the brain's depth, to large, swirling gray matter bands from deep brain folds. There should be genetic and developmental causes

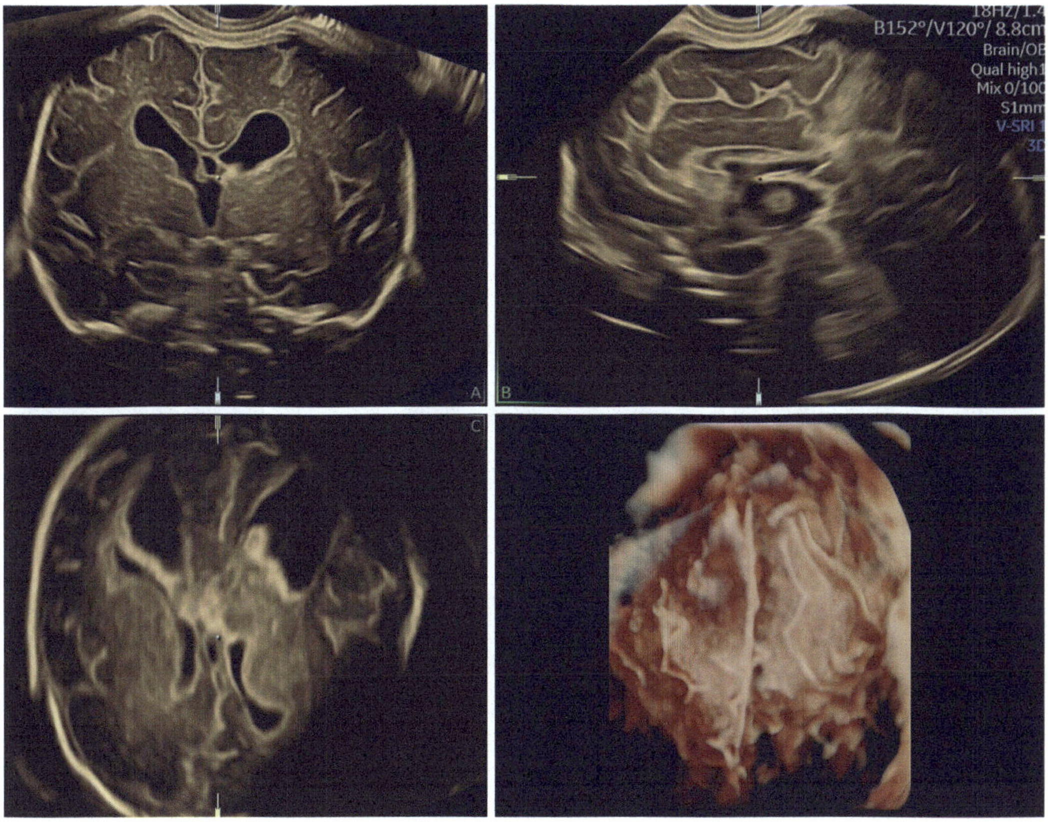

Fig. 15 Cortical dysgyria due to *TUBB3* variant at 33 weeks of gestation. Transvaginal 3D orthogonal views and 3D surface rendering image of brain surface (right lower). In the three orthogonal view showing the coronal plane (upper left), sagittal plane (upper right), and axial plane (lower left), is noted the asymmetrical structure of the brain, cortical dysgyria with deep sulci in the coronal plane, thin/short CC in the coronal and sagittal planes, and abnormal SF in the coronal plane

behind these complex forms. These conditions, where neurons scatter from the inner ventricle to the brain surface, are considered malformations from incorrect neuronal migration [16]. Gray matter heterotopia is categorized into three types according to their clinical presentations and imaging features: subependymal, subcortical, and band heterotopia [99, 100]. However, it is important to note that subcortical heterotopia may exhibit a range of morphological appearances. Figure 16 shows a rare case of cortical dysplasia at 16 weeks with abnormal early gyrification. Detection of heterotopia by neuroimaging is still challenging, but histology findings exhibit various types of heterotopia, as shown in Fig. 16.

PNH, with its unique embryogenesis and often known genetic causes, is classified differently in the MCD subcategory under neuroependymal malformations [16]. In PNH, certain neurons do not migrate toward the developing cerebral cortex but instead form nodules that adhere to the ventricular surface. Figure 17 shows PNH in MCD cases.

4.11 Schizencephaly

Schizencephaly is characterized by a cleft lined by polymicrogyria gray matter and/or heterotopia extending from the ventricular surface to the brain's mantle [101–103]. This malformation likely results from early prenatal focal brain injury, mostly of the germinal matrix, of ischemic or hemorrhagic origin [101, 102]. Schizencephaly

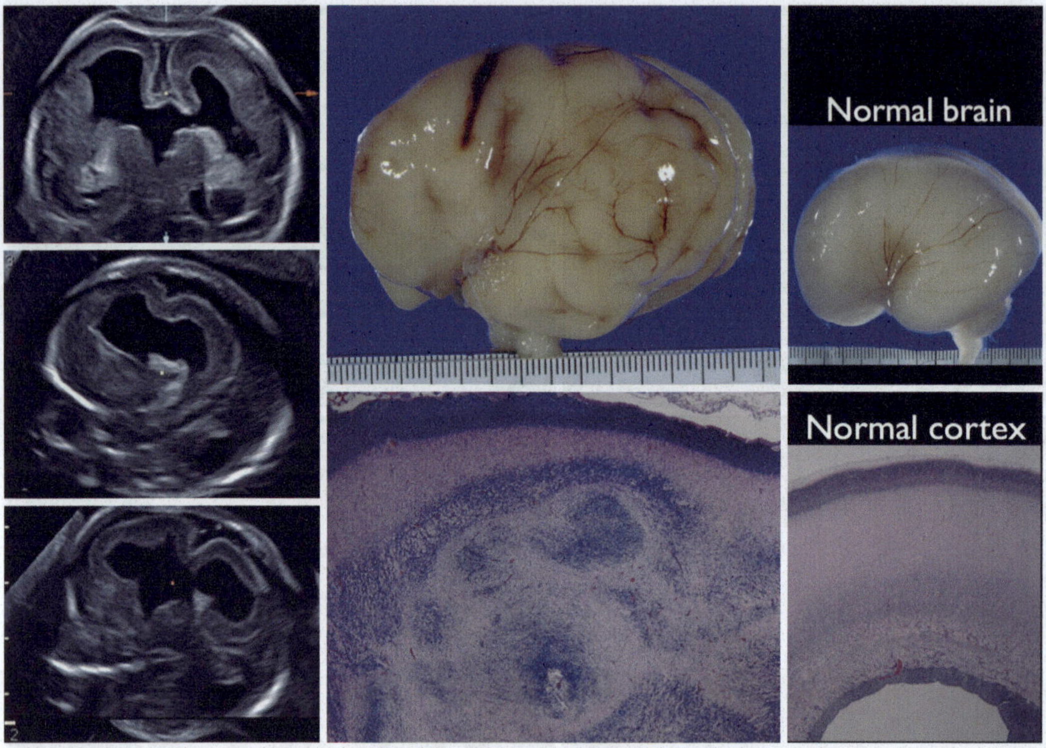

Fig. 16 Heterotopia with cortical maldevelopment at 16 weeks of gestation. The left column shows transvaginal 3D neurosonographic images in the coronal, parasagittal of the left brain, and parasagittal of the right brain from top to bottom. Note the asymmetric brain parenchyma with kinking and asymmetric ventricles with abnormal early gyrification. The middle upper picture is the macroscopic brain after the termination of pregnancy at 20 weeks. Note the abnormal early gyrification on the brain surface. The middle lower picture shows histological findings with various types of heterotopia. The right column shows normal pathology at the same gestation, which is in comparison with abnormal histology in the middle column

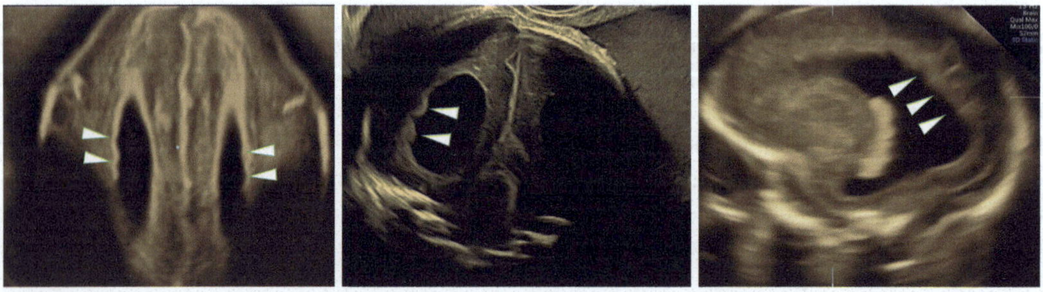

Fig. 17 Periventricular nodular heterotopia (PNH). In some MCD cases, PNH is visible, as shown here (arrowheads). In PNH, certain neurons do not migrate toward the developing cerebral cortex but instead form nodules that adhere to the ventricular surface

may be considered a severe variant of acquired PMG [16, 104] and is associated with young maternal age, poor prenatal care, alcohol abuse, and non-CNS anomalies that are likely secondary to vascular disruption [105, 106], while genetic causes seem to be very rare. However, the *COL4A1* variant was reported as a genetic causal factor [107, 108]. It is divided into open and

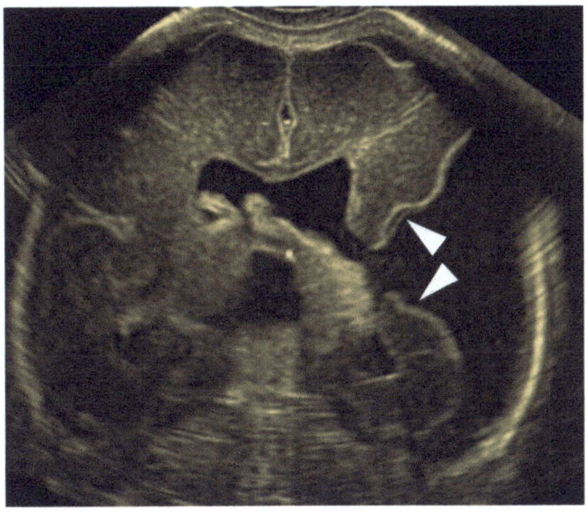

Fig. 18 Unilateral schizencephaly at 27 weeks of gestation. Open lips in schizencephaly are obviously demonstrated (arrowheads). In this case, no other brain abnormalities were found, and the postnatal prognosis has been favorable for 10 years

closed lip forms, depending on whether the cleft is fully patent or sealed by cortical margins, respectively [104]. On imaging, differentiation from clastic lesions like porencephaly is based on the features of the gray matter lining the cleft [40]. Schizencephalic clefts are often multiple and may be associated with contralateral polymicrogyria, as well as abnormalities of the fornices and septum pellucidum, sometimes part of the septo-optic dysplasia spectrum [109]. Figure 18 shows neurosonography image in the case of unilateral schizencephaly at 27 weeks of gestation.

5 Conclusions

Progress in ultrasound technology has facilitated the detection of MCDs during the fetal period. Additionally, advances in molecular genetics are constantly unfolding, with the discovery of novel pathogenic genes causing MCD. However even with the same genetic mutations, the morphologic characteristics of MCD may be profoundly different, indicating that the relationship between phenotype and genotype is influenced by environmental or epigenetic factors.

References

1. Pugash D, Hendson G, Dunham CP, Dewar K, Money DM, Prayer D. Sonographic assessment of normal and abnormal patterns of fetal cerebral lamination. Ultrasound Obstet Gynecol. 2012;40(6):642–51.
2. Kaas JH. The evolution of brains from early mammals to humans Jon. Wiley Interdiscip Rev Cogn Sci. 2013;4(1):33–45.
3. Markov NT, Ercsey-ravasz M, Van Essen DC, Knoblauch K, Toroczkai Z, Kennedy H. Cortical high-density counterstream architectures nikola. Science (80-). 2013;342(6158):1238406.
4. Rakic P. Confusing cortical columns. PNAS. 2008;105(34):12099–100.
5. Lui JH, Hansen DV, Kriegstein AR. Development and evolution of the human neocortex. Cell. 2011;146(1):18–36.
6. Oh SW, Harris JA, Ng L, Winslow B, Cain N, Mihalas S, et al. A mesoscale connectome of the mouse brain. Nature. 2014;508(7495):207–14.
7. Zingg B, Hintiryan H, Gou L, Song MY, Bay M, Bienkowski MS, et al. Neural networks of the mouse neocortex. Cell. 2014;156(5):1096–111. https://doi.org/10.1016/j.cell.2014.02.023.
8. Pinson A, Xing L, Namba T, Kalebic N, Peters J, Oegema CE, et al. Human TKTL1 implies greater neurogenesis in frontal neocortex of modern humans than Neanderthals. Science (80-). 2022;377(6611):eabl6422.
9. Kosik KS. MicroRNAs and cellular phenotypy. Cell. 2010;143(1):21–6. https://doi.org/10.1016/j.cell.2010.09.008.
10. Arcila ML, Betizeau M, Cambronne XA, Guzman E, Doerflinger N, Bouhallier F, et al. Novel primate miRNAs coevolved with ancient target genes in germinal zone-specific expression patterns. Neuron. 2014;81(6):1255–62.
11. Dehay C, Kennedy H, Kosik KS. The outer subventricular zone and primate-specific cortical complexification. Neuron. 2015;85(4):683–94. https://doi.org/10.1016/j.neuron.2014.12.060.
12. Barkovich AJ. Complication begets clarification in classification. Brain. 2013;136(2):368–70.
13. Barkovich AJ, Kuzniecky RI, Dobyns WB, Jackson GD, Becker LE, Evrard P. A classification scheme for malformations of cortical development. Neuropediatrics. 1996;27(2):59–63.
14. Barkovich AJ, Kuzniecky RI, Jackson GD, Guerrini R, Dobyns WB. Classification system for malformations of cortical development: update 2001. Neurology. 2001;57(12):2168–78.
15. Barkovich AJ, Kuzniecky RI, Jackson GD, Guerrini R, Dobyns WB. A developmental and genetic classification for malformations of cortical development. Neurology. 2005;65:1873–87.
16. Barkovich AJ, Guerrini R, Kuzniecky RI, Jackson GD, Dobyns WB. A developmental and genetic

classification for malformations of cortical development: update 2012. Brain. 2012;135:1348–69.

17. Astick M, Vanderhaeghen P. From human pluripotent stem cells to cortical circuits [internet]. In: Current topics in developmental biology, vol. 129. 1st ed. Elsevier Inc.; 2018. p. 67–98. https://doi.org/10.1016/bs.ctdb.2018.02.011.
18. Silva CG, Peyre E, Nguyen L. Cell migration promotes dynamic cellular interactions to control cerebral cortex morphogenesis. Nat Rev Neurosci. 2019;20(6):318–29. https://doi.org/10.1038/s41583-019-0148-y.
19. Lian G, Sheen VL. Cytoskeletal proteins in cortical development and disease: actin associated proteins in periventricular heterotopia. Front Cell Neurosci. 2015;9:1–13.
20. Di Donato N, Chiari S, Mirzaa GM, Aldinger K, Parrini E, Olds C, et al. Lissencephaly: expanded imaging and clinical classification. Am J Med Genet A. 2017;173(6):1473–88.
21. Budday S, Raybaud C, Kuhl E. A mechanical model predicts morphological abnormalities in the developing human brain. Sci Rep. 2014;4:1–7.
22. Budday S, Steinmann P, Kuhl E. Physical biology of human brain development. Front Cell Neurosci. 2015;9:1–17.
23. Manzini MC, Walsh CA. What disorders of cortical development tell us about the cortex: one plus one does not always make two. Curr Opin Genet Dev. 2011;21(3):333–9.
24. Juric-Sekhar G, Hevner RF. Malformations of cerebral cortex development: molecules and mechanisms. Annu Rev Pathol Mech Dis. 2019;14:293–318.
25. Guerrini R, Dobyns WB. Malformations of cortical development: clinical features and genetic causes. Lancet Neurol. 2014;13(7):710–26. https://doi.org/10.1016/S1474-4422(14)70040-7.
26. Toi A, Lister WS, Fong KW. How early are fetal cerebral sulci visible at prenatal ultrasound and what is the normal pattern of early fetal sulcal development? Ultrasound Obstet Gynecol. 2004;24:706–15.
27. Mittal P, Gonçalves LF, Kusanovic JP, Espinoza J, Lee W, Nien JK, et al. Objective evaluation of sylvian fissure development by multiplanar 3-dimensional ultrasonography. J Ultrasound Med. 2007;26(3):347–53.
28. Quarello E, Stirnemann J, Ville Y, Guibaud L. Assessment of fetal Sylvian fissure operculization between 22 and 32 weeks: a subjective approach. Ultrasound Obstet Gynecol. 2008;32(1):44–9.
29. Pooh RK. Fetal neuroimaging of neural migration disorder. Ultrasound Clin. 2008;3(4):541–52.
30. Poon LC, Sahota DS, Chaemsaithong P, Nakamura T, Machida M, Naruse K, et al. Transvaginal three-dimensional ultrasound assessment of Sylvian fissures at 18–30 weeks' gestation. Ultrasound Obstet Gynecol. 2019;54(2):190–8.
31. Pooh RK, Machida M, Nakamura T, Uenishi K, Chiyo H, Itoh K, et al. Increased Sylvian fissure angle as early sonographic sign of malformation of cortical development. Ultrasound Obstet Gynecol. 2019;54(2):199–206.
32. Del Bigio MR. Cell proliferation in human ganglionic eminence and suppression after prematurity-associated haemorrhage. Brain. 2011;134(5):1344–61.
33. Stuempflen M, Taymourtash A, Kienast P, Schmidbauer VU, Schwartz E, Mitter C, et al. Ganglionic eminence: volumetric assessment of transient brain structure utilizing fetal magnetic resonance imaging. Ultrasound Obstet Gynecol. 2023;62(3):405–13.
34. Righini A, Frassoni C, Inverardi F, Parazzini C, Mei D, Doneda C, et al. Bilateral cavitations of ganglionic eminence: a fetal MR imaging sign of halted brain development. Am J Neuroradiol. 2013;34(9):1841–5.
35. Prefumo F, Petrilli G, Palumbo G, Sartori E, Izzi C, Pinelli L. Prenatal ultrasound diagnosis of cavitation of ganglionic eminence. Ultrasound Obstet Gynecol. 2019;54(4):558–60.
36. Goergen SK, Alibrahim E, Christie J, Dobrotwir A, Fahey M, Fender L, et al. The fetus with ganglionic eminence abnormality: head size and extracranial sonographic findings predict genetic diagnoses and postnatal outcomes. Am J Neuroradiol. 2021;42(8):1528–34.
37. Contro E, Volpe N, Larcher L, Dall'Asta A, Penas Da Costa MA, Vairo G, et al. Normal and abnormal appearance of fetal ganglionic eminence on second-trimester three-dimensional ultrasound. Ultrasound Obstet Gynecol. 2023;62(3):398–404.
38. Ashwal S, Michelson D, Plawner L, Dobyns WB. Practice parameter : diagnostic assessment of the child with report of the quality standards Subcommittee of the American Academy of Neurology and the Practice Committee of the Child Neurology Society. Neurology. 2009;73(11):887–97.
39. Woods CG, Parker A. Investigating microcephaly. Arch Dis Child. 2013;98(9):707–13.
40. Raybaud C, Widjaja E. Development and dysgenesis of the cerebral cortex: malformations of cortical development. Neuroimaging Clin N Am. 2011;21(3):483–543. https://doi.org/10.1016/j.nic.2011.05.014.
41. Seltzer LE, Paciorkowski AR. Genetic disorders associated with postnatal microcephaly. Am J Med Genet Part C Semin Med Genet. 2014;166(2):140–55.
42. Jean F, Stuart A, Tarailo-Graovac M. Dissecting the genetic and etiological causes of primary microcephaly. Front Neurol. 2020;11:570830.
43. Von der Hagen M, Pivarcsi M, Liebe J, von Bernuth H, Didonato N, Hennermann JB, et al. Diagnostic approach to microcephaly in childhood: a two-center study and review of the literature. Dev Med Child Neurol. 2014;56(8):732–41.
44. Desir J, Cassart M, David P, Van Bogaert P, Abramowicz M. Primary microcephaly with ASPM mutation shows simplified cortical gyration with

antero-posterior gradient pre- and post-natally. Am J Med Genet A. 2008;146(11):1439–43.
45. Naveed M, Kazmi SK, Amin M, Asif Z, Islam U, Shahid K, et al. Comprehensive review on the molecular genetics of autosomal recessive primary microcephaly (MCPH). Genet Res (Camb). 2018;100:e7.
46. Vermeulen RJ, Wilke M, Horber V, Krägeloh-Mann I. Microcephaly with simplified gyral pattern: MRI classification. Neurology. 2010;74(5):386–91.
47. Adachi Y, Poduri A, Kawaguch A, Yoon G, Salih MA, Yamashita F, et al. Congenital microcephaly with a simplified gyral pattern: associated findings and their significance. Am J Neuroradiol. 2011;32(6):1123–9.
48. Valence S, Garel C, Barth M, Toutain A, Paris C, Amsallem D, et al. RELN and VLDLR mutations underlie two distinguishable clinico-radiological phenotypes. Clin Genet. 2016;90(6):545–9.
49. Pavone P, Praticò AD, Rizzo R, Corsello G, Ruggieri M, Parano E, et al. A clinical review on megalencephaly. Medicine (Baltimore). 2017;96(26):e6814.
50. Severino M, Geraldo AF, Utz N, Tortora D, Pogledic I, Klonowski W, et al. Definitions and classification of malformations of cortical development: practical guidelines. Brain. 2020;143(10):2874–94.
51. Mirzaa GM, Poduri A. Megalencephaly and hemimegalencephaly: breakthroughs in molecular etiology. Am J Med Genet Part C Semin Med Genet. 2014;166(2):156–72.
52. Winden KD, Yuskaitis CJ, Poduri A. Megalencephaly and macrocephaly. Semin Neurol. 2015;35(3):277–87.
53. Keppler-Noreuil KM, Rios JJ, Parker VER, Semple RK, Lindhurst MJ, Sapp JC, et al. PIK3CA-related overgrowth spectrum (PROS): diagnostic and testing eligibility criteria, differential diagnosis, and evaluation. Am J Med Genet A. 2015;167A:287–95.
54. Mirzaa G, Roy A, Dobyns WB, Millen K, Hevner RF. Hemimegalencephaly and dysplastic megalencephaly. Dev Neuropathol. 2018:55–61.
55. Pooh RK, Machida M, Imoto I, Arai EN, Ohashi H, Takeda M, et al. Fetal megalencephaly with cortical dysplasia at 18 gestational weeks related to paternal UPD mosaicism with PTEN mutation. Genes (Basel). 2021;12(3):358. https://www.mdpi.com/2073-4425/12/3/358
56. Sato N, Ota M, Yagishita A, Miki Y, Takahashi T, Adachi Y, et al. Aberrant midsagittal fiber tracts in patients with hemimegalencephaly. Am J Neuroradiol. 2008;29(4):823–7.
57. D'Gama AM, Woodworth MB, Hossain AA, Bizzotto S, Hatem NE, LaCoursiere CM, et al. Somatic mutations activating the mTOR pathway in dorsal telencephalic progenitors cause a continuum of cortical dysplasias. Cell Rep. 2017;21(13):3754–66.
58. Mirzaa GM, Conway RL, Gripp KW, Lerman-Sagie T, Siegel DH, deVries LS, et al. Megalencephaly-capillary malformation (MCAP) and megalencephaly-polydactyly-polymicrogyria-hydrocephalus (MPPH) syndromes: two closely related disorders of brain overgrowth and abnormal brain and body morphogenesis. Am J Med Genet A. 2012;158 A(2):269–91.
59. Mirzaa GM, Rivière JB, Dobyns WB. Megalencephaly syndromes and activating mutations in the PI3K-AKT pathway: MPPH and MCAP. Am J Med Genet Part C Semin Med Genet. 2013;163C:122–30.
60. Crino PB. mTORopathies: a road well-traveled. Epilepsy Curr. 2020;20(6_suppl):64S–6S.
61. Lee DY. Roles of mTOR signaling in brain development. Exp Neurobiol. 2015;24(3):177–85.
62. Takei N, Nawa H, Tarassishin L, Einstein A. mTOR signaling and its roles in normal and abnormal brain development. Geisel Sch Med. 2014; www.frontiersin.org
63. Bockaert J, Marin P. mTOR in brain physiology and pathologies. Physiol Rev. 2015;95(4):1157–87.
64. Morleo M, Brillante S, Formisano U, Ferrante L, Carbone F, Iaconis D, et al. Regulation of autophagosome biogenesis by OFD1-mediated selective autophagy. EMBO J. 2021;40(4):1–14.
65. Mühlebner A, Bongaarts A, Sarnat HB, Scholl T, Aronica E. New insights into a spectrum of developmental malformations related to mTOR dysregulations: challenges and perspectives. J Anat. 2019;235(3):521–42.
66. Dobyns WB. The clinical patterns and molecular genetics of lissencephaly and subcortical band heterotopia: malformations of cortical development—genetics. Epilepsia. 2010;51(SUPPL. 1):5–9.
67. Li S, Jin Z, Koirala S, Bu L, Xu L, Hynes RO, et al. GPR56 regulates pial basement membrane integrity and cortical lamination. J Neurosci. 2008;28(22):5817–26.
68. Vandervore L, Stouffs K, Tanyalçin I, Vanderhasselt T, Roelens F, Holder-Espinasse M, et al. Bi-allelic variants in COL3A1 encoding the ligand to GPR56 are associated with cobblestone-like cortical malformation, white matter changes and cerebellar cysts. J Med Genet. 2017;54(6):432–40.
69. Di Donato N, Timms AE, Aldinger KA, Mirzaa GM, Bennett JT, Collins S, et al. Analysis of 17 genes detects mutations in 81% of 811 patients with lissencephaly. Genet Med. 2018;20(11):1354–64.
70. Barth PG, Mullaart R, Stam FC, Slooff JL. Familial lissencephaly with extreme neopallial hypoplasia. Brain and Development. 1982;4(2):145–51.
71. Sztriha L, Al-Gazali I, Várady E, Nork M, Varughese M. Microlissencephaly. Pediatr Neurol. 1998;18(4):362–5.
72. Dobyns WB, Stratton RF, Greenberg F. Syndromes with lissencephaly. I: Miller-Dieker and Norman-Roberts syndromes and isolated lissencephaly. Am J Med Genet. 1984 Jul;18(3):509–26.
73. Bahi-buisson N, Maillard C. Tubulinopathies overview 1. Clinical characteristics of tubulinopathies. 2021;1–15.

74. Bahi-Buisson N, Poirier K, Fourniol F, Saillour Y, Valence S, Lebrun N, et al. The wide spectrum of tubulinopathies: what are the key features for the diagnosis? Brain. 2014;137(6):1676–700.
75. Hebebrand M, Hüffmeier U, Trollmann R, Hehr U, Uebe S, Ekici AB, et al. The mutational and phenotypic spectrum of TUBA1A-associated tubulinopathy. Orphanet J Rare Dis. 2019;14(1):1–13.
76. Harding BN, Moccia A, Drunat S, Soukarieh O, Tubeuf H, Chitty LS, et al. Mutations in citron kinase cause recessive microlissencephaly with multinucleated neurons. Am J Hum Genet. 2016;99:511–20.
77. Juric-Sekhar G, Kapur RP, Glass IA, Murray ML, Parnell SE, Hevner RF. Neuronal migration disorders in microcephalic osteodysplastic primordial dwarfism type I/III. Acta Neuropathol. 2011;121(4):545–54.
78. Vigliano P, Dassi P, Di Blasi C, Mora M, Jarre L. LAMA2 stop-codon mutation: Merosin-deficient congenital muscular dystrophy with occipital polymicrogyria, epilepsy and psychomotor regression. Eur J Paediatr Neurol. 2009;13(1):72–6.
79. Stutterd CA, Leventer RJ. Polymicrogyria: a common and heterogeneous malformation of cortical development. Am J Med Genet Part C Semin Med Genet. 2014;166(2):227–39.
80. Barkovich AJ. Current concepts of polymicrogyria. Neuroradiology. 2010;52(6):479–87.
81. Barkovich JA. MRI analysis of sulcation morphology in polymicrogyria. Epilepsia. 2010;23(1):1–15. https://www.ncbi.nlm.nih.gov/pmc/articles/PMC3624763/pdf/nihms412728.pdf
82. Blümcke I, Thom M, Aronica E, Armstrong DD, Harry V, Palmini A, et al. The clinico-pathological spectrum of focal cortical dysplasias: a consensus classification proposed by an ad hoc task force of the ILAE diagnostic methods commission. Epilepsia. 2011;52(1):158–74.
83. Najm IM, Sarnat HB, Blümcke I. Review: the international consensus classification of focal cortical dysplasia—a critical update 2018. Neuropathol Appl Neurobiol. 2018;44(1):18–31.
84. Vanhaesebroeck B, Stephens L, Hawkins P. PI3K signalling: the path to discovery and understanding. Nat Rev Mol Cell Biol. 2012;13(3):195–203.
85. Pirozzi F, Berkseth M, Shear R, Gonzalez L, Timms AE, Sulc J, et al. Erratum: profiling PI3K-AKT-MTOR variants in focal brain malformations reveals new insights for diagnostic care. Brain. 2022;145(3):925–38. https://doi.org/10.1093/brain/awab376. Brain 2023;146(1):E7–8
86. Saxton RA, Sabatini DM. mTOR signaling in growth, metabolism, and disease. Cell. 2017;168(6):960–76.
87. Inglis-Broadgate SL, Thomson RE, Pellicano F, Tartaglia MA, Pontikis CC, Cooper JD, et al. FGFR3 regulates brain size by controlling progenitor cell proliferation and apoptosis during embryonic development. Dev Biol. 2005;279(1):73–85.
88. Hevner RF. The cerebral cortex malformation in thanatophoric dysplasia: neuropathology and pathogenesis. Acta Neuropathol. 2005;110(3):208–21.
89. Bosakova MK, Varecha M, Hampl M, Duran I, Nita A, Buchtova M, et al. Regulation of ciliary function by fibroblast growth factor signaling identifies FGFR3-related disorders achondroplasia and thanatophoric dysplasia as ciliopathies. Hum Mol Genet. 2018;27(6):1093–105.
90. Blaas HGK, Vogt C, Eik-Nes SH. Abnormal gyration of the temporal lobe and megalencephaly are typical features of thanatophoric dysplasia and can be visualized prenatally by ultrasound. Ultrasound Obstet Gynecol. 2012;40(2):230–4.
91. Wang DC, Shannon P, Toi A, Chitayat D, Mohan U, Barkova E, et al. Temporal lobe dysplasia: a characteristic sonographic finding in thanatophoric dysplasia. Ultrasound Obstet Gynecol. 2014;44(5):588–94.
92. Itoh K, Pooh R, Kanemura Y, Yamasaki M, Fushiki S. Brain malformation with loss of normal FGFR3 expression in thanatophoric dysplasia type I. Neuropathology. 2013;33(6):663–6.
93. Krsek P, Maton B, Korman B, Pacheco-Jacome E, Jayakar P, Dunoyer C, et al. Different features of histopathological subtypes of pediatric focal cortical dysplasia. Ann Neurol. 2008;63(6):758–69.
94. Aronica E, Mühlebner A. Neuropathology of epilepsy. Handb Clin Neurol. 2018;145(1):193–216.
95. Mutch CA, Poduri A, Sahin M, Barry B, Walsh CA, Barkovich AJ. Disorders of microtubule function in neurons: imaging correlates. Am J Neuroradiol. 2016;37(3):528–35.
96. Oegema R, Cushion TD, Phelps IG, Chung SK, Dempsey JC, Collins S, et al. Recognizable cerebellar dysplasia associated with mutations in multiple tubulin genes. Hum Mol Genet. 2015;24(18):5313–25.
97. Blumkin L, Leibovitz Z, Krajden-Haratz K, Arad A, Yosovich K, Gindes L, et al. Autosomal dominant TUBB3-related syndrome: fetal, radiologic, clinical and morphological features. Eur J Paediatr Neurol. 2020;2020(26):46–60. https://doi.org/10.1016/j.ejpn.2020.03.001.
98. Ramirez Zegarra R, Casati D, Volpe N, Lanna M, Dall'Asta A, Chiarelli A, et al. The "cortical invagination sign": a midtrimester sonographic marker of unilateral cortical focal dysgyria in fetuses with complete agenesis of the corpus callosum. Am J Obstet Gynecol MFM. 2023;5(12):1–7.
99. Barkovich AJ. Morphologic characteristics of subcortical heterotopia: MR imaging study. Am J Neuroradiol. 2000;21(2):290–5.
100. Barkovich AJ, Guerrini R, Battaglia G, Kalifa G, N'Guyen T, Parmeggiani A, et al. Band heterotopia: correlation of outcome with magnetic resonance imaging parameters. Ann Neurol. 1994;36(4):609–17.
101. Yakovlev PI, Wadsworth R. Schizencephalies: a study of the congenital clefts in the cerebral mantle,

I: clefts with fused lips. J Neuropathol Exp Neurol. 1964;5:116–30.

102. Yakovlev PI, Wadsworth R. Schizencephalies; a study of the congenital clefts in the cerebral mantle; II. Clefts with hydrocephalus and lips separated. J Neuropathol Exp Neurol. 1964;5(3):169–206.
103. Byrd SE, Osborn RE, Bohan TP, Naidich TP. The CT and MR evaluation of migrational disorders of the brain part II. Schizencephaly, heterotopia and polymicrogyria. Pediatr Radiol. 1989;19: 219–22.
104. Barkovich AJ, Kjos B. Schizencephaly: correlation of clinical findings with MR characteristics thought to be an extremely rare developmental of this study was to correlate clinical data with anatomic data as assessed by MR in an attempt to find those MR characteristics that a. Am J Neuro-Radiol. 1992;13:85–94.
105. Curry CJ, Lammer EJ, Nelson V, Shaw GM. Schizencephaly: heterogeneous etiologies in a population of 4 million California births. Am J Med Genet. 2005;137 A(2):181–9.
106. Dies KA, Bodell A, Hisama FM, Guo CY, Barry B, Chang BS, et al. Schizencephaly: association with young maternal age, alcohol use, and lack of prenatal care. J Child Neurol. 2013;28(2):198–203.
107. Sato Y, Shibasaki J, Aida N, Hiiragi K, Kimura Y, Akahira-Azuma M, et al. Novel COL4A1 mutation in a fetus with early prenatal onset of schizencephaly. Hum Genome Var. 2018;5:4.
108. Shannon P, Hum C, Parks T, Schauer GM, Chitayat D, Chong K, et al. Brain and placental pathology in fetal COL4A1 related disease. Pediatr Dev Pathol. 2021;24(3):175–86.
109. Griffiths PD. Schizencephaly revisited. Neuroradiology. 2018;60(9):945–60.

Destructive Lesions of the Brain: Intracranial Hemorrhage and Stroke

Simona Boito, Grazia Volpe, Margherita Scarrone, and Nicola Persico

Abstract

Both intracranial hemorrhage (ICH) and stroke may lead to parenchymal damage with different mechanisms. ICH usually originates from the germinal matrix which may then rupture into the ventricular system. In some cases, the hemorrhagic event may extend at the level of the medullary venous plexus causing venous stroke, which results in parenchymal damage. Venous stroke may also occur as an isolated lesion, not associated with ICH. On the other hand, arterial stroke leads to major cortical damage through an arterial ischemic/ hypoxic event.

Supplementary Information The online version contains supplementary material available at https://doi.org/10.1007/978-3-031-70192-4_9.

S. Boito · G. Volpe · M. Scarrone · N. Persico (✉)
Prenatal Diagnosis and Fetal Surgery Unit, Fondazione IRCCS Cà Granda, Ospedale Maggiore Policlinico, Milan, Italy
e-mail: Simona.Boito@policlinico.mi.it; Grazia.Volpe@policlinico.mi.it; Margherita.Scarrone@unimi.it; Nicola.Persico@unimi.it

Keywords

Destructive lesions · Intracranial hemorrhage · Ischemic stroke · Porencephaly · Hydranencephaly

1 Intracranial Hemorrhage

- **Incidence:** Rare (1:1000–10,000 pregnancies) [1–5].
- **Causes:** Can be broadly categorized into maternal and fetal causes (see Table 1).
  Maternal factors include abdominal trauma, seizures, hypoxia, immune thrombocytopenia (ITP), infections (cytomegalovirus, toxoplasmosis), febrile disease, anticoagulant therapy (e.g., warfarin), coagulation disorders, drugs (cocaine), maternal complications of pregnancy (preeclampsia, placental abruption), and maternal vitamin K deficiency.
  Fetal factors include congenital coagulopathies (e.g., deficiency of Factor V and X, single-gene disorders interfering with vitamin K absorption), cerebral arteriovenous malformations, *COL4A1/COL4A2 mutations* (see Box 1) [6, 7], twin-to-twin or maternal-fetal transfusion, death of a co-twin in monochorionic pregnancy, fetal thrombophilia (factor V Leiden, protein C gene mutation), thrombosis of the umbilical cord, cord entanglement, and severe fetal growth restriction (potentially associated with parenchymal hemorrhage).

P. Volpe, T. Ghi (eds.), *Fetal Neurosonography*, Ultrasound in Obstetrics and Gynecology,
https://doi.org/10.1007/978-3-031-70192-4_9

Table 1 Maternal and fetal factors contributing to fetal intracranial hemorrhage

Maternal	Fetal
Abdominal trauma	Coagulopathy (e.g., deficiency of factor V and X, single-gene disorders interfering with vitamin K absorption)
Anticoagulant therapy (e.g., warfarin)	Cerebral arteriovenous malformations
Coagulation disorders	COL4A1/COL4A2 mutations
Hyperpyrexia	CMV infection (parenchymal, cerebellar)
Feto-maternal alloimmune thrombocytopenia (FMAIT)	Severe FGR (parenchymal)

Box 1: COL4A1/COL4A2 mutations

- Genes encoding alpha1 and alpha2 chains of type IV collagen (key component of basement membrane).
- Mode of transmission: autosomal dominant.
- Clinical presentation: cerebral angiopathy with severe and/or multifocal hemorrhagic or ischemic-hemorrhagic cerebral lesions, with or without schizencephaly (SCZ) or porencephaly.
- Associated findings: cataract.

The most important determinant of fetal ICH is represented by *feto-maternal alloimmune thrombocytopenia (FMAIT)* (see Box 2) [1]. However, a maternal or fetal predisposing condition for fetal ICH is only identified in 20–45% of the cases while in the majority of cases, etiology remains unknown [3, 5, 8].

1.1 Types of ICH

Based on the anatomic location, ICH can be categorized into two main groups: **extracerebral** and **intracerebral** hemorrhage. The **extracerebral** group includes subdural and subarachnoid hemorrhage. The **intracerebral** group can be further subdivided into *subependymal/intraventricular* (IVH), *intraparenchymal and infratentorial* hemorrhages [5, 8]. In the fetus (as well as in the preterm neonate), the subependymal/intraventricular hemorrhage is the most common type of ICH. The initial bleeding episode occurs in the germinal matrix, which is a highly vascularized region with thin-walled vessels. Due to this structural fragility, the germinal matrix is prone to profuse hemorrhage [9].

Box 2: Feto-maternal alloimmune thrombocytopenia (FMAIT)

- Incidence: 1:1000–1:5000 pregnancies.
- Pathogenesis: maternal alloimmunization against fetal Human Platelet Antigens (HPA) of paternal origin (HPA1a in 80–85% of cases) leading to fetal platelet destruction.
- Clinical presentation: fetal hemorrhage (both intra- and extra-cranial). It usually occurs during the first pregnancy (60% of cases).
- Possible antenatal treatment: Intravenous immunoglobulins (IV IG), intrauterine platelet transfusion.
- No screening program or prophylaxis available (ongoing research).

1.1.1 Subdural, Subarachnoid, and Epidural Hemorrhage

Supratentorial extra-axial (subdural, subarachnoid, and epidural) hemorrhage may occur after maternal trauma. Subdural hemorrhage may also be caused by bleeding diathesis such as autoimmune thrombocytopenia or maternal warfarin intake. Reverse flow on Doppler ultrasound may be detected, possibly due to raised intracranial pressure [1].

1.1.2 Posterior Fossa Hemorrhage

Infratentorial fetal hemorrhages include subdural and intracerebellar bleeding. These types of hemorrhage can be diagnosed in utero, even if they are often recognized only in the neonatal period. It may have different etiologies including CMV, vascular factors, or hypoxic factors. They may also be caused by hemorrhagic diathesis, intrauterine transfusion (for fetal anemia), and acute hypertension in case of eclampsia, even though evidence for the latter case is limited. Posterior fossa hemorrhage may lead to destructive lesions of the cerebellum, which are often associated with poor neurodevelopmental outcomes [1].

1.2 Ultrasound Diagnosis and Grading

The diagnosis of ICH most often occurs late in pregnancy as an incidental finding, with a mean gestational age of 30–31 weeks at the time of diagnosis [3, 8].

1.2.1 Sonographic Features of ICH

Fetal ICH has an extremely variable sonographic appearance which mainly depends on the site, the severity, and the time elapsed since the lesion occurred [10]. A recent hemorrhage will appear as a homogeneous echogenic mass without posterior shadowing within the brain parenchyma or ventricles that is distinct from the choroid plexus [5]. Following reorganization and lysis of the clot, the mass will develop an external echogenic rim and an internal anechoic area (see Fig. 5c) [3]. ICH can either spontaneously resolve, or it may lead to ventriculomegaly (VM) secondary to obstruction of the cerebrospinal fluid circulation [3]. Obstruction can occur at the level of the aqueduct of Sylvius (see Fig. 4a) or at the level of the foramina of Monro (see Fig. 4b–d), resulting in bilateral or unilateral ventriculomegaly, respectively. Impaired reabsorption of the cerebrospinal fluid secondary to inflammation of the subarachnoid villi by blood may also contribute to the development of ventriculomegaly. Furthermore, ventricular lining will appear hyperechoic or nodular, due to ventriculitis secondary to hemosiderin deposits (*clearly visible on the axial plane in* Fig. 1c) [2].

The hemorrhage can extend into the periventricular white matter leading to parenchymal necrosis and resorption secondary to venous stroke [1]. Usually, 2 weeks after the hemorrhagic event, necrotic brain parenchyma will be substituted by porencephalic cysts (*visible on coronal and sagittal planes in* Figs. 5, 6, and 7) [3]. Periventricular leukomalacia (PVL) usually occurs in the area around the frontal horns as a result of a reperfusion injury of ischemic periventricular white matter (*visible on the sagittal view in* Figs. 1d, 6b, and 7a) [3, 5, 8].

Ultrasonographic Features of ICH

- Zone of increased echogenicity or subependymal cysts at the level of the caudate nucleus (*visible on coronal transcaudate plane*).
- Homogeneous echogenic mass without posterior shadowing (recent hemorrhage).
- Mass with external echogenic rim and an internal anechoic area (old hemorrhage).
- Ventriculomegaly.
- Bright echogenic ventricular lining.
- Porencephalic cysts.
- Periventricular multiple small cysts (*periventricular leukomalacia*).

1.2.2 Grading of IVH

A grading system (Papile's grading [11]) has been developed for premature neonates, and it has subsequently been adapted to fetal IVH [3] (Fig. 1):

1. *Grade I:* Limited to subependymal matrix. At neurosonography, a subtle hyperechogenicity of the germinal matrix on the coronal transcaudate plane can be appreciated (Fig. 2a). On MRI T2-weighted sequences, a small area of hypointensity can be seen at the level of the germinal matrix (Fig. 2b).
2. *Grade II*: Clear spillover into the ventricles, but filling less than 50% of the lateral ventricle and without severe ventriculomegaly (transverse diameter of the lateral ventricular atrium <15 mm). The blood clot filling the

lateral ventricles can be appreciated on axial, coronal, and sagittal planes of neurosonography (Fig. 1b) and MRI (Fig. 3).

3. *Grade III*: Spillover into the ventricle, with filling of 50% or more of one or both lateral ventricles and severe ventriculomegaly (transverse diameter of the lateral ventricular atrium >15 mm). On the axial transventricular plane, dilatation of both lateral ventricles and third ventricle can be appreciated in case of obstruction of the Sylvius aqueduct (Fig. 4a). Selective obstruction of one Monro foramen is evident on axial, coronal, and parasagittal planes at MRI T2-weighted sequences showing severe unilateral ventriculomegaly associated with the presence of an intraventricular hypointense blood clot, adjacent to the foramen of Monro (Fig. 4b–d).
4. *Grade IV*: Grades I, II, or III with hemorrhage involving also a large part of the periventricular parenchyma Figs. 5, 6, and 7). In grade IV, parenchymal necrotic lesions are secondary to venous stroke of the medullary veins' plexus. If the ependymal lining ruptures, the necrotic lesion is then passively filled with CSF leading to the formation of porencephalic cysts. They are defined as cystic lesions of the brain due to an encephaloclastic insult (hemorrhage + venous stroke), lined by white matter (unlike schizencephaly, lined by polymicrogyria), which communicate with the ventricular system (see Figs. 5d, 6d, and 7a, b).

The majority of IVH are classified as Grade 3 and 4, with a range reported in the literature between 70% and 100%. A more recent classification does not include grade IV, as parenchymal involvement is not considered a direct consequence of the bleeding but rather a result of parenchymal infarction due to impaired medullary venous drainage. Consequently, it is now more correct to refer to IVH grade IV as periventricular hemorrhagic infarction (PVHI) [12].

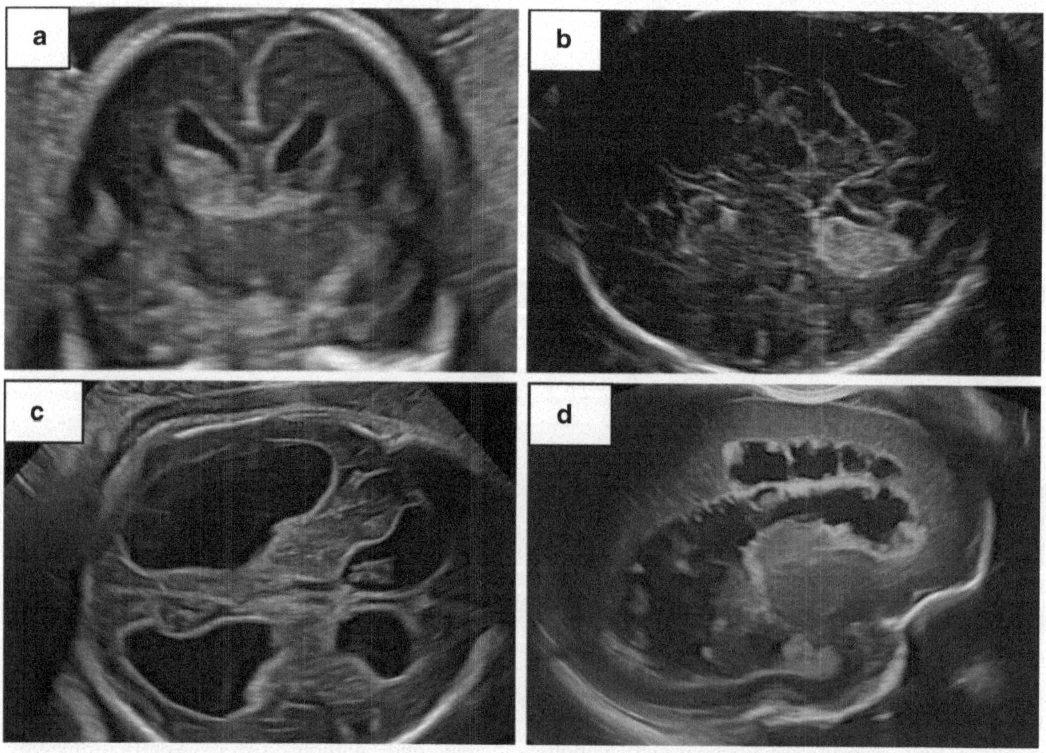

Fig. 1 Papile's grading of fetal IVH. (**a**) Grade I: limited to the germinal matrix; (**b**) grade II: spillover to ventricles with atrial width < 15.0 mm; (**c**) grade III: spillover to ventricles with severe VM (atrial width ≥ 15.0 mm); (**d**) grade IV: grades I, II, or III + porencephalic cysts

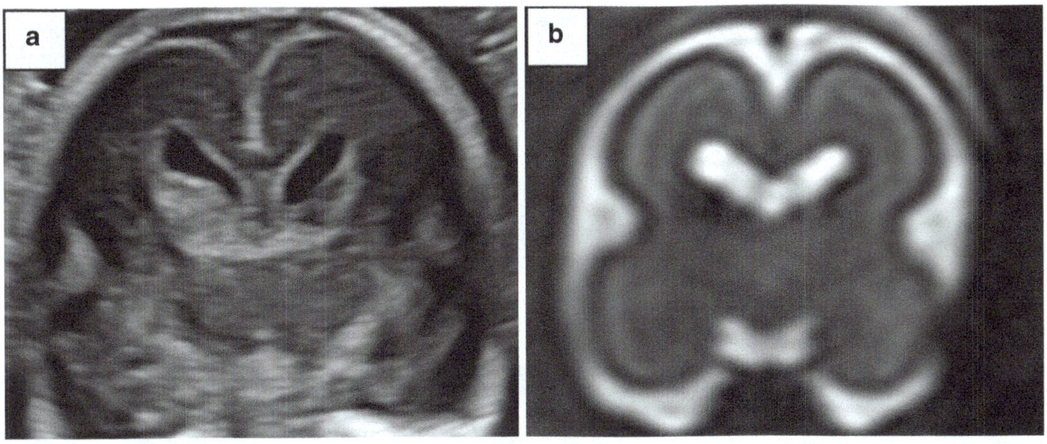

Fig. 2 IVH grade I at 22 gestational weeks. (**a**) On transvaginal neurosonography (coronal transcaudate plane), a small hyperechogenic clot can be seen at the level of the germinal matrix. Note absence of ventricular spillover. (**b**): At MRI T2-weighted images, a small area of hypointensity can be observed at the level of the germinal matrix level

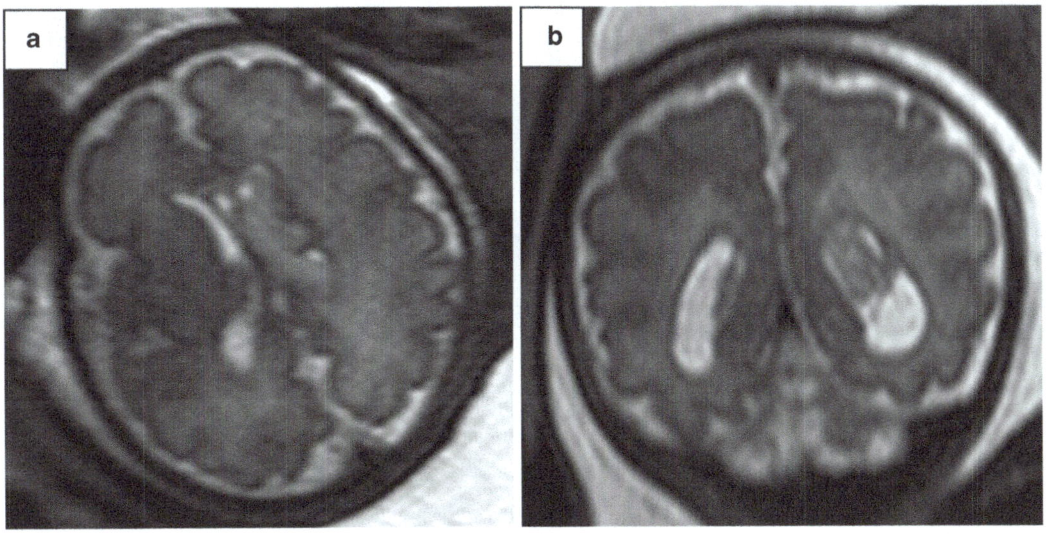

Fig. 3 IVH grade II at 34 gestational weeks. MRI T2-weighted images: unilateral ventriculomegaly due to the presence of IVH which occupies the middle cell and the frontal horn of the lateral ventricle; modest irregularity of the ventricular profile at the middle cell level; altered signal of the ipsilateral parietal white matter due to edema secondary to impairment of the venous drainage. (**a**) Axial view. (**b**) Coronal view

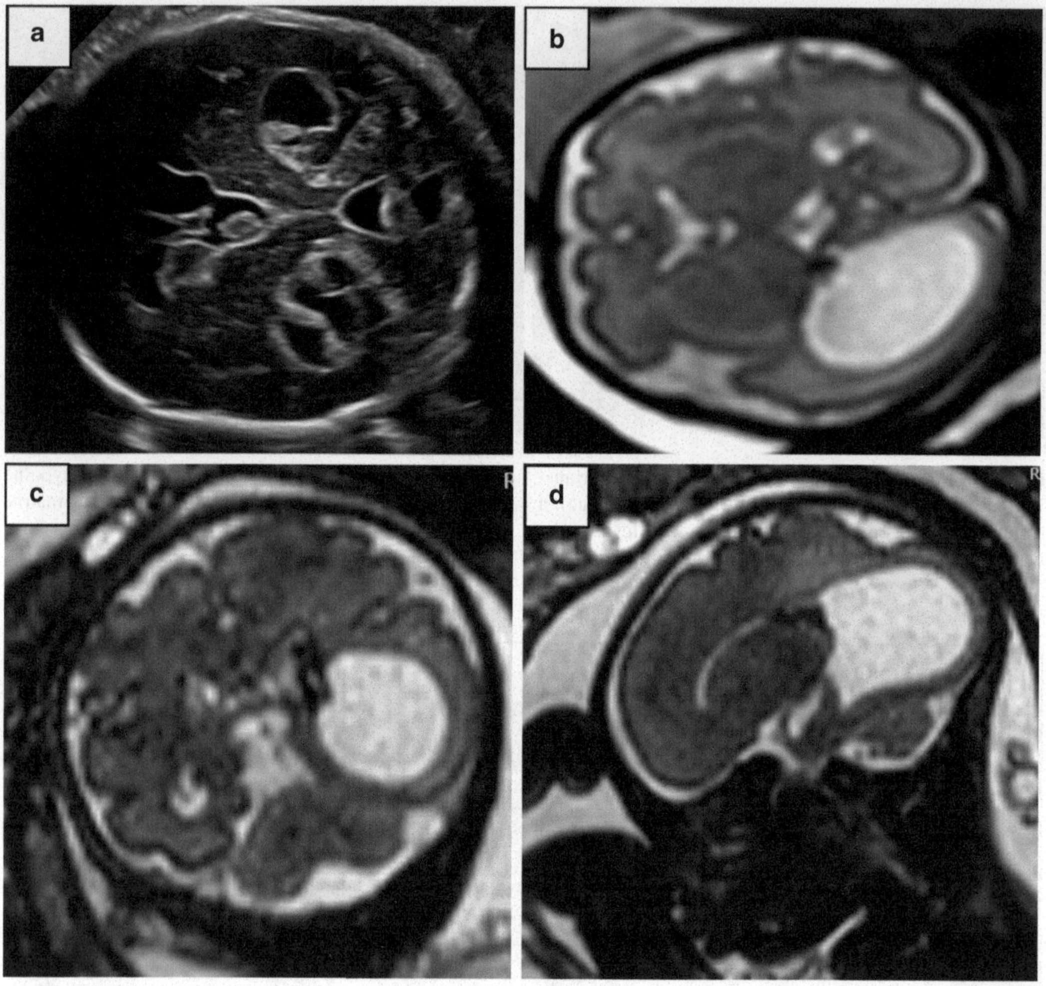

Fig. 4 IVH grade III. (**a**) Axial transventricular plane at 30 gestational weeks showing dilatation of the frontal and the occipital horns of the lateral ventricles as well as of the third ventricle (secondary to aqueduct of Sylvius obstruction); note the hyperechogenicity of ventricular lining. MRI T2-weighted images on (**b**) transventricular, (**c**) coronal, and (**d**) parasagittal planes showing IVH grade III at 33 gestational weeks with selective obstruction of one Monro foramen where a severe unilateral ventriculomegaly (31 mm) associated with the presence of an intraventricular hypointense blood clot, adjacent to the foramen of Monro is observed. The adjacent brain parenchyma appears markedly thinned with associated smoothing of the cortical sulci and reduced representation of the perien-cephalic subarachnoid spaces

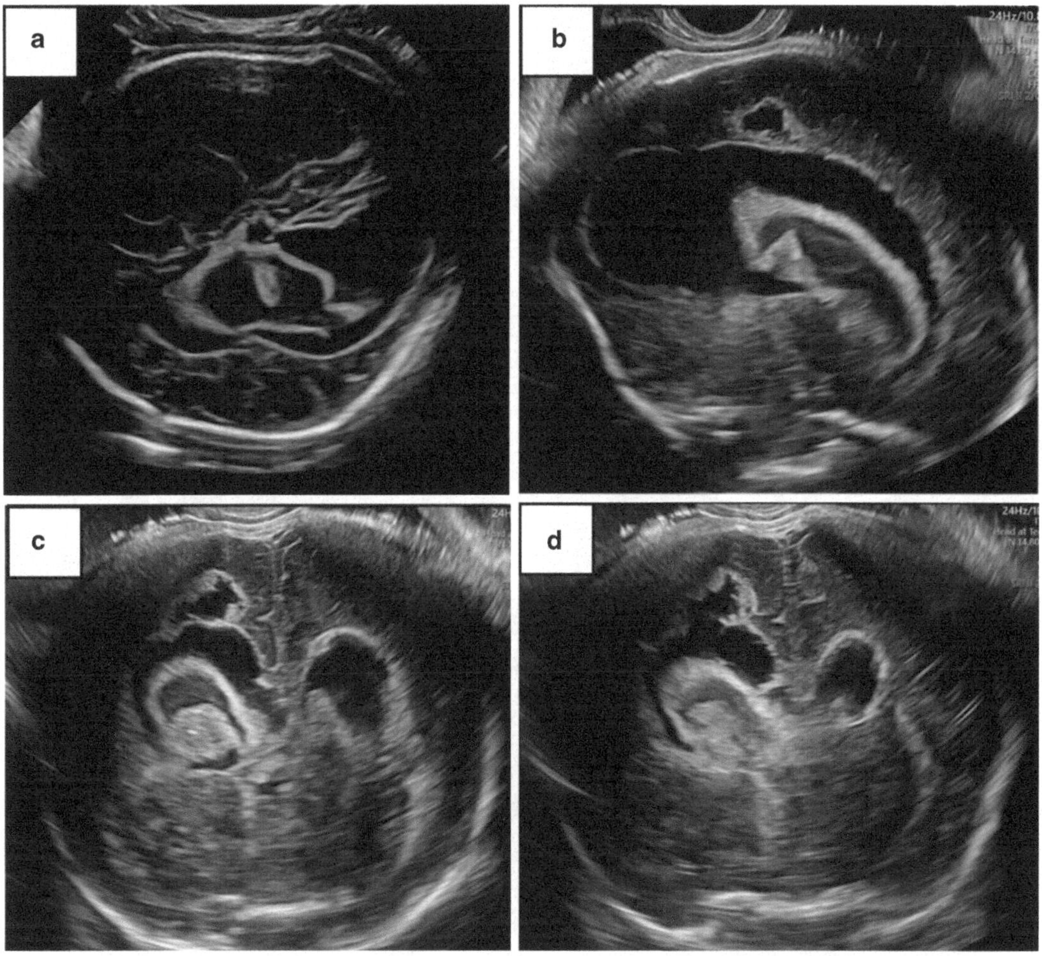

Fig. 5 IVH grade IV at 34 gestational weeks, with moderate parenchymal destruction. (**a**) Axial view demonstrating severe bilateral ventriculomegaly and the intraventricular clot with the hyperechoic margins and the hypoechoic core; (**b**) parasagittal plane of the ventricle demonstrating the parenchymal lesion and the intraventricular clot. (**c**) Coronal transthalamic plane of the same case; note the intraventricular clot with the hyperechoic margins and the hypoechoic core; (**d**) note the porencephalic cyst communicating with the ventricular lumen

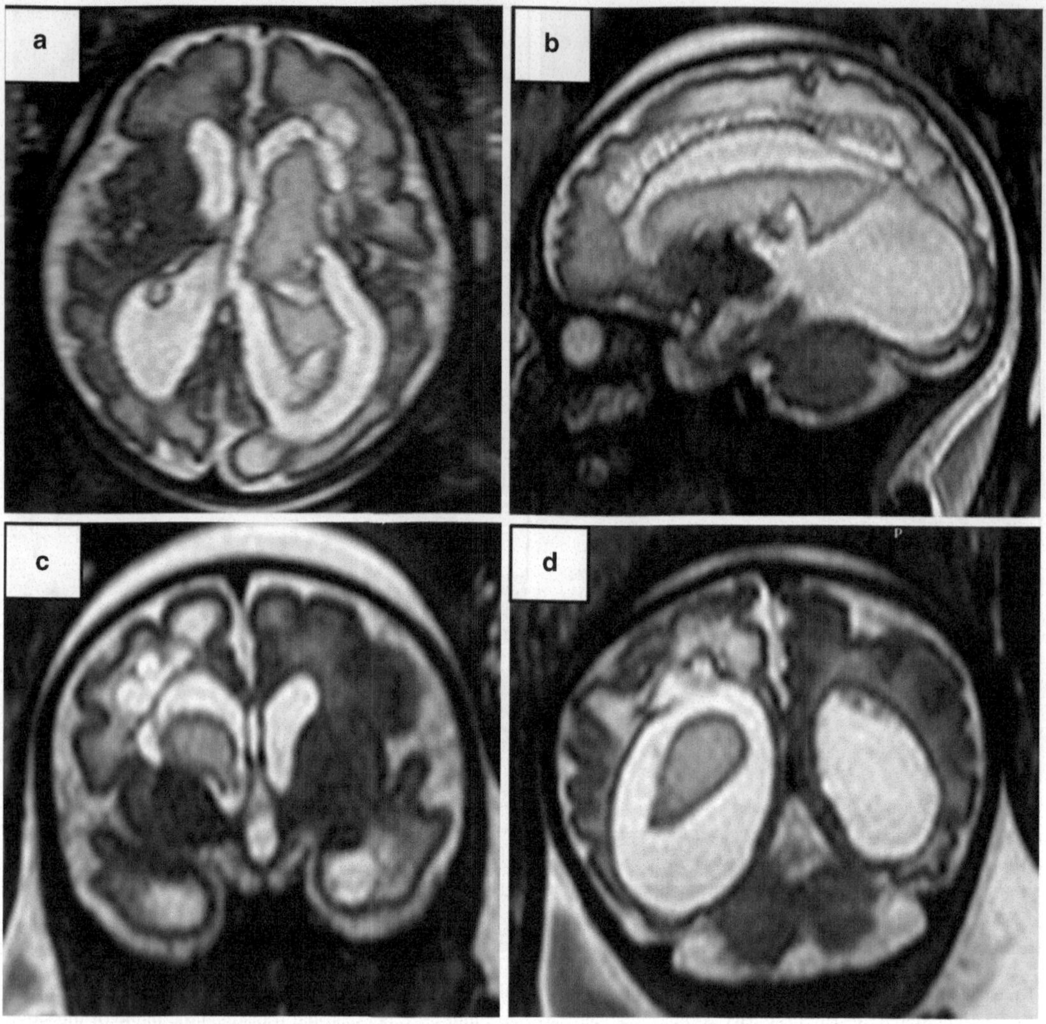

Fig. 6 IVH grade IV at 35 gestational weeks. MRI images of the same case of Fig. 5. (**a**) Endoventricular hemorrhage which occupies more than 50% of the left lateral ventricle. Endoventricular hemorrhage causes supratentorial hydrocephalus (ventricular diameter measured at the atria is 35 mm on the left and 21 mm on the right). The parenchyma of the left hemisphere is diffusely thinned, particularly in the occipital area. (**b**) Associated diffuse cortical T2 hyperintensity with small cavitations in the fronto-parietal white matter of the left hemisphere is visible on the left parasagittal plane. (**c**) Damage with loss of substance of the thalamus, the posterior portion of the lenticular nucleus and the posterior arm of the ipsilateral internal capsule is visible on the coronal plane. (**d**) A porencephalic cyst communicating with the ventricular lumen is evident on the transcerebellar coronal plane

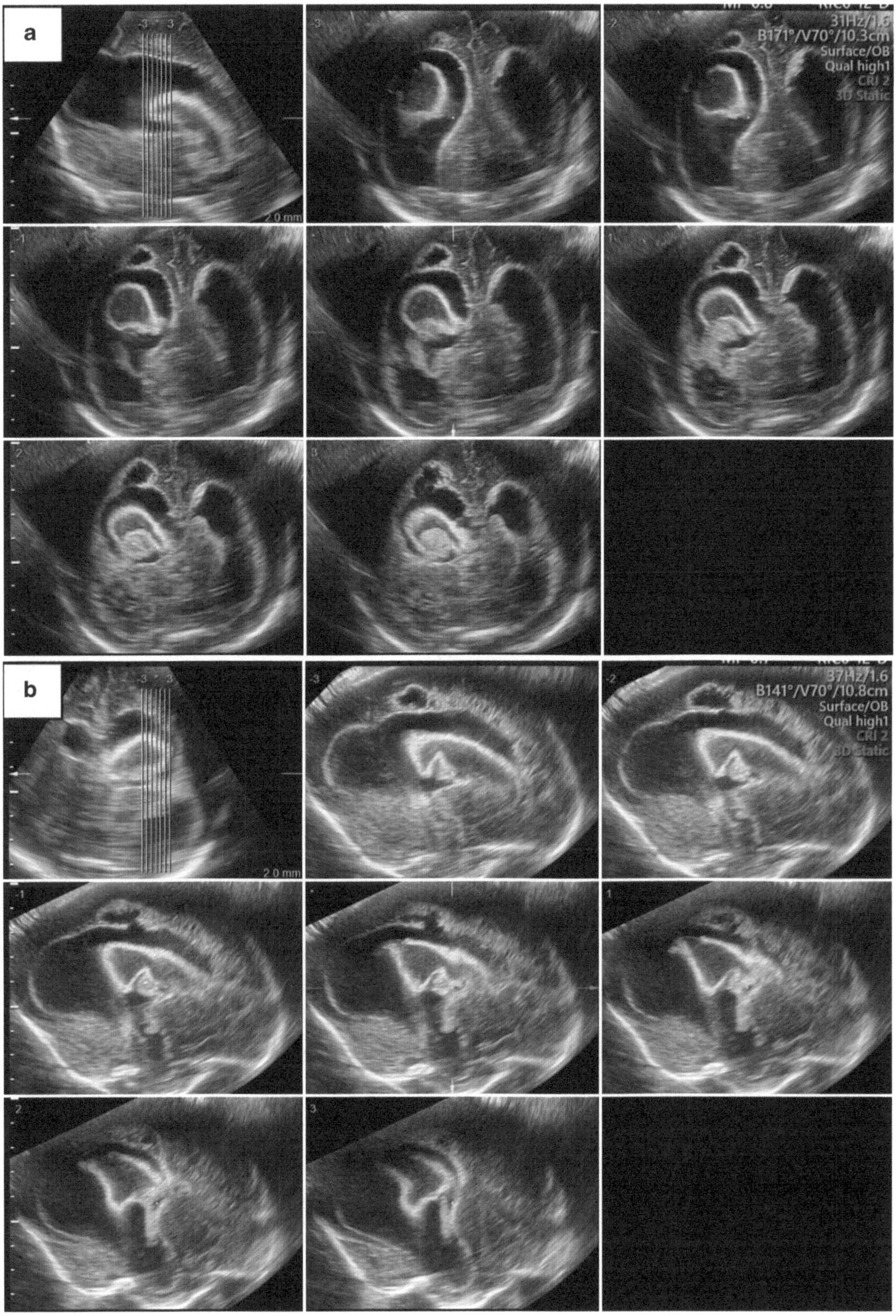

Fig. 7 Tomographic images of coronal (**a**) and sagittal (**b**) planes of the fetal brain in a case of grade IV ICH at 34 gestational weeks (same case of Figs. 5 and 6)

Table 2 Papile's grading system of IVH hemorrhage

Grade	Frequency (%)	US features	Prognosis
I	10	Subtle hyperechogenicity of the germinal matrix/ganglionic eminence area (absence of ventricular spillover)	Good
II	2	Clear spillover to ventricles with atrial width < 15.0 mm	Good
III	43	Spillover to ventricles with severe ventriculomegaly (VM) (atrial width ≥ 15.0 mm)	Intermediate
IV (PVHI)	45	Grades I, II, or III + parenchymal hemorrhage/porencephalic cyst	Poor

1.2.3 Parenchymal Hemorrhage

It may occur as a primary hemorrhagic event (not associated with intraventricular hemorrhage) due to venous stroke of the medullary plexus. Parenchymal hemorrhage may be secondary to vascular insults, but it can also be associated with severe fetal growth restriction (FGR) and CMV infection. As for all types of hemorrhage, the ultrasonographic features depend on the time since it occurred: a recent hemorrhage appears as a hyperechoic mass, while older hemorrhages develop a hypo/anechoic core due to colliquation of the clot (Fig. 8).

1.2.4 Subdural Hemorrhage

In this case, a blood clot or fluid blood is evident in the subdural spaces. When fluid blood is visible, it is more likely caused by coagulopathy. Subdural hematomas are often associated with midline displacement and compression of the cerebral hemispheres evident on the axial transventricular view (Fig. 9).

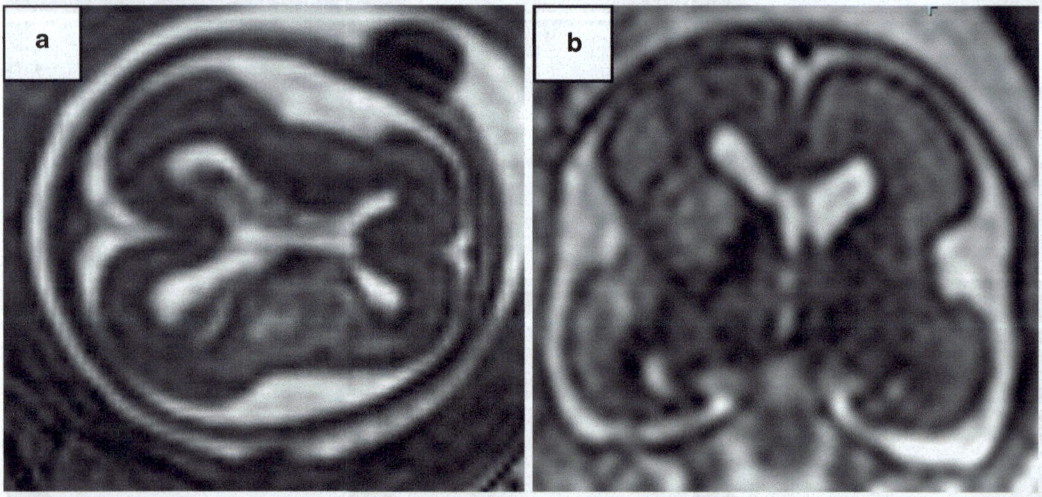

Fig. 8 Parenchymal hemorrhage at 21 gestational weeks. A deep hemorrhagic lesion in the supratentorial basal nuclei area, characterized by inhomogeneous T2 signal, predominantly hyperintense with hypointense margins. The MRI appearance of the hemorrhagic lesion is suggestive of an organization phase with probable associated perilesional edema component. (**a**) Modest enlargement of the ipsilateral ventricular temporo-occipital horn is present on the transventricular plane. (**b**) On the transcaudate plane, the lesion imprints the adjacent ventricle but does not cause deviation of median structures

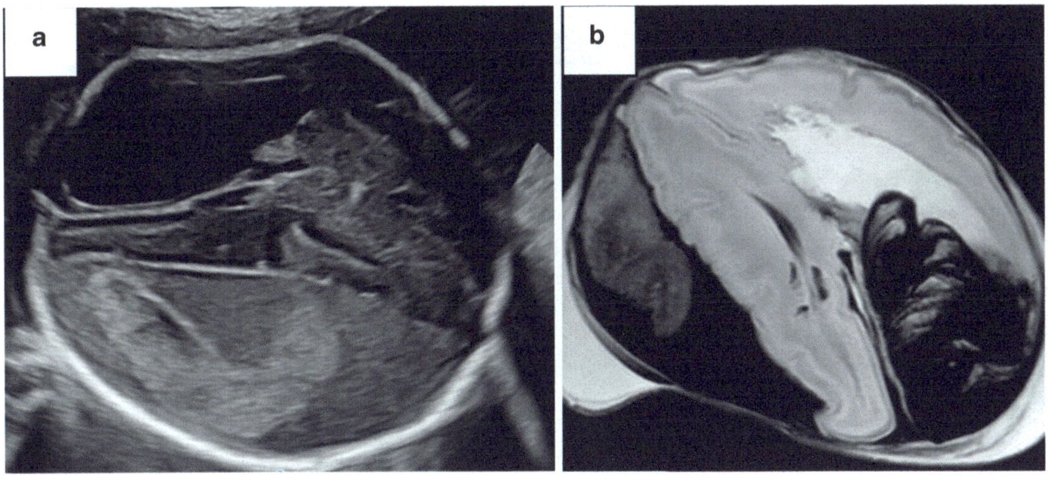

Fig. 9 Subdural hematoma at 30 gestational weeks. (**a**) On the trans-ventricular plane, note the hypoechoic collection of blood in the subdural space, associated with midline shift and compression of adjacent cerebral structures. (**b**) MRI performed after intrauterine death shows extensive right subdural hematoma associated with compression of the right cerebral hemisphere. Concomitant left parietal intraparenchymal hemorrhage extending into the extra-axial space and the endoventricular area is also evident. The midline deviates to the left

1.2.5 Cerebellar Hemorrhage

It can be isolated or may be associated with severe, multifocal hemorrhage. On ultrasound, a hyperechoic lesion can be detected at the level of the cerebellar parenchyma, often leading to cerebellar hemispheres and/or vermis hypoplasia (visible on the midsagittal view). On axial and coronal views, cerebellar hemispheres may have an irregular profile (Fig. 10) and cystic formations can develop within the cerebellar parenchyma, as a consequence of the hemorrhagic event. Ultrasound diagnosis is rather challenging since an extensive collection of blood in the posterior fossa significantly impairs the neurosonographic assessment. In these cases, MRI may add valuable clinical information (Fig. 10b–d).

1.3 Associated Anomalies

ICH is usually isolated. However, some associated anomalies related to the underlying etiology may be seen. For example, if ICH is the result of *COL4A1/COL4A2 mutations*, cataract may be found [6]. Conversely, if ICH is caused by a fetal infection, such as CMV or toxoplasmosis, other features typical of fetal infection may be evident (e.g., intracranial or liver calcification, hydrops, fetal growth restriction). Large ICH resulting in fetal anemia can lead to the development of nonimmune hydrops [5]. ICH can also be associated with fetal growth restriction, and it may rarely be associated with aneurysm of the vein of Galen. In this case, the high blood pressure due to arteriovenous malformation may cause hemorrhage and parenchymal damage (see Chap. 12)

- **Risk of aneuploidy:** Very low.
- **Risk of genetic diseases:** Association with COL4A1/COL4A2 mutations.
- **Risk of syndromic conditions:** Low. ICH may be associated with a Binder phenotype in some cases related to genetic or acquired vitamin K deficiency.

1.4 Differential Diagnosis

The most relevant differential diagnosis is with *intracranial tumors*. Particularly, a recent intraparenchymal hemorrhage closely resembles some cerebral tumors since they both appear as hyperechoic round lesions (Figs. 8 and 11).

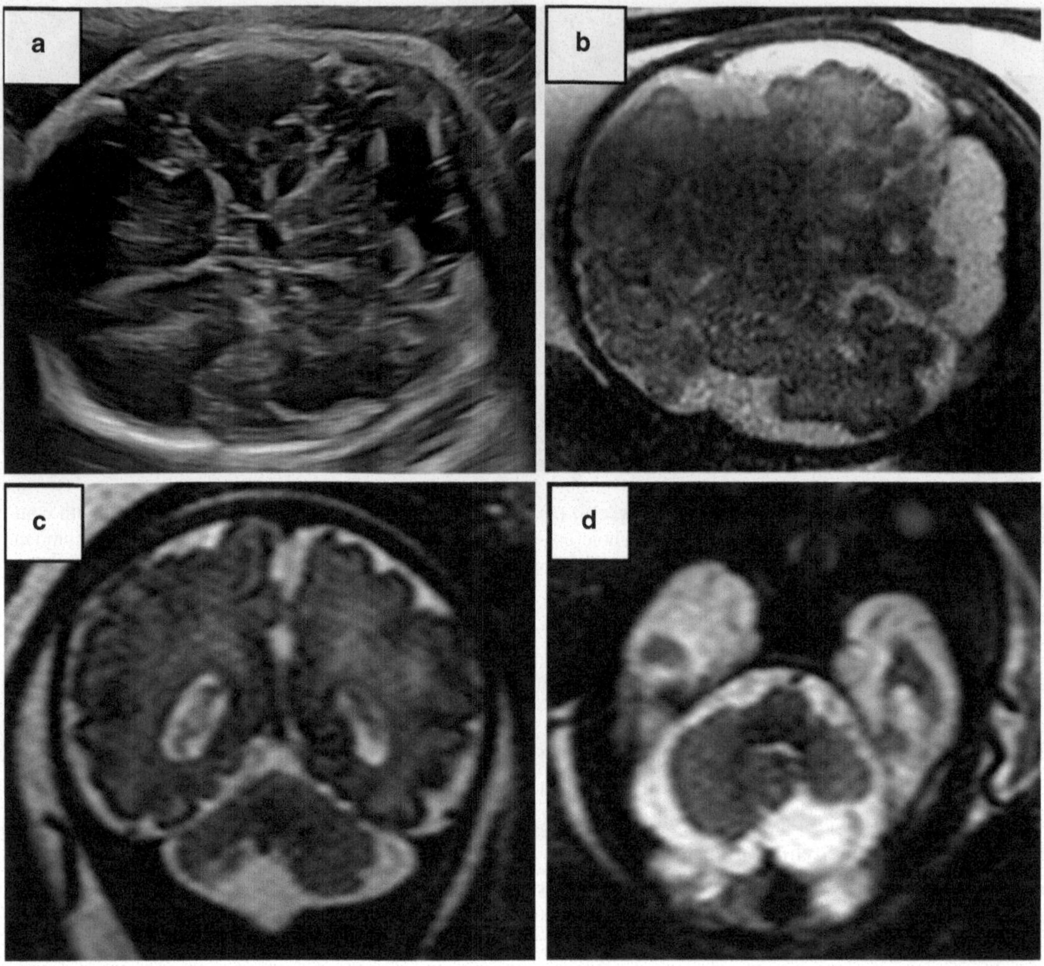

Fig. 10 Cerebellar hemorrhage. (**a**) 30 weeks' gestation. At axial transcerebellar plane, two hyperechoic lesions are present in the cerebellar hemispheres, which present an irregular profile. At MRI T2-weighted sequences of the same case (**b**) on the axial plane, the cerebellar hemispheres appear irregular with a reduced transcerebellar diameter. In another case of cerebellar hemorrhage at 31 gestational weeks on (**c**) coronal and (**d**) axial planes, there is an evident loss of substance on the lower margin, especially on one side, with associated small hypointensities suggestive for hemosiderin deposits

However, tumors generally tend to have a heterogeneous appearance, a rapid growth, and an intense vascularity. Hemorrhages may have more irregular boundaries than that of the tumor. A rare tumor of the choroid plexus, called *choroid plexus papilloma*, may mimic a blood clot. Differential diagnosis may be supported by the use of by *Color Doppler* as tumors usually show an increased vascular flow, while no blood flow is evidenced in ICH. In cases of ventriculomegaly, if the clot has dissolved completely, the recognition of the hemorrhagic origin of a VM may be challenging. In these cases, MRI can help in the differential diagnosis with other etiologies of VM, as it can detect hemosiderin depositions on T2-weighted images.

1.5 Diagnostic Work-Up and Antenatal Management

A thorough past medical history and family history should be conducted to identify possible risk factors and/or family members with bleeding disorders or other lesions of the central nervous system.

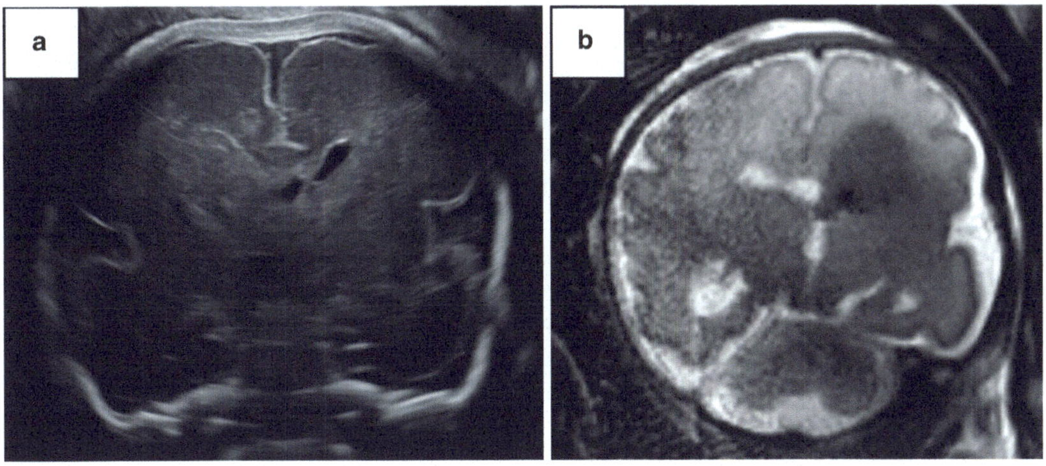

Fig. 11 Large neurofibroma at 29 gestational weeks. (**a**) At fetal neurosonography, the subependymal hyperechoic area can resemble a grade I IVH. (**b**) At MRI T2 sequence along the middle cell of the right lateral ventricle an oval lesion, hypointense on T2 is evident; the lesion however has not specific features and differential diagnosis includes IVH or hamartoma

Genetic counseling should be offered, even if association with chromosomal and genetic conditions is rare. Testing for a COL4A1 mutation can be considered in instances where cataract is also present or in cases of unknown ICH etiology. All patients with fetal ICH should be screened for feto-maternal alloimmune thrombocytopenia (FMAIT) [8]. Maternal serologic studies for cytomegalovirus, rubella, toxoplasmosis, parvovirus B19 infections should be performed. Fetal magnetic resonance imaging (MRI) can be helpful in the differential diagnosis with intracranial tumors and for a better characterization of the intracranial hemorrhage. It has been demonstrated that MRI, given the ability to detect hemosiderin debris and areas of parenchymal infarction, can often provide additional information to ultrasound imaging. Several studies have shown that MRI is more accurate than ultrasound in diagnosing parenchymal lesions and grading ICH, usually upgrading severity of lesions [3, 8]. Follow up with serial ultrasound evaluations is indicated in the third trimester of pregnacy, to assess progression of the lesions and of ventriculomegaly. In low-grade ICH, progressive resolution of abnormal sonographic findings can occur and these cases are usually associated with a normal postnatal outcome. Conversely, hemorrhage can progress from a low to high grade in utero. Termination of pregnancy is an option that should be offered, in accordance with legal limits.

1.6 Mode and Time of Delivery

Timing and indications for cesarean delivery should take into account the etiology of the ICH and the sonographic findings. Cesarean delivery is generally indicated for ICH, especially in FMAIT given the likely severe fetal thrombocytopenia. Delivery should occur in a tertiary center with availability of a neonatal intensive care unit, pediatric neurology, and neurosurgery [5].

1.7 Prognostic Factors

The grade of the hemorrhage represents the main prognostic indicator in case of ICH. Grade IV IVH which is associated with parenchymal damage has the worse prognosis, as illustrated in the next paragraph. Etiology is also important in determining the prognosis: FMAIT or COL4A1/COL4A2 mutations are associated with a much worse prognosis, as these lesions are often multiple and may relapse throughout pregnancy. Prematurity and/or FGR are other prognostic factors impacting on neurodevelopmental outcome of neonates with ICH.

1.8 Prognosis

1.8.1 Intraventricular Hemorrhage

Data on neurodevelopmental outcomes in infants with fetal IVH is limited. Mortality and neurodevelopmental outcomes mainly depend on the grade of IVH and the presence and severity of associated brain injury. In mild cases, resolution of the hemorrhagic lesion without residual deficit may occur, but in high-grade IVHV about half of fetuses die, and among the survivors, more than half show a neurodevelopmental impairment at short-term follow-up [3]. Neonates with grade I and II IVH have a good prognosis, comparable with preterm neonates without IVH. Survival rates are reported at 100%, with mild neurologic sequelae occurring in 10% of neonates. In grade III, despite a survival rate of about 95%, approximately two-thirds of the neonates have mild (31.6%) or severe (31.6%) neurologic impairment. In neonates with grade IV mortality rate reaches 16.6%. In the surviving infants, a normal outcome is reported in approximately 15%, mild neurologic sequelae in 25%, and severe neurologic sequelae in 60% [8].

A recent systematic review has reported a neonatal mortality rate of 12%, with 80% of these occurring premature neonates with FGR. The need for ventriculo-peritoneal shunt was 0% in grade I-II, 19% in non-progressing VM, and 71% in fetuses with progressing VM. Neurodevelopmental delay (NDD) was present in 0% of neonates with IVH grade I-II, 21% in grade III IVH, and 57% in grade IV IVH.

Motor impairment was evident in 24% of neonates with IVH grade III-term, 48% of IVH grade III-premature, and 78% of IVH grade IV [13]. Epilepsy is present in 25% of neonates showing parenchymal damage. A recent retrospective study showed a lower proportion of normal neurodevelopmental outcomes with increasing grade of both unilateral and bilateral IVH. In unilateral IVH, neonates had a normal neurological outcome in 70%, 50%, and 20% of grade II, III, IV respectively. In bilateral IVH, a normal neurological outcome was present in 100% of neonates with grade II and III, while only in 25% of grade IV IVH. These results indicate a more favorable outcome compared to that described in previous literature regarding grade III IVH [14]. The disparity in outcomes may be attributed to the fact that grade III and IV are often grouped in the literature, which does not allow for a finer distinction of the prognoses between these two distinct IVH entities. Additionally, in the literature, there is rarely any specification of the laterality (whether unilateral or bilateral) of the hemorrhage and the gestational week at the time of diagnosis, factors that could significantly impact the prognosis of the fetus.

1.8.2 Cerebellar Hemorrhage

The available data on the prognosis of cerebellar hemorrhage is limited. In a review of the literature, two-thirds of the neonates who had an antenatal diagnosis of cerebellar hemorrhage were defined as neurologically normal after birth [3]. In cases where the cerebellar hemorrhage is not lethal in utero, the prognosis is generally described as favorable, particularly when the injury is unilateral and does not affect the vermis [15–17]. Nevertheless, various outcomes have been described, encompassing a broad spectrum of neurological impairments, ranging from normal functionality to severe disability [18, 19]. Some of the reported neurocognitive impairments include dyspraxia, speech disorders, and difficulties in visuo-perceptual processing [15]. However, given the high number of cases where intrauterine fetal demise or termination of pregnancy is observed, information on postnatal outcomes has been limited. Consequently, there remains a considerable level of uncertainty regarding the neurodevelopmental prognosis for children born with isolated cerebellar hemorrhage, which represents a substantial obstacle in the context of prenatal counseling [20].

1.8.3 Subdural Hemorrhage

A recent meta-analysis suggested that subdural hemorrhage leads to perinatal death in 32% of the cases. Normal neurological outcome was observed in 58% of the survivors, whereas the remaining 42% had neurological morbidity [21].

2 Ischemic Stroke

- *Definition:* Perinatal ischemic stroke can be defined as a group of heterogeneous conditions in which there is a focal disruption of cerebral blood flow secondary to arterial or cerebral venous thrombosis or embolization between 20 weeks of fetal life through twenty-eight postnatal day confirmed by neuroimaging or neuropathologic studies [20].
- *Incidence*: 1:2300–1:5000 live births [22].
- *Pathogenesis*: Prenatal ischemic stroke can be the result of an arterial ischemic event or a venous thrombosis.

2.1 Venous Stroke

- *Etiology*: Venous stroke at the level of the medullary veins' plexus may occur secondary to IVH (grade IV). Venous stroke may also occur as an isolated lesion, not associated with ICH.
- *Ultrasound diagnosis*:
- Venous stroke secondary to intraventricular hemorrhage: see grade IV IVH.
- Isolated venous stroke resulting in parenchymal hemorrhage (see "parenchymal hemorrhage").
- *Periventricular leukomalacia* (PVL): Hemorrhagic lesion developing as a result of a venous stroke at the level of the medullary plexus. In US, it presents with several small cysts, along the course of the medullary veins, corresponding to focal necrosis of the parenchyma.

2.2 Arterial Stroke

- *Etiology*: Transient blood pressure imbalance or vascular disruption. Thrombophilias (factor V Leiden and antiphospholipid syndrome) may play an important role in the pathogenesis of perinatal stroke, even if their role is unclear [23].
- *Ultrasound diagnosis*: Wide range of parenchymal lesions including the hypoxic/ischemic lesions that may be present in monochorionic twins, polymicrogyria (PMG) (see Chap. 8), schizencephaly (SCZ) (see Chap. 8), focal cortical dysplasia, and hydranencephaly. These types of lesions may be isolated with no sign of intracranial bleeding or associated with classic ICH. Parenchymal lesions resulting from arterial stroke with no signs of associated ICH cannot be graded according to ICH grading system and should be anatomically described.

3 Focus on Porencephaly

- *Etiology:* Depends on the underlying cause of porencephaly.
- *Pathogenesis*: Porencephaly represents the end-stage lesion of different insults to the fetal brain including hemorrhage, ischemic stroke (following either an arterial or venous infarction), infection, or trauma. These insults result in focal or multifocal areas of brain necrosis, which are subsequently reabsorbed forming fluid-filled cavities [24]. Fetal brain is prone to undergo dissolution and eventually cavitation due to several anatomic factors. The majority of fetal neurons have unmyelinated fibers with a high-water content, which is released upon neurons' necrosis and contributes to dissolution. Furthermore, deficient glial response is responsible for the cavitation [2].
- *Porencephaly of Venous Origin*: Venous medullary infarcts (usually in type IV IVH) undergo cystic degeneration, typically resulting in a single porencephalic cyst along the frontal, parietal, or temporal horns that communicates with the ventricular cavity. This is often associated with ventriculomegaly. Instead, small ischemic lesions usually evolve into periventricular leukomalacia. In most of these cases, this process does not involve the cortical mantle and the cysts take the shape of the infarcted area [24].
- *Porencephaly of Arterial Origin or Clastic Porencephaly*: This can be caused by occlusion of any cerebral arteries, including the middle cerebral (most common), anterior

cerebral, posterior cerebral, or anterior choroidal artery. It occurs most commonly on the left side of the brain (55% of cases), along the path of the MCA [24, 25].

- *Ultrasound diagnosis*: Cystic lesion that communicates with the lateral ventricles. Usually associated with dilatation of the ipsilateral ventricle (see Figs. 5d, 6d, and 7a, b).
- *Differential diagnosis*: Includes all cystic brain lesions (see Chap. 10), most importantly arachnoid cysts and unilateral schizencephaly. Arachnoid cysts are collections of cerebrospinal fluid (CSF) that do not communicate with the ventricles, but they may communicate with the subarachnoid space. In unilateral schizencephaly, the cyst is lined by gray matter and, unlike porencephaly, it communicates with the subarachnoid space.

4 Focus on Hydranencephaly

- *Incidence*: 1 in 10,000 to 1 in 5000 (0.01–0.02%) of pregnancies.
- *Etiology*: Unknown. Possible causes of the vascular insult include ischemic arterial stroke (most common), infections, hypoxia, single-gene mutations, monochorionic pregnancies, and syndromic conditions.
- *Pathogenesis*: The most commonly proposed mechanism involves infarction of cerebral hemispheres secondary to bilateral occlusion of the internal carotid artery (ICA) and, in some cases, the middle cerebral artery (MCA). This leads to the absence of structures perfused by the ICA/MCA and preserved structures perfused by the posterior cerebral artery and the basilar artery.
- *Ultrasound diagnosis*: Most often, the diagnosis is performed in the second or early third trimester, even if some cases can be detected as early as 13 weeks of gestation. There is a complete absence of the cerebral hemispheres, which are replaced by cerebrospinal fluid (CSF) which fills the whole cranial cavity. The falx can be present. The meninges, thalami, basal ganglia, brain stem, and cerebellum may be normal. It can be associated with macrocephaly or it can also progress from hydranencephaly to microcephaly, due to skull collapse (fetal brain disruption sequence).
- *Differential diagnosis*: (1) Alobar holoprosencephaly (HPE): the thalami are fused and residual cortex is visible. (2) Severe hydrocephalus: a thin layer of cortex and the falx can be seen.
- *Prognosis:* Most patients with hydranencephaly die in utero. Neonates with hydranencephaly may appear completely normal at birth or present with evident symptoms such as seizures, myoclonus, and respiratory difficulty. Months after birth patients start developing seizures and hydrocephalus. Hearing is usually preserved, while most of the children have cortical visual impairment. Other symptoms/signs may include growth retardation, spastic diplegia, and cognitive delay [26].

References

1. Kirkham FJ, Zafeiriou D, Howe D, Czarpran P, Harris A, Gunny R, et al. Fetal stroke and cerebrovascular disease. Eur J Paediatr Neurol. 2018;22:989–1005. https://doi.org/10.1016/j.ejpn.2018.08.008.
2. Monteagudo A, Pilu G, Malinger G, Buyukkurt S, Jadhav A. Intrauterine insults: fetal stroke and destructive processes. In: Timor-Tritsch IE, Monteagudo A, Pilu G, Malinger G, editors. Ultrasonography of the prenatal brain, 3e. New York, NY: McGraw-Hill Education; 2017.
3. Ghi T, Simonazzi G, Perolo A, Savelli L, Sandri F, Bernardi B, et al. Outcome of antenatally diagnosed intracranial hemorrhage: case series and review of the literature. Ultrasound Obstet Gynecol. 2003;22:121–30. https://doi.org/10.1002/uog.191.
4. Elchalal U, Yagel S, Gomori JM, Porat S, Beni-Adani L, Yanai N, et al. Fetal intracranial hemorrhage (fetal stroke): does grade matter? Ultrasound Obstet Gynecol. 2005;26:233–43. https://doi.org/10.1002/uog.1969.
5. Monteagudo A. Intracranial hemorrhage. Am J Obstet Gynecol. 2020;223:B34–7. https://doi.org/10.1016/j.ajog.2020.08.183.
6. Colin E, Sentilhes L, Sarfati A, Mine M, Guichet A, Ploton C, et al. Fetal intracerebral hemorrhage and cataract: think COL4A1. J Perinatol. 2014;34:75–7. https://doi.org/10.1038/jp.2013.135.
7. Coste T, Vincent-Delorme C, Stichelbout M, Devisme L, Gelot A, Deryabin I, et al. *COL4A1/COL4A2* and

inherited platelet disorder gene variants in fetuses showing intracranial hemorrhage. Prenat Diagn. 2022;42:601–10. https://doi.org/10.1002/pd.6113.
8. Adiego B, Martínez-Ten P, Bermejo C, Estévez M, Recio Rodriguez M, Illescas T. Fetal intracranial hemorrhage. Prenatal diagnosis and postnatal outcomes. J Matern Fetal Neonatal Med. 2019;32:21–30. https://doi.org/10.1080/14767058.2017.1369521.
9. Egesa WI, Odoch S, Odong RJ, Nakalema G, Asiimwe D, Ekuk E, et al. Germinal matrix-intraventricular hemorrhage: a tale of preterm infants. Int J Pediatr. 2021;2021:1–14. https://doi.org/10.1155/2021/6622598.
10. Carletti A, Colleoni GG, Perolo A, Simonazzi G, Ghi T, Rizzo N, et al. Prenatal diagnosis of cerebral lesions acquired in utero and with a late appearance. Prenat Diagn. 2009;29:389–95. https://doi.org/10.1002/pd.2244.
11. Papile LA, Burstein J, Burstein R, Koffler H. Incidence and evolution of subependymal and intraventricular hemorrhage: a study of infants with birth weights less than 1,500 gm. J Pediatr. 1978;92:529–34. https://doi.org/10.1016/s0022-3476(78)80282-0.
12. Dudink J, Lequin M, Weisglas-Kuperus N, Conneman N, van Goudoever JB, Govaert P. Venous subtypes of preterm periventricular haemorrhagic infarction. Arch Dis Child Fetal Neonatal Ed. 2008;93:F201–6. https://doi.org/10.1136/adc.2007.118067.
13. Dunbar MJ, Woodward K, Leijser LM, Kirton A. Antenatal diagnosis of fetal intraventricular hemorrhage: systematic review and meta-analysis. Develop Med Child Neurol. 2021;63:144–55. https://doi.org/10.1111/dmcn.14713.
14. Gupta V, Schlatterer SD, Bulas DI, du Plessis AJ, Mulkey SB. Pregnancy and child outcomes following fetal intracranial hemorrhage. Pediatr Neurol. 2023;140:68–75. https://doi.org/10.1016/j.pediatrneurol.2022.12.014.
15. Massoud M, Cagneaux M, Garel C, Varene N, Moutard M-L, Billette T, et al. Prenatal unilateral cerebellar hypoplasia in a series of 26 cases: significance and implications for prenatal diagnosis. Ultrasound Obstet Gynecol. 2014;44:447–54. https://doi.org/10.1002/uog.13217.
16. Bolduc M-E, Limperopoulos C. Neurodevelopmental outcomes in children with cerebellar malformations: a systematic review. Dev Med Child Neurol. 2009;51:256–67. https://doi.org/10.1111/j.1469-8749.2008.03224.x.
17. Pinchefsky EF, Accogli A, Shevell MI, Saint-Martin C, Srour M. Developmental outcomes in children with congenital cerebellar malformations. Dev Med Child Neurol. 2019;61:350–8. https://doi.org/10.1111/dmcn.14059.
18. Poretti A, Limperopoulos C, Roulet-Perez E, Wolf NI, Rauscher C, Prayer D, et al. Outcome of severe unilateral cerebellar hypoplasia. Dev Med Child Neurol. 2010;52:718–24. https://doi.org/10.1111/j.1469-8749.2009.03522.x.
19. Abdelkader MA, Ramadan W, Gabr AA, Kamel A, Abdelrahman RW. Fetal intracranial hemorrhage: sonographic criteria and merits of prenatal diagnosis. J Matern Fetal Neonatal Med. 2017;30:2250–6. https://doi.org/10.1080/14767058.2016.1245283.
20. Hayashi M, Poretti A, Gorra M, Farzin A, Graham EM, Huisman TAGM, et al. Prenatal cerebellar hemorrhage: fetal and postnatal neuroimaging findings and postnatal outcome. Pediatr Neurol. 2015;52:529–34. https://doi.org/10.1016/j.pediatrneurol.2015.01.011.
21. Cheung KW, Tan LN, Seto MTY, Moholkar S, Masson G, Kilby MD. Prenatal diagnosis, management, and outcome of fetal subdural haematoma: a case report and systematic review. Fetal Diagn Ther. 2019;46:285–95. https://doi.org/10.1159/000496202.
22. Raju TNK, Nelson KB, Ferriero D, Lynch JK, and the NICHD-NINDS Perinatal Stroke Workshop Participants. Ischemic Perinatal Stroke: Summary of a Workshop Sponsored by the National Institute of Child Health and Human Development and the National Institute of Neurological Disorders and Stroke. Pediatrics. 2007;120:609–16. https://doi.org/10.1542/peds.2007-0336.
23. Simchen MJ, Goldstein G, Lubetsky A, Strauss T, Schiff E, Kenet G. Factor V Leiden and antiphospholipid antibodies in either mothers or infants increase the risk for Perinatal arterial ischemic Stroke. Stroke. 2009;40:65–70. https://doi.org/10.1161/STROKEAHA.108.527283.
24. Govaert P. Prenatal stroke. Semin Fetal Neonatal Med. 2009;14:250–66. https://doi.org/10.1016/j.siny.2009.07.008.
25. Benders MJNL, Groenendaal F, De Vries LS. Preterm arterial ischemic stroke. Semin Fetal Neonatal Med. 2009;14:272–7. https://doi.org/10.1016/j.siny.2009.07.002.
26. Sandoval JI, De Jesus O. Hydranencephaly. [Updated 2023 Aug 23]. In: StatPearls [Internet]. Treasure Island, FL: StatPearls Publishing; 2024. https://www.ncbi.nlm.nih.gov/books/NBK558991/.

Fetal Intracranial Cysts and Tumors

Elisa Montaguti, Sara Doroldi,
Emiliana Angilletta, and Gianluigi Pilu

Abstract

Fetal intracranial cysts are fluid collections reported at prenatal ultrasound examination in the context of the cerebral parenchyma or in the ventricular system. They appear as anechoic formations of varying size. The prognosis is determined by the location, the dimensions, and the etiology of the formation itself. Usually choroid plexus cysts, when isolated, have a good outcome and often regress during pregnancy. Arachnoid cysts, cavum vergae, and cavum veli interpositi fluid collections are benign as well, without relevant impact on postnatal life. Paraventricular and germinolytic cysts require a careful evaluation of fetal brain, because of the challenging differential diagnosis with periventricular leukomalacia, which is related to brain hypoxic damage.

Intracranial tumors appear as complex masses, causing a remarkable distortion of normal brain architecture. A histological diagnosis is not possible at prenatal ultrasound, and the prognosis is usually poor.

Keywords

Intracranial cyst · Choroid plexus · Arachnoid cyst · Periventricular cyst · Fetal brain · Tumors

1 Fetal Intracranial Cysts

Intracranial cysts represent a frequent finding during prenatal ultrasound examination of fetal brain, appearing as anechoic rounded formations of varying sizes in the context of the cerebral parenchyma or in the ventricular system. Most of these fluid collections, such as arachnoid cysts and choroid plexus cysts, are usually benign and often regress spontaneously in the postnatal life, having no impact on the child neurodevelopment [1–3]. When not associated with other fetal anomalies, they generally do not interfere with normal life, whether or not postnatal treatment is required. The correct diagnosis of their nature is of crucial importance to exclude the presence of other kind of lesions, such as cystic neoplasms or intracranial hemorrhage, which carry a worse prognosis and negatively affect neurodevelopment after birth [3].

The typical ultrasound characteristics of intracranial cysts are those of a hypoechoic mass of variable volume, shifting or lifting up the adjacent brain and/or ventricles. If possible, a precise assessment of the fetal brain performed with

E. Montaguti (✉) · S. Doroldi · E. Angilletta · G. Pilu
Obstetric Unit, IRCCS Azienda Ospedaliero-Universitaria di Bologna, Bologna, Italy
e-mail: gianluigi.pilu@aosp.bo.it

P. Volpe, T. Ghi (eds.), *Fetal Neurosonography*, Ultrasound in Obstetrics and Gynecology,
https://doi.org/10.1007/978-3-031-70192-4_10

Table 1 Classification of fetal intracranial cystic formation

Extra-axial cysts	Intraventricular cysts	Intraparenchymal cysts
Arachnoid cyst	Choroid plexus cyst	Periventricular pseudocyst
Glioependymal cyst	Choroid plexus hemorrhage	Cystic periventricular leukomalacia
Endodermal cyst		Porencephalic cyst
Dural separation		Cystic brain tumor
Cystic tumors (teratoma)		

transvaginal ultrasound is advisable, providing detailed information about location, size, relationship to the ventricular system and midline structures of those formations. This imaging also enables the identification of solid components, as seen in brain tumors, or hemorrhage (i.e., blood clots) and facilitates Doppler studies to assess blood flow patterns in cases of vascular malformations like aneurysms of the vein of Galen. In selected case, in utero magnetic resonance imaging (MRI) can be considered to better define the content of those formations and the presence of cortical disruption [4]. However, despite the progress of imaging techniques, some lesions may still require histological examination of the cyst wall for a definitive diagnosis.

This chapter classifies intracranial cysts into three groups according to their location within the brain: extra-axial cysts, with arachnoid cysts being the most prevalent; intraparenchymal cysts, primarily periventricular pseudocysts and porencephalic cysts, and intraventricular cysts, with choroid plexus cysts being the most common (Table 1).

2 Arachnoid Cysts

2.1 Definition

Arachnoid cysts are collections of cerebrospinal fluid (CSF) between the dura and the brain substance.

2.2 Epidemiology

They represent approximately 1% of all intracranial masses in children [2] and often occur as isolated lesions, with a slight predilection for the left side of the brain, while the occurrence of multiple and bilateral arachnoid cysts is uncommon. They show up with a male-to-female ratio of 2:1, and family presentation has been reported in only a few cases [5–7].

2.3 Etiology and Pathogenesis

Arachnoid cysts can be classified as primary or acquired (secondary) lesions, depending on the absence or presence of prior pathological insults as in utero hemorrhage, infection, or traumas.

At histological examination, the wall of arachnoid cysts is observed to be lined with collagen and cells derived from the arachnoid matter, specifically meningothelial cells. In contrast to normal arachnoid membranes, arachnoid cysts contain a thick layer of collagen and hyperplastic arachnoid cells in the cyst wall, but fewer trabecular processes within the cyst [1, 3]. Electron microscopic analysis and immunohistochemical markers may help in differentiating these cells from epithelium, showing lack of cilia and no staining with antibodies targeting GFAP, S-100, transthyretin, and CEA (common characteristics of epithelial cells).

The leading theory about the pathogenesis of arachnoid cysts suggests that they may result from aberrant subarachnoid development: a disruption in the mesencephalic neural crest is thought to lead to a splitting of the primordial membrane, creating a space where fluid accumulates. Sometimes the CSF accumulates only in advanced stages, making it impossible to diagnose them as early as in the second trimester of pregnancy. The enlargement of these cysts could be attributed to various mechanisms, such as the presence of one-way valve connecting the cyst and the subarachnoid space, the difference in osmotic pressure between the cystic content and cerebrospinal fluid (CSF), or the generation of fluid by the cells lining the cyst walls [6].

2.4 Ultrasound Diagnosis

Most arachnoid cysts can be detected during routine prenatal ultrasonography. Prenatal diagnosis before 20 weeks of gestation is unusual, as reported in one of the largest series evaluating fetuses with arachnoid cysts [8]: they are generally detected during the late second or third trimester of pregnancy [9]. Nonetheless, there have been instances of first-trimester sonographic diagnosis, complemented by histological confirmation of an arachnoid cyst [10, 11].

The characteristic sonographic appearance of arachnoid cysts is that of an anechoic cystic mass with a thin, smooth wall, whose limits are well defined compared to the surrounding parenchyma (Figs. 1, 2, and 3). There might be internal segmentations and usually they have no blood flow on color Doppler imaging [2].

Unlike some intraparenchymal cysts or lesions such as porencephaly, dorsal cysts of holoprosencephaly and schizencephaly, arachnoid cysts do not communicate with lateral ventricles [12]. Nonetheless, ventriculomegaly may appear in up to one-third of cases, especially in advanced stages, sometimes leading to the occurrence of hydrocephalus, due to the obstruction of CSF flow because of the compression caused by the mass itself.

The majority of arachnoid cysts are located in the supratentorial region of the brain: according to the largest series published by Pierre-Kahn, which included 54 patients with arachnoid cysts, 63% of the cysts were supratentorial, predominantly interhemispheric (30%), with a few in the base, suprasellar, or interventricular area and only 22% of the cysts were located infratentorially [13].

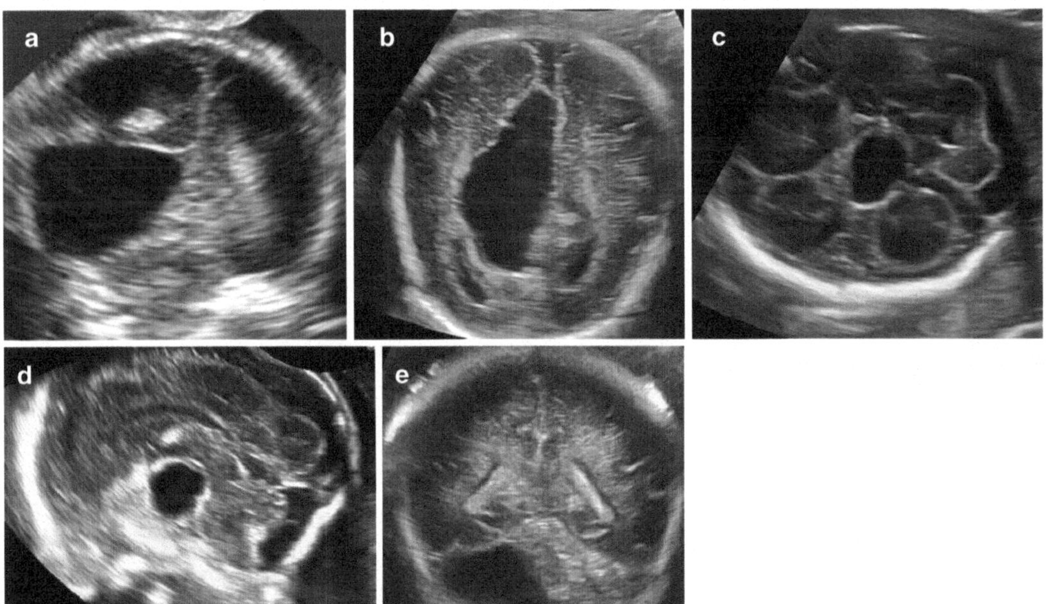

Fig. 1 Examples of arachnoid cysts. The lesions appear as anechoic structures with thin walls fulfilled with cerebrospinal fluid within the arachnoid layer and not communicating with the ventricles. They can be located close to the brain surface (**a**), near the midline (**b**, **c**) or the brainstem (**d**), or in the posterior fossa (**e**)

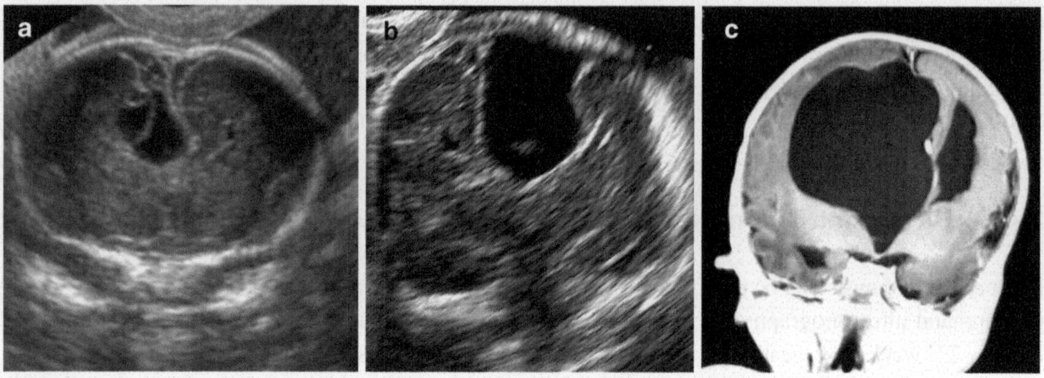

Fig. 2 Examples of arachnoid cysts of increasing size at prenatal ultrasound (**a**, b). Appearance of a big arachnoid fluid collection at postnatal imaging with compression of the brain parenchyma (**c**)

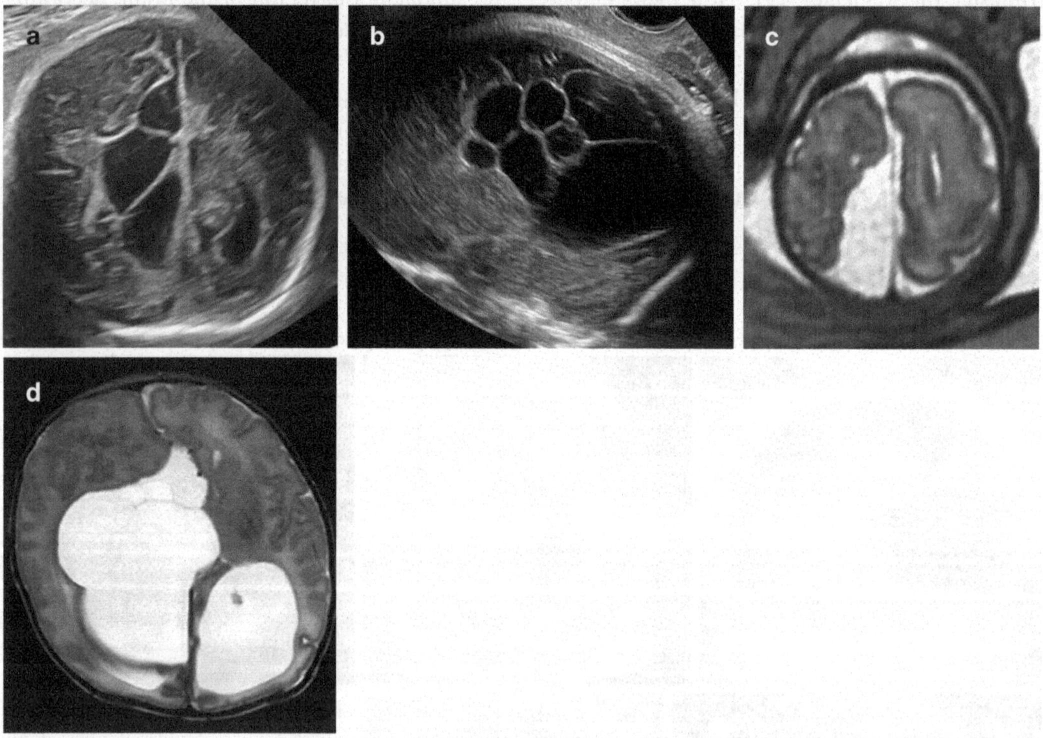

Fig. 3 Complex multilocular arachnoid cyst at prenatal ultrasound (**a**, **b**) and its corresponding at prenatal (**c**) and postnatal (**d**) MRI

2.5 Associated Anomalies

Arachnoid cysts typically manifest as isolated lesions; however, they have been associated with various central nervous system anomalies [14]. These include ventriculomegaly, agenesis of the corpus callosum or other callosal anomalies [11], absent cavum septum pellucidi, vermian abnormalities (including Dandy–Walker malformation) and alobar holoprosencephaly [9], Arnold-Chiari type I malformation, malformations of cortical development, and arteriovenous malformation [15]. No extra-CNS malformations have been found to be strongly linked with arachnoid cysts, anyway it is worth noting that this condition might coexist with abnormalities in other organs, such as shortened femur length, cleft lip and palate, and heart anomalies.

2.6 Risk of Chromosomal Anomalies and Non-chromosomal Syndromes

Most arachnoid cysts are not associated with chromosomal abnormalities [14]. According to previous reports, chromosomal anomalies were reported in 6–10% of the fetuses with arachnoid cysts, and all of these were accompanied by multiple structural abnormalities. Chromosomal abnormalities that have been reported in relation to arachnoid cysts include partial trisomy 9q and partial monosomy Xq [16], unbalanced reciprocal translocation of chromosomes 14q and 20p [17] and trisomy 18 [18].

Few case reports suggest a potential association of arachnoid cysts with non-chromosomal syndromes like distichiasis-lymphedema and Mohr syndrome. However, it is important to note that the strength of this association is low because of the limited number of cases described [14].

2.7 Risk of Recurrence

The discovery of an arachnoid cyst is not generally considered to indicate an elevated risk for future pregnancies. However, there are a few hereditary conditions associated with arachnoid cysts that may increase the likelihood of recurrence, often following an autosomal recessive or X-linked pattern. One example is Aicardi syndrome, a rare X-linked dominant syndrome characterized by agenesis of the corpus callosum, interhemispheric cyst, choroidal anomalies, and infantile seizures [14].

2.8 Obstetrical Management

After the diagnosis of an arachnoid cyst is made, it is reasonable to conduct a targeted and detailed neurosonographic examination and, eventually, a fetal brain MRI. Those exams are useful to determine the exact location and size of the cyst, assessing its impact on nearby brain structures and the presence of any associated intracranial malformations or secondary anomalies [9]. Fetal MRI can be valuable in identifying additional anomalies, particularly cortical migration disorders, providing further reassurance [19].

A comprehensive evaluation of fetal anatomy is recommended, in order to identify extracranial associated anomalies as well as a genetic counseling to discuss possible fetal karyotype assessment [20]. These cases need a sonographic longitudinal follow-up to identify changes in size during pregnancy and to exclude the onset of complications (ventriculomegaly, hydrocephalus, compression of surrounding parenchyma).

There are some reports about experimental interventions, specifically utilizing fetoscopy, when there is a rapid increase in the size of arachnoid cysts. Chalouhi et al [21] documented a successful fetocisternoscopy with fenestration of the cystic wall performed at 31 weeks in a fetus with a rapidly enlarging cyst. The infant was delivered at 36 weeks, underwent an additional neurosurgery after birth with good outcomes. Even if the authors propose fetoscopic surgery as a potential option for cases with rapidly growing intracranial arachnoid cysts, it is essential to note that in utero treatment is not actually a standard of care.

The presence of an arachnoid cyst typically does not impact the mode of delivery unless the presence of hydrocephalus precludes vaginal delivery due to cephalopelvic disproportion.

2.9 Postnatal Therapy

Confirmation of arachnoid cysts should be conducted after birth through MRI or ultrasonography, as certain cysts may either regress after delivery: notably, in 10–40% of patients, cysts are not detectable after birth [19]. Furthermore, a meticulous examination is essential to identify potential congenital anomalies, macrocephaly, intracranial abnormalities, as well as visual and neuroendocrine symptoms.

The management varies depending on the symptoms and the presence of hydrocephalus: while incidentally discovered arachnoid cysts often have a favorable outcome and can be managed expectantly, symptomatic cases are considered candidates for surgical intervention. According to a recent systematic review, surgical interventions were carried out in 44% of patients within the first month, 40% between 1 a d 6 months, and 15% after 6 months. The decision for surgery is influenced by various factors, including ventriculomegaly or hydrocephalus (47%), cystic expansion (15%), and the presence of mass effect or elevated intracranial pressure. Notably, in 87% of cases where cyst progression occurred during fetal development, surgery was necessary shortly after birth [11].

Surgical options for treatment encompass ventriculoperitoneal and cystoperitoneal shunting, open or endoscopic fenestration, and stereotactic aspiration. According to the above cited review, among the patients who underwent surgery, 30% required a second surgery and 5% required a third neurosurgical procedure.

2.10 Prognosis, Survival, and Quality of Life

The presence of clinical manifestations of arachnoid cysts is directly correlated with their size and location within the brain. Small cysts are typically asymptomatic, while larger cysts may have symptoms resulting from the mass effect (seizures, headache, or neurological signs and even motor or behavior anomalies) although it is noteworthy that even large cysts exerting pressure on brain structures may remain asymptomatic. In infants, severe cases of hydrocephalus can manifest with increased head circumference and calvarial asymmetry. Overall, the prognosis is generally favorable, even in cases necessitating drainage in the neonatal or infancy period. Neurodevelopmental outcomes are more closely related to genetic factors and the concomitance of central nervous system (CNS) or extra-CNS abnormalities rather than to the gestational age at diagnosis, cyst size, location, or the necessity for surgery. Furthermore, cases of visual impairment and growth hormone deficits have been reported in connection with large suprasellar cysts.

2.11 Differential Diagnosis

The differential diagnosis of arachnoid cysts should encompass lesions presenting as intracranial hypoechoic formations, including porencephalic cysts, glioependymal cysts, aneurysms of the vein of Galen, schizencephaly, cystic neoplasms, and intracranial hemorrhage [18].

- Porencephalic cysts are characterized by parenchymal loss and lined by white matter and are supposed to be the effect of a localized cerebral insult, most frequently during late gestation (intraparenchymal hemorrhage, ischemia, trauma, or infections); they communicate with the ventricular system or with the subarachnoid space, without mass effect, a distinctive feature in the differential diagnosis of arachnoid cysts [22].
- Glioependymal cysts are uncommon cysts found in various locations. When present extra-axially, distinguishing them from arachnoid cysts can be challenging. Both types appear fulfilled by cerebrospinal fluid on MRI and exhibit no contrast enhancement, necessitating histological examination for an accurate differential diagnosis [23].
- Aneurysms of the vein of Galen present as an elongated anechoic lesion at the level of the cistern of the vein of Galen. They can be differentiated from arachnoid cysts by color and spectral Doppler evidence of intraluminal blood flow [18].
- Schizencephaly is a primitive cortical abnormality resulting in a brain cleft lined by heterotopic gray matter [24]. The cleft can be "open-lip" with separated walls or "closed-lip" with apposed walls and fulfilled with CSF, harder to be distinguished from arachnoid cysts.
- Cystic neoplasms like teratomas and astrocytomas with a cystic component can be differentiated from arachnoid cysts because of the presence of solid irregular portions [25].

- Fetal intracranial hemorrhage: its appearance varies according to the time elapsed from the bleeding. In recent hemorrhages, the blood clot is usually echogenic, while in the older ones the clot is ipo-anechoic and cavitations may occur. The MRI is more reliable in differentiating fetal intracranial hemorrhage from other intracranial lesions [26] thanks to the characteristic T1 MRI signal of hemosiderin deposits.

3 Periventricular Pseudocysts/ Germinolytic Cysts

3.1 Definition

Periventricular pseudocysts (also called "germinolytic cysts") are small intraparenchymal periventricular cystic lesions which can result from different brain insults such as hemorrhages, ischemia, infection, or tumors. The prognosis depends on the underlying cause of the cyst and on the presence of associated anomalies.

3.2 Epidemiology

This finding is quite uncommon in prenatal ultrasound, however the incidence after birth is about 1% in general population and about 3% in the newborns admitted to intensive care unit [27].

3.3 Etiology and Pathogenesis

These cerebral lesions have been commonly named "pseudocysts" since they do not completely fulfill the criteria of cysts, as they do not show an epithelial wall around the fluid collection. Instead, they are surrounded with immature undifferentiated cells, occasionally bordered by a dense glial meshwork [28]. These pseudocysts are normally found within the residual germinative zone, typically situated at the upper external angle of the lateral ventricle, anterior to or at the level of the foramen of Monro [29], in the region of the wall of the caudate nucleus or in the caudothalamic groove. According to their origin, they are also called "germinolytic cysts."

Histologically, the cystic cavity is surrounded by a pseudo-capsule, which comprises aggregates of germinal cells and glial tissue, but no epithelium can be identified in this lining. The origin of germinolytic cysts remains unclear. They can be primitive or acquired; when primitive probably are the result of a persistence of the germinal matrix: this explains why they are more often found in preterm infants [30].

When they are acquired, they are derived by a prenatal disruption of undifferentiated germinal matrix cells. This can result from various factors such as vascular, metabolic, toxic, or teratogenic insults. In particular, viral infections, mainly cytomegalovirus, are commonly diagnosed when the pseudocysts are multilocular and associated with other characteristics abnormalities of the central nervous system [29, 31].

3.4 Ultrasound Diagnosis

They usually appear as unilocular hypoechoic cystic formations with thin wall typically located to the side of lateral ventricles in the germinal matrix (Fig. 4), caudothalamic grove, caudate nucleus, on the lateral side of frontal horns below the level of the roof of the lateral ventricle [32–35]. They can be unilateral or bilateral, uni- or multilocular and show no vascularization on color Doppler. Germinolytic cysts can be detected on the axial planes, but maybe the coronal approach is the most informative, allowing the differential diagnosis with the periventricular leukomalacia, in which the cysts are located superior to the lateral ventricle and are the result of white matter necrosis. Periventricular leukomalacia is more common in preterm infants, as occur after hypoxic-ischemic insults. Transvaginal approach is very useful in those cases.

The role of MRI is quite unclear; because of the typical small size of the lesions, they can be missed by MRI [36]. On the other hand, an MRI should be offered to patient when a periventricular pseudocyst is detected because it could better depict a cortex migration anomaly which may coexist.

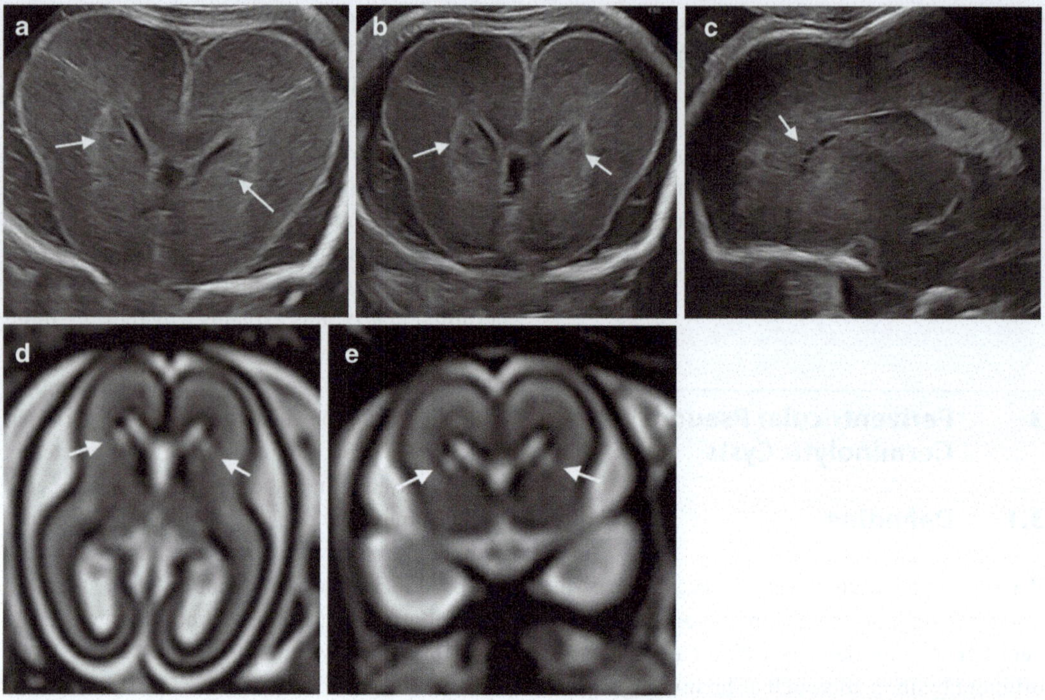

Fig. 4 Ultrasound characteristics of germinolytic cysts by transvaginal approach. They appear as small hypoechoic cystic formations with thin wall located to the side of lateral ventricles in the germinal matrix below the level of the roof of the lateral ventricle (arrow, **a–c**). The same formations at MRI imaging (**d**, **e**)

3.5 Differential Diagnosis

The most challenging differential diagnosis is the distinction between germinolytic cyst, paraventricular cyst, and periventricular leukomalacia, which has a significantly worse prognosis (Fig. 5) [33].

- Leukomalacia is due to white matter necrosis, typically associated with prematurity in preterm newborns but also in fetuses with hypoxic-ischemic insults or as a result of intraamniotic infection/inflammation. These neonates are more likely to develop cerebral palsy and visual impairment. The ultrasound characteristics of periventricular leukomalacia are very similar to those of pseudocysts, but the location is different. Leukomalacia is commonly above the external angle of lateral ventricle and not by its side as periventricular pseudocysts. Coronal views allow this differential diagnosis.

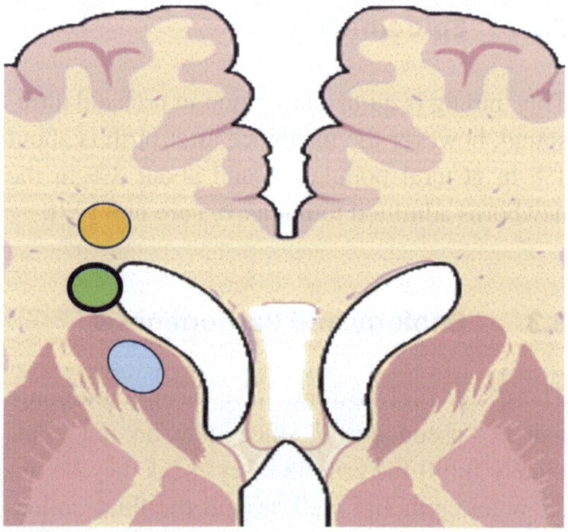

Fig. 5 Differential diagnosis of paraventricular cystic brain formation according to the location in relation of frontal horn of lateral ventricle. Germinolytic pseudocysts (blue) are typically found on the lateral side of frontal horns below the level of the roof of the ventricle in the context of germinal matrix. They have thin wall without epithelium. Periventricular cysts (also called connatal cysts, green) are located on the superior lateral side of frontal horns, with well-defined walls. Periventricular leukomalacia (orange) is the result of white matter necrosis and is located above the external angle of lateral ventricle

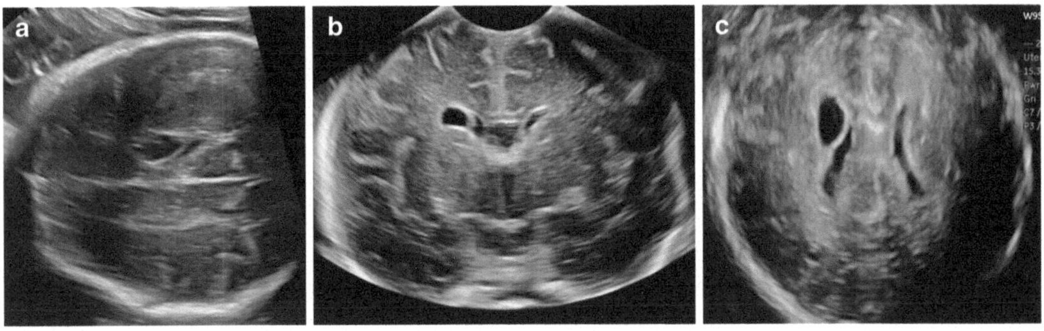

Fig. 6 Periventricular pseudocysts diagnosed in the third trimester of pregnancy (**a–c**) on the superior lateral side of frontal horns. They are supposed to be the result of the juxtaposition the lateral ventricle walls

- Periventricular cysts (or connatal cysts, Fig. 6) are cystic areas adjacent to the superolateral margins of the body and frontal horns of lateral ventricles. They are a quite rare finding, detected in less than 1% of fetuses examined (range 0.4–6%) [37, 38]. They were believed to be a consequence of an insult to the developing brain, but nowadays they are supposed to be a normal variant caused by the juxtaposition of the lateral ventricle walls. Those formations appear as walled cyst located in the superior and lateral aspect of the frontal horn of lateral ventricle, anteriorly to the foramina of Monro. They can be single or multiple ("string of pearl" appearance). The differential diagnosis from leukomalacia or pseudocyst of the germinal matrix is possible on the coronal view, analyzing the location of the cystic formations in relation to the frontal horn. The prognosis of periventricular cysts is usually good, with spontaneous regression at follow-up.

3.6 Associated Anomalies

Germinolytic pseudocysts can be found in association with other brain anomalies, including callosal anomalies, ventriculomegaly, and abnormalities in the cortex development [30]. Signs which may suggest a cytomegalovirus infection can be noted.

3.7 Risk of Chromosomal Anomalies

Pseudocysts are usually sporadic but there are cases associated with metabolic or hereditary disorder; in those cases, the risk of recurrence could be higher and a genetic evaluation should be offered. Those cysts may be a marker of chromosomal deletions associated with impaired neuronal migration, such as Del q6 and Del p4 [39, 40].

3.8 Risk of Nonchromosomal Syndromes

Pseudocysts are likewise identified in metabolic disorders characterized by compromised neuronal migration, including Zellweger syndrome [41], cerebro–hepato–renal syndrome, generalized peroxisomal disorder, and holocarboxylase synthetase deficiency. Notably, in the case of holocarboxylase synthetase deficiency, the administration of biotin supplementation to neonates has shown to be linked to the resolution of pseudocysts within a span of 6 months [42].

3.9 Obstetric Management

When a germinolytic cyst is suspected, it is advisable to perform a focused and comprehensive neurosonographic examination, and if necessary, consider a fetal brain MRI for a more detailed assessment and to identify the presence of associated anomalies, in particular cortex anomaly. MRI typically shows a high intensity in T1-weighted sequences and a low signal in T2-weighted sequences [43]. They do not usually change their aspect during the pregnancy but a longitudinal follow-up is anyway recommended.

The transvaginal ultrasound approach is preferable, as it allows a better evaluation of the periventricular zone.

Since they can represent an acquired lesion, a good practice includes also screening for viral maternal infections (especially CMV, toxoplasmosis, and rubella), assessment of parental platelet compatibility to exclude one of the most common causes of intracranial hemorrhage such as alloimmune thrombocytopenia, and counseling regarding invasive prenatal diagnosis.

When no other clinical indications for a cesarean delivery are present, vaginal birth is recommended.

3.10 Postnatal Therapy

Postnatal therapy for germinolytic cysts identified during prenatal ultrasound typically involves a multidisciplinary approach tailored to the specific clinical scenario. In cases where isolated pseudocysts are detected, the prognosis is good and spontaneous regression is expected [30, 44]. However, if atypical large pseudocysts are identified or if there are associated anomalies or underlying conditions, the prognosis is a less favorable [45, 46] and a multidisciplinary evaluation with pediatric neurology and neurosurgery is needed. Other differential diagnoses are with porencephalic cyst, brain tumor, and arachnoid cyst.

3.11 Prognosis, Survival, and Quality of Life

Isolated pseudocysts generally exhibit a favorable prognosis, with spontaneous regression occurring in up to 93.5% of cases within 1–12 months after birth. The prognosis for atypical pseudocysts, instead, is influenced by the underlying conditions and associated anomalies [32, 47].

4 Choroid Plexus Cysts

4.1 Definition

Choroid plexus cysts are small round sonolucent areas in the atrium of lateral ventricles with a diameter of more than 3 mm; they are typically considered as normal variants and, in most cases, appear after 14 weeks' gestation and typically disappear in the third trimester. When their characteristics or locations are atypical, a detailed neurosonogram and a karyotype analysis may be considered [48].

4.2 Incidence

The real incidence is probably dependent upon the resolution of the ultrasound equipment, the attention of the operator, and the use of transvaginal probe during screening ultrasound. The reported incidence is about 1% of all fetuses scanned [48]. However, some studies reported a incidence as high as 3.6% [49].

4.3 Pathology

The choroid plexus starts its development at about 6 weeks of pregnancy in the roof of the fourth ventricle, then in the lateral and third ventricles, filling the lateral ventricles by 9 weeks of gestation. The choroid plexus is responsible to produce cerebrospinal liquid, and the plexus cysts are the result of a collection of this fluid within the neuroepithelial fold. Fetal cysts of the choroid plexuses are typically a benign and transient finding, and therefore there is a lack of pathological studies, as most of those formation detected during a midtrimester ultrasound will resolve within the third trimester. The ultrasound appearance suggests that those cysts are a collection of fluid surrounded by choroid plexus tissue.

4.4 Diagnosis

Choroid plexus cysts appear as anechoic spaces within the choroid plexus, with well-defined walls (Fig. 7). The cyst may be unilateral or bilateral, and occasionally multiple. At high-resolution ultrasound, the choroid plexus of lateral ventricle appears slightly inhomogeneous: to be defined as cyst, the formation should measure at least 3 mm in diameters [50]. Choroid plexus cysts can be divided in typical and atypical depending on their ultrasound characteristics. Typical cysts are found at the level of the atrium of lateral ventricles, have regular borders, and measure less than 10 mm, without any enlargement of the ventricle cavity. Atypical cysts, instead, can be larger in diameter and usually contain internal segmentations; they can be located not only in the atrium of ventricles, but also at the level of the bodies or the frontal horns.

4.5 Differential Diagnosis

The diagnosis of a choroid plexus cyst is straightforward and is based on the sonographic detection of a simple rounded fluid-filled formation within the atria of lateral ventricles, with normal appearance of the fetal brain. In the minority of case, the differentiation between a large choroid plexus cyst (i.e., distending the cavity of the ventricle) from a primary ventriculomegaly, other intracranial cysts, such as arachnoid cyst, or intracranial hemorrhage can be challenging. Demonstrating the presence of the echogenic wall of the choroid plexus may facilitate the differential diagnosis. In dubious cases, a follow-up scan may be useful, as most choroid plexus cysts will decrease in size and eventually disappear with advancing gestation, while an intraventricular bleeding present with an echogenic clot if recently occurred, and undergo a

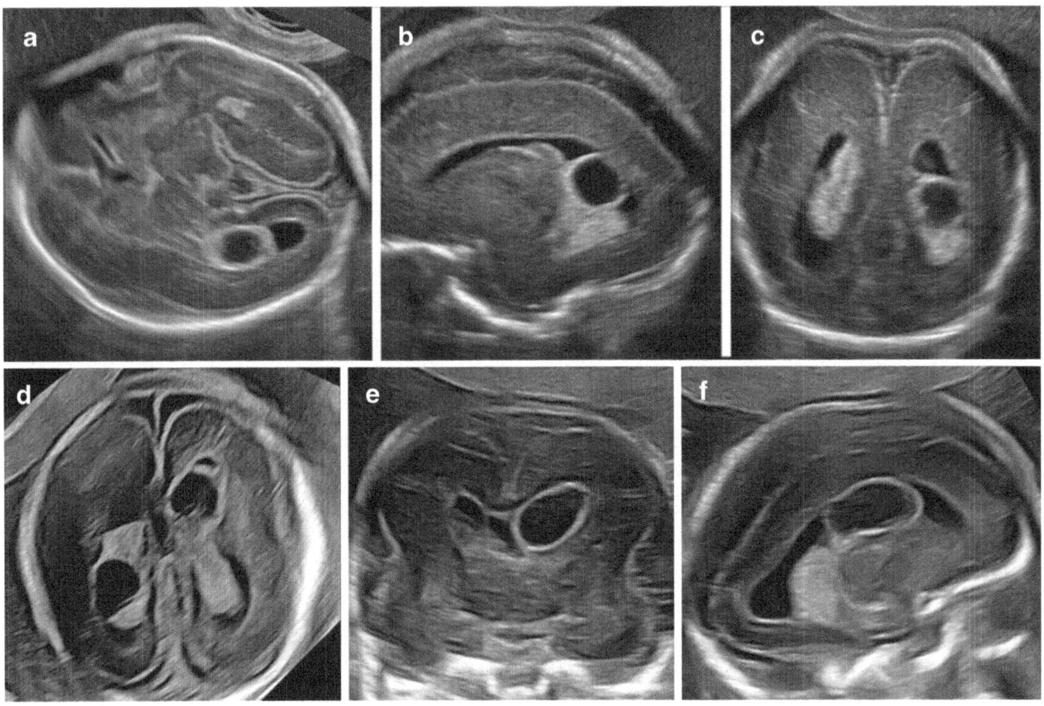

Fig. 7 Typical aspect of a choroid plexus cyst in axial, sagittal, and coronal view during second trimester scan (**a–c**): it appears as an anechoic space within the choroid plexus of lateral ventricles, with well-defined walls, measuring less than 10 mm, without ventriculomegaly. Choroid plexus cysts may be bilateral (**d**) or with atypical features, such as internal segmentations or peculiar locations within the bodies or frontal horns of lateral ventricles (**e**, **f**)

progressive irregular cavitation. In those cases, MRI may be helpful because of its ability to identify hemosiderin deposits typical of hemorrhages [51].

4.6 Associated Anomalies

Most choroid plexus cysts occur as isolated findings in fetuses without any other anomaly detected and with a low risk at first-trimester aneuploidy screening. There have been reports associating choroid plexus cysts with abnormal karyotype, in particular trisomy 18 (85% of cases), but in those cases other anomalies are detected, such as heart defects, skeletal, facial or kidney anomalies, single umbilical artery, thickened nuchal fold, or cystic hygroma. The incidence of trisomy 18 in fetuses without sonographic evidence of associated anomalies was only 0.36%, and it may be lower with a reassuring combined test or NIPT (noninvasive prenatal test). There is no evidence of an association between choroid plexus cysts and any other aneuploidy but trisomy 18 [52, 53].

4.7 Prognosis

When isolated, typical choroid plexus cysts should be considered as normal anatomic variants [48–50]. They are typically seen around midgestation, decrease rapidly in size and tend to disappear by the third trimester. The significance of plexus cysts with atypical appearance or location is uncertain [54]. Some authors report a higher percentage of chromosomal anomalies or deletions/duplications, so in these cases genetic counseling and determination of the fetal karyotype with CGH array can be discussed, although this data needs to be further investigated and the postnatal prognosis is usually good. Euploid children with prenatal diagnosis of choroid plexus cysts have not worse neurocognitive ability, motor function, or behavior than others. The recurrence risk is not known to be increased.

4.8 Obstetrical Management

Isolated choroid plexus cysts with typical appearance and location should not modify standard obstetrical management. Ultrasound atypical features of the cysts such as large size, segmentations, atypical location, and persistence throughout pregnancy have been reported to confer a higher risk of chromosomal abnormalities, but from the available evidence this data are still uncertain and should not be used to modify the counseling [55].

5 Cystic Lesions of Midline Structures

5.1 Cavum Veli Interpositi

5.1.1 Definition

The cavum veli interpositi (CVI) is the space between the double-layered tela choroidea of the third ventricle and occasionally it is fluid-filled and sonographically detected as an interhemispheric anechoic cyst, usually with regular borders.

5.1.2 Etiology/Pathogenesis

The cavum veli interpositi is a space within the double layer of the choroidal tissue of the third ventricle [55]. The tela choroidea is composed of a dual-layer loose connective tissue of pia mater surmounted by the ependyma. It is located antero-inferior to the splenium of the corpus callosum; the columns of the fornix separate it from the septum pellucidum and from the cavum vergae. This space may occasionally be filled with fluid and visible as an interhemispheric anechoic cyst. Embryologically, the CVI originates from the diencephalon by an extension of the pia mater, which protrudes into the primitive neural tube during the third month of gestation.

5.1.3 Sonographic Findings and Differential Diagnosis

At ultrasound, CVI cyst appears as a round-shaped lesion with regular borders within the interhemispheric scissure (Figs. 8 and 9); in axial

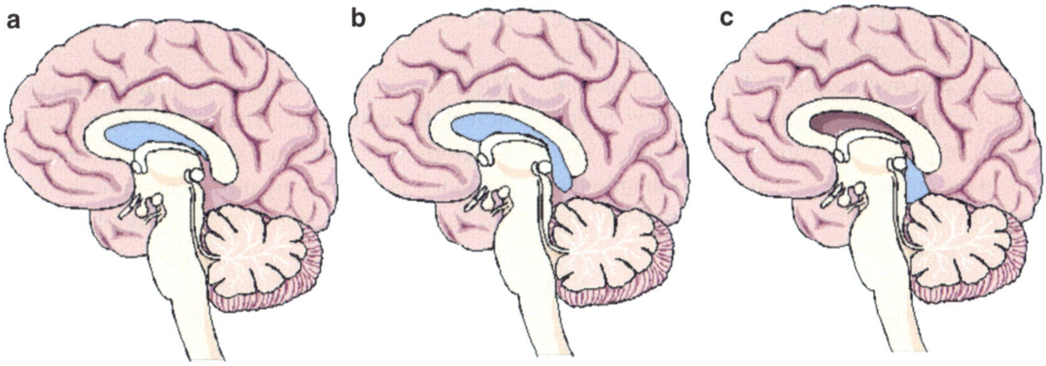

Fig. 8 Median sagittal plane of a normal brain (**a**): the "cavum septi pellucidi" is the cavity between the two leaflets of the septum pellucidum (blue) and it is delimited anteriorly and superiorly by the corpus callosum, inferiorly by the fornix and posteriorly by the splenium of the corpus callosum. The "cavum vergae" (**b**) is a posterior extension of the cavum septum pellucidum itself, lying between the splenium of the corpus callosum and the posterior columns of the fornix. A cavum veli interpositi cyst (**c**) is located under the splenium of the corpus callosum, over the thalamus and is separated from the cavum septi pellucidi

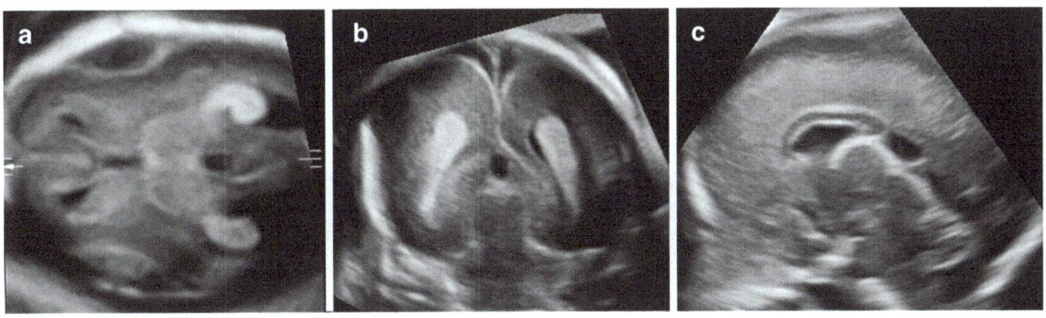

Fig. 9 Typical aspect at 3D ultrasound of a cavum veli interpositi cyst. In axial planes (**a**), it appears as a small round-shaped lesion with regular borders within the interhemispheric scissure, posteriorly to the thalamus. In coronal (**b**) and sagittal plane (**c**), CVI cyst can be seen under the splenium of the corpus callosum above the thalamus. It is separated from the cavum septum pellucidum

scan is located posteriorly to the thalamus [55–57]. In the midsagittal view, CVI cyst can be seen under the splenium of the corpus callosum, over the thalamus; the columns of the fornix constitute the superolateral walls of the cyst, separating it from the septum pellucidum and the cavum vergae. Sometimes CVI cysts may be larger in size and with irregular walls. The differential diagnosis is with a dilation of the septum pellucidum or cavum vergae and with an arachnoid cyst of the quadrigeminal cistern. The sagittal scan is useful in distinguishing between these lesions: the dilation of cavum vergae is superior and anterior to the columns of the fornix, in continuity with the corpus callosum; CVI cyst instead is separated from the corpus callosum and from the ventricular system.

5.1.4 Prognosis

Those formations are classified separately from arachnoid cysts, due to their different prognostic significance. It is difficult to distinguish by ultrasound a true cyst of the CVI from a para-physiological accumulation of fluid within this space, which tends to disappear during pregnancy or after birth. Neonatal outcome appears to be mainly related to the size of the cyst at birth; the prognosis is good in most cases when no other malformations are demonstrated [14].

At birth, CVI cysts are mostly asymptomatic, but psychotic disorders, motor abnormalities, epilepsy, and hydrocephalus have been reported, although rare, in those children with big formations. The postnatal treatment, if required, consists in the collapse of the cavity, the shunting, or the endoscopic ventricular fenestration and has almost always a good prognosis [56].

5.1.5 Obstetrics Management

Progression of the cysts in utero is quite rare, while the regression may occur in 25% of cases. When a CVI cyst is reported, a careful examination of the fetal brain and of the extracerebral anatomy should be performed. The incidence of other associated intracranial and extracranial anomalies has been reported in 31% and 6% of the cases, respectively [14]. In the isolated cases, the fetal karyotype is usually normal. Routine obstetric management is not modified by the finding of a CVI cyst.

5.2 Cavum Vergae

The cavum vergae is a posterior fluid-filled extension of the septi pellucidi cavity. It communicates anteriorly with the cavum septi pellucidi, and it is delimited posteriorly by the splenium of the corpus callosum, superiorly by the body of the corpus callosum and inferiorly by the columns of fornix (Figs. 8 and 10). It has also been referred to as the sixth ventricle, but this definition was abandoned because of the lack of any direct communication between the cavum vergae and the ventricular system [57–59].

In some fetuses, this cavity is fluid-filled and therefore detectable at ultrasound as the persistence of the embryological space between the leaflets of the septum pellucidum. In axial planes, the cavum septi pellucidi appears elongated posteriorly. The differential diagnosis is between a CVI cyst or an interhemispheric arachnoid cyst: in sagittal planes, the diagnosis is easily made by

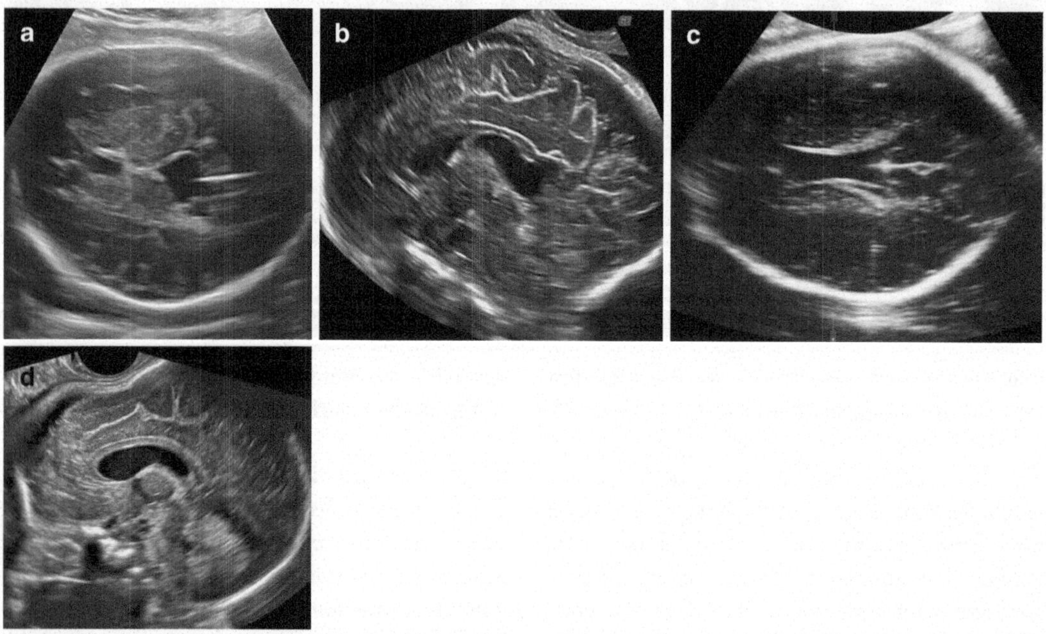

Fig. 10 Axial (**a**) and sagittal (**b**) view of a large cavum veli interpositi cyst, with irregular shape and borders; it is located at the inferior part of the splenium of the corpus callosum. Axial (**c**) and midsagittal (**d**) view of a large cavum vergae: in axial planes is seen as an elongated cavum speti pellucidi; the diagnosis is confirmed by sagittal evaluation, where a posterior prolongation beyond the corpus callosum splenium communicating with the cavum septi pellucidi itself is demonstrated

demonstrating this posterior prolongation of the cavum septi pellucidi beyond the corpus callosum splenium. The use of color Doppler helps to exclude a Galen vein aneurism. In the absence of any other brain or extra-brain anomaly, the prognosis is usually good and in isolated cases the risk of chromosomal anomalies is not increased.

By term cavum vergae and cavum septi pellucidi will progressively obliterate and are not detectable after 37 weeks in most fetuses; in the remaining cases, they will close by 6 months of age and only in sporadic cases this dilatation may persist in adulthood but is usually asymptomatic.

6 Intracranial Tumors

6.1 Definition

Fetal intracranial tumors are rare intracranial formations with an incidence of 0.34 per million live births; at ultrasound they appear as complex vascularized masses distorting the normal intracranial anatomy. Their histological differential diagnosis is quite challenging in prenatal life.

6.2 Pathology and Ultrasound Characteristics

The etiology of fetal brain tumors is unknown, but they are thought to derive from embryologically dysplastic cells. In animals, those formations are induced by chemical or viral teratogens but in human brain, the role of these agents in inducing brain neoplasm is still uncertain (Figs. 11 and 12).

The anatomical origin of tumors diagnosed in utero is frequently difficult to ascertain, given the large dimensions of the mass at the time of sonographic diagnosis. Most of the lesions are however supratentorial, in contrast to the more frequent infratentorial location of brain tumors occurring in pediatric population. The most frequent fetal brain tumor is teratoma (62%), while

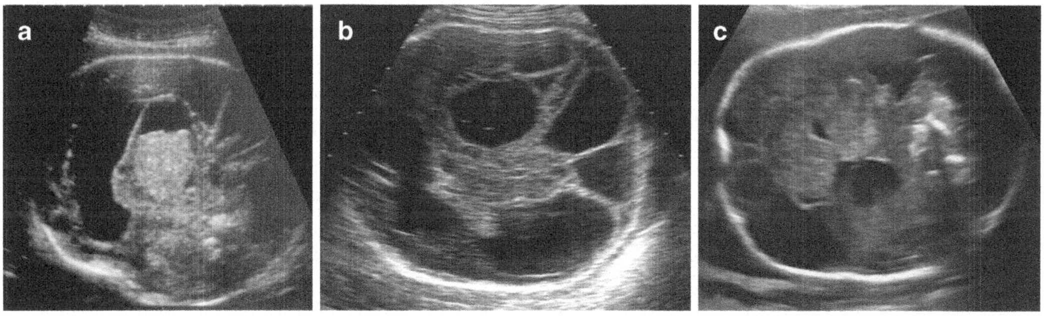

Fig. 11 Sonographic characteristics of three cases of fetal teratomas (**a–c**), appearing as complex masses with mixed solid and fluid content, causing major distortion of fetal brain

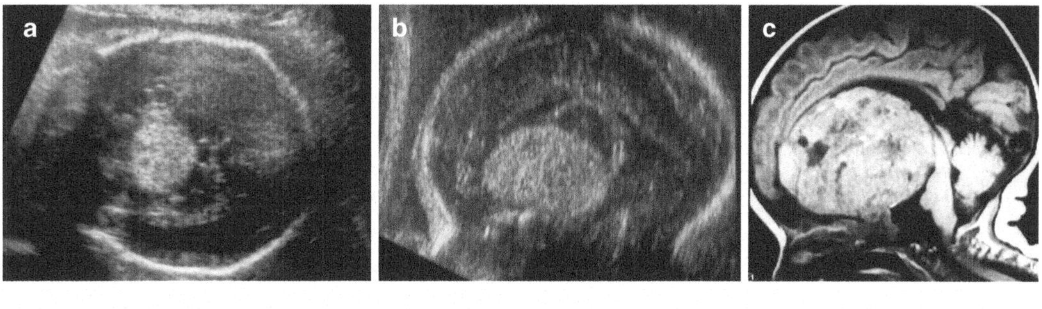

Fig. 12 Axial (**a**) and sagittal (**b**) view of a fetal craniopharyngioma: this case presents a prevalent solid component and is located in the suprasellar region. Postnatal MRI appearance of the same case (**c**)

neuroepithelial tumors represent the 15%, lipomas 15%, and craniopharyngiomas 6% [60] of the cases.

There are several classifications of congenital brain tumors (Table 2).

The most frequent are as follows [61]:

– **Teratoma:** It is the most frequent variant of intracranial neoplasms diagnosed antenatally (48%). They usually appear as complex masses with mixed solid and fluid content, causing major distortion of the surrounding brain and often associated with macrocrania because of the rapid growth especially during the third trimester of pregnancy. Teratomas may contain well-differentiated structures (hair, bone, or muscle) or undifferentiated structures: in the latter case, the tendency to malignancy is higher. The regions where they are more frequently detected are the pineal region, the suprasellar region, or within the fourth ventricle [60–63]. From the brain, teratomas may expand toward extracranial region, through orbits, mouth, or occipital bone. The prognosis is typically poor, with a 93% mortality during the first year of life.
– **Epidermoid tumors:** Derive from epithelial cells and appear as cystic lesions which contain an inhomogeneous material originating by the desquamation of the internal epithelial lining. They are mostly located at the level of the cerebellopontine angle, suprasellar region, and temporal lobe.
– **Dermoid tumors** contain desquamated epithelium, sebaceous secretions and hair and are usually connected with the skin surface by a dermal sinus. The most frequent location is the posterior fossa.
– **Germinomas** originate from germ cells. They are solid mass located in the pineal and suprasellar regions.
– Tumors originating from differentiated germ cells include **choriocarcinoma** (trophoblastic cells), **endodermal sinus tumor** (yolk sac), and **embryonal carcinoma**.
– **Medulloblastoma** only arises in the posterior fossa. It is a highly malignant lesion that appears as a soft, friable mass often inhomogeneous in its content because of the presence of necrosis.
– **Craniopharyngioma** is the most frequent supratentorial tumor in children. It originates from the craniopharyngeal duct and consists of both cystic and solid components located in the suprasellar region. It appears as a complex mass distorting the brain architecture and can be associated with intracranial calcification, ventriculomegaly, and macrocephaly.
– **Choroid plexus tumors** appear as echogenic masses within the ventricle; their differentiation from intraventricular hemorrhages is challenging at ultrasound, as well as the distinction between benign formations (papilloma) or malignant mass (carcinoma) because the sonographic appearance is similar. They can lead to ventriculomegaly and subarach-

Table 2 Classification of congenital intracranial tumors

Classification
Embryonic tumors
Teratoma
Epidermoid
Dermoid
Germinal tumors
Germinoma
Embryonal carcinoma
Choriocarcinoma
Endodermal sinus tumor
Neuroblastic tumors
Medulloblastoma
Neuroblastoma
Retinoblastoma
Tumors related to embryonal remnant tissues
Craniopharyngioma
Chordoma
Tumors of ependymal origin
Ependymoma
Subependymal mixed glioma
Choroid plexus papilloma
Multiform glioblastoma
Malignant astrocytoma
Tumors associated with genetic diseases
Tuberous sclerosis (Bourneville's disease)
Neurofibromatosis (von Recklinghausen's disease)
Systemic angiomatosis of the CNS and eye (Von Hippel–Lindau disease)
Colloid cyst of the third ventricle
Heterotopia and hamartoma
Lipoma
Vascular tumors: Hemangioblastoma

noid space enlargement [64]. Papillomas are by far more frequent in the neonatal period than in prenatal life [65].
- **Multiform glioblastoma** (also called hemorrhagic glioblastoma) is the most frequent neoplasm originating from glial cells of the cerebral hemispheres, less frequently of the brainstem or the spinal cord. The differential diagnosis from an intracranial hemorrhage can benefit from a MRI evaluation.
- **Lipomas:** They are a relatively frequent finding and appear as a well-defined echogenic area, usually located in the midline, in the position normally occupied by the corpus callosum, and/or within the bodies of lateral ventricles. They are quite frequently associated with callosal anomalies (complete or partial agenesis). The prognosis is usually good, even if the patients can develop epilepsy during the second decade of life.

Tuberous sclerosis, neurofibromatosis, and systemic angiomatosis of the CNS and eye are autosomal dominant diseases characterized by the presence of intracranial tumors. Neurofibromatosis is associated with acoustic neurinoma, multiple meningioma, and glioma. Systemic angiomatosis of the CNS and eye is characterized by cerebellar hemangioblastoma. In tuberous sclerosis, multiple neuroglial nodules are detected within the brain, together with single or multiple cardiac rhabdomyomas.

6.3 Associated Anomalies

Fetal intracranial tumors are frequently associated with macrocephaly, ventriculomegaly because of the obstruction of cerebrospinal fluid circulation, intracranial calcifications, or hemorrhages. A quite frequent finding is polyhydramnios (40% of cases), probably related to a neurological insult and a subsequent failure of swallowing or because of a pharynx mechanical obstruction. Hydrops has also been described as a consequence of arteriovenous shunting within the mass and high-output cardiac failure. Attention must be paid to face and neck because some neoplasm can extend out of the cranial skull. The relationship between interhemispheric lipomas and agenesis of the corpus callosum is well established. The risk of chromosomal aberrations is usually not increased.

6.4 Diagnosis

An intracranial tumor is suspected when a mass is seen within the fetal brain, both with cystic and solid components [60, 61, 63, 66]. The suspicion is raised also when a change in the shape or size of the head is seen, as well as a shift in the midline or a distortion of normal brain structures. The ultrasound characteristics, however, usually do not allow a specific diagnosis of the histologic type. Frequently, the aspect of these neoplasms is not easy to be differentiated from brain hemorrhages or hydrocephalus. Magnetic resonance is helpful to characterize better the normal cerebral parenchyma from the tumor mass as well as its extracranial extension.

6.5 Differential Diagnosis

The differential diagnosis of intracranial tumors includes other occupying space intracranial lesions: it can be particularly challenging to distinguish between a tumor and a recent intraparenchymal hemorrhage, with the blood clot resembling the solid neoplasm component. In these cases, serial sonograms or antenatal MRI may enable a specific diagnosis.

6.6 Prognosis

The prognosis of congenital brain tumors is frequently poor, especially for those cases diagnosed in utero. The mortality rate is 77% overall [60], and the neurological impairment in survivors is expected to be high as well. The histologic type of tumor is a major prognostic factor: in postnatal series, the one-year survival rate of teratomas was 7%, 44% of astrocytomas [67], while choroid plexus papillomas or lipomas have a better outcome. Unfortunately, the antenatal diagnosis of the specific type of tumor is not possible in most cases.

6.7 Obstetrical Management

Pregnancy termination can be offered to the parents according to country law; however, a large proportion of cases are diagnosed at late gestation when this option is mostly not permitted. In the presence of large complex masses distorting cerebral anatomy, the prognosis is generally poor and a conservative management should be offered to the couple, without modifying the current obstetrical care.

References

1. Malinger G, Sereño EC, Lerman-Sagie T. The differential diagnosis of fetal intracranial cystic lesions. Ultrasound Clinics. 2008;3(4):553–8.
2. Pierre-Kahn A, Sonigo P. Malformative intracranial cysts: diagnosis and outcome. Childs Nerv Syst. 2003;19(7–8):477–83.
3. Pappalardo EM, Militello M, Rapisarda G, Imbruglia L, Recupero S, Ermito S, Dinatale A, Carrara S, Cavaliere A. Fetal intracranial cysts: prenatal diagnosis and outcome. J Prenat Med. 2009;3(2):28–30.
4. Rossi AC, Prefumo F. Additional value of fetal magnetic resonance imaging in the prenatal diagnosis of central nervous system anomalies: a systematic review of the literature. Ultrasound Obstet Gynecol. 2014;44(4):388–93.
5. Galassi E, Tognetti F, Gaist G, Fagioli L, Frank F, Frank G. CT scan and metrizamide CT cisternography in arachnoid cysts of the middle cranial fossa: classification and pathophysiological aspects. Surg Neurol. 1982;17(5):363–9.
6. Gosalakkal JA. Intracranial arachnoid cysts in children: a review of pathogenesis, clinical features, and management. Pediatr Neurol. 2002;26(2):93–8.
7. Sato K, Shimoji T, Yaguchi K, Sumie H, Kuru Y, Ishii S. Middle fossa arachnoid cyst: clinical, neuroradiological, and surgical features. Childs Brain. 1983;10(5):301–16.
8. Yeaton-Massey A, Monteagudo A. Intracranial cysts. Am J Obstet Gynecol. 2020;223(6):B42–b6.
9. Yin L, Yang Z, Pan Q, Zhang J, Li X, Wang F, Ye Y, Deng X, Hu C. Sonographic diagnosis and prognosis of fetal arachnoid cysts. J Clin Ultrasound. 2018;46(2):96–102.
10. Bretelle F, Senat MV, Bernard JP, Hillion Y, Ville Y. First-trimester diagnosis of fetal arachnoid cyst: prenatal implication. Ultrasound Obstet Gynecol. 2002;20(4):400–2.
11. Beresford C, Hall S, Smedley A, Mathad N, Waters R, Chakraborty A, Sparrow OC, Tsitouras V. Prenatal diagnosis of arachnoid cysts: a case series and systematic review. Childs Nerv Syst. 2020;36(4):729–41.
12. Chuang S, Harwood-Nash D. Tumors and cysts. Neuroradiology. 1986;28(5–6):463–75.
13. Pierre-Kahn A, Hanlo P, Sonigo P, Parisot D, McConnell RS. The contribution of prenatal diagnosis to the understanding of malformative intracranial cysts: state of the art. Childs Nerv Syst. 2000;16(10–11):619–26.
14. Youssef A, D'Antonio F, Khalil A, Papageorghiou AT, Ciardulli A, Lanzone A, Rizzo G, Thilaganathan B, Pilu G. Outcome of fetuses with supratentorial extra-axial intracranial cysts: a systematic review. Fetal Diagn Ther. 2016;40(1):1–12.
15. Malinger G, Kidron D, Schreiber L, Ben-Sira L, Hoffmann C, Lev D, Lerman-Sagie T. Prenatal diagnosis of malformations of cortical development by dedicated neurosonography. Ultrasound Obstet Gynecol. 2007;29(2):178–91.
16. Hogge WA, Schnatterly P, Ferguson JE 2nd. Early prenatal diagnosis of an infratentorial arachnoid cyst: association with an unbalanced translocation. Prenat Diagn. 1995;15(2):186–8.
17. Souter VL, Glass IA, Chapman DB, Raff ML, Parisi MA, Opheim KE, Disteche CM. Multiple fetal anomalies associated with subtle subtelomeric chromosomal rearrangements. Ultrasound Obstet Gynecol. 2003;21(6):609–15.
18. Pilu G, Falco P, Perolo A, Sandri F, Cocchi G, Ancora G, Bovicelli L. Differential diagnosis and outcome of fetal intracranial hypoechoic lesions: report of 21 cases. Ultrasound Obstet Gynecol. 1997;9(4):229–36.
19. Yahal O, Katorza E, Zvi E, Berkenstadt M, Hoffman C, Achiron R, Bar-Yosef O. Prenatal diagnosis of arachnoid cysts: MRI features and neurodevelopmental outcome. Eur J Radiol. 2019;113:232–7.
20. Hong S, Pae J, Ko HS. Fetal arachnoid cyst: characteristics, management in pregnancy, and neurodevelopmental outcomes. Obstet Gynecol Sci. 2023;66(2):49–57.
21. Chalouhi GE, Marangoni M, Zerah M, Ville Y. P09.24: Intrauterine treatment of a suprasellar interhemispheric arachnoid cyst by feto-cisternoscopy. Ultrasound Obstetr Gynecol. 2012;40(S1):210.
22. Abergel A, Lacalm A, Massoud M, Massardier J, des Portes V, Guibaud L. Expanding porencephalic cysts: prenatal imaging and differential diagnosis. Fetal Diagn Ther. 2017;41(3):226–33.
23. Robles LA, Paez JM, Ayala D, Boleaga-Duran B. Intracranial glioependymal (neuroglial) cysts: a systematic review. Acta Neurochir (Wien). 2018;160(7):1439–49.
24. Halabuda A, Klasa L, Kwiatkowski S, Wyrobek L, Milczarek O, Gergont A. Schizencephaly-diagnostics and clinical dilemmas. Childs Nerv Syst. 2015;31(4):551–6.

25. Chen CP, Chang TY, Wang W. Third-trimester ultrasound evaluation of arachnoid cysts. Taiwan J Obstet Gynecol. 2007;46(4):427–8.
26. Adiego B, Martínez-Ten P, Bermejo C, Estévez M, Recio Rodriguez M, Illescas T. Fetal intracranial hemorrhage. Prenatal diagnosis and postnatal outcomes. J Matern Fetal Neonatal Med. 2019;32(1):21–30.
27. Ramenghi LA, Domizio S, Quartulli L, Sabatino G. Prenatal pseudocysts of the germinal matrix in preterm infants. J Clin Ultrasound. 1997;25(4):169–73.
28. De León GA, Girling DJ. Cystic degeneration of the telencephalic subependymal germinal layer in newborn infants. J Neurol Neurosurg Psychiatry. 1975;38(3):265–71.
29. Rademaker KJ, De Vries LS, Barth PG. Subependymal pseudocysts: ultrasound diagnosis and findings at follow-up. Acta Paediatr. 1993;82(4):394–9.
30. Bats AS, Molho M, Senat MV, Paupe A, Bernard JP, Ville Y. Subependymal pseudocysts in the fetal brain: prenatal diagnosis of two cases and review of the literature. Ultrasound Obstet Gynecol. 2002;20(5):502–5.
31. Achiron R, Pinhas-Hamiel O, Lipitz S, Heiman Z, Reichman B, Mashiach S. Prenatal ultrasonographic diagnosis of fetal cerebral ventriculitis associated with asymptomatic maternal cytomegalovirus infection. Prenat Diagn. 1994;14(7):523–6.
32. Makhoul IR, Zmora O, Tamir A, Shahar E, Sujov P. Congenital subependymal pseudocysts: own data and meta-analysis of the literature. Isr Med Assoc J. 2001;3(3):178–83.
33. Malinger G, Lev D, Ben Sira L, Kidron D, Tamarkin M, Lerman-Sagie T. Congenital periventricular pseudocysts: prenatal sonographic appearance and clinical implications. Ultrasound Obstet Gynecol. 2002;20(5):447–51.
34. Malinger G, Lev D, Lerman-Sagie T. Imaging of fetal cytomegalovirus infection. Fetal Diagn Ther. 2011;29(2):117–26.
35. Malinger G, Lev D, Zahalka N, Ben Aroia Z, Watemberg N, Kidron D, Sira LB, Lerman-Sagie T. Fetal cytomegalovirus infection of the brain: the spectrum of sonographic findings. AJNR Am J Neuroradiol. 2003;24(1):28–32.
36. Qiu L, Chen N, Luo H. Fetal periventricular pseudocysts: is MRI evaluation needed? What is the long-term neurodevelopmental outcome? Systematic review and meta-analysis. Arch Gynecol Obstet. 2023;307(6):1697–711.
37. T. R, D. B, H. K. Connatal cyst. Reference article, Radiopaedia.org
38. Scelsi CL, Rahim TA, Morris JA, Kramer GJ, Gilbert BC, Forseen SE. The lateral ventricles: a detailed review of anatomy, development, and anatomic variations. AJNR Am J Neuroradiol. 2020;41(4):566–72.
39. De Keersmaecker B, Albert M, Hillion Y, Ville Y. Prenatal diagnosis of brain abnormalities in Wolf-Hirschhorn (4p-) syndrome. Prenat Diagn. 2002;22(5):366–70.
40. Rohrbach M, Chitayat D, Maegawa G, Shanske S, Davidzon G, Chong K, Clarke JT, Toi A, Tarnopolsky M, Robinson B, Blaser S. Intracerebral periventricular pseudocysts in a fetus with mitochondrial depletion syndrome: an association or coincidence. Fetal Diagn Ther. 2009;25(2):177–82.
41. Russel IM, van Sonderen L, van Straaten HL, Barth PG. Subependymal germinolytic cysts in Zellweger syndrome. Pediatr Radiol. 1995;25(4):254–5.
42. Squires L, Betz B, Umfleet J, Kelley R. Resolution of subependymal cysts in neonatal holocarboxylase synthetase deficiency. Dev Med Child Neurol. 1997;39(4):267–9.
43. Sun C, Zhang X, Chen X, Wei X, Chen Y, Yang A, Zhu J, Wang G. Evaluation of MRI features and neurodevelopmental outcomes for prenatally diagnosed periventricular pseudocysts. Front Pediatr. 2021;9:681999.
44. Lu JH, Emons D, Kowalewski S. Connatal periventricular pseudocysts in the neonate. Pediatr Radiol. 1992;22(1):55–8.
45. Esteban H, Blondiaux E, Audureau E, Sileo C, Moutard ML, Gelot A, Jouannic JM, Ducou le Pointe H, Garel C. Prenatal features of isolated subependymal pseudocysts associated with adverse pregnancy outcome. Ultrasound Obstet Gynecol. 2015;46(6):678–87.
46. Cooper S, Bar-Yosef O, Berkenstadt M, Hoffmann C, Achiron R, Katorza E. Prenatal evaluation, imaging features, and neurodevelopmental outcome of prenatally diagnosed periventricular pseudocysts. AJNR Am J Neuroradiol. 2016;37(12):2382–8.
47. Levy M, Lev D, Leibovitz Z, Kashanian A, Gindes L, Tamarkin M, Shalev J, Sira LB, Mizrachi Y, Borovich A, Birnbaum R, Lerman-Sagie T, Malinger G, Haratz KK. Periventricular pseudocysts of noninfectious origin: Prenatal associated findings and prognostic factors. Prenat Diagn. 2020;40(8):931–41.
48. Gupta JK, Cave M, Lilford RJ, Farrell TA, Irving HC, Mason G, Hau CM. Clinical significance of fetal choroid plexus cysts. Lancet. 1995;346(8977):724–9.
49. Chinn DH, Miller EI, Worthy LM, Towers CV. Sonographically detected fetal choroid plexus cysts. Frequency and association with aneuploidy. J Ultrasound Med. 1991;10(5):255–8.
50. Chitty LS, Chudleigh P, Wright E, Campbell S, Pembrey M. The significance of choroid plexus cysts in an unselected population: results of a multicenter study. Ultrasound Obstet Gynecol. 1998;12(6):391–7.
51. Shah N. Prenatal diagnosis of choroid plexus cyst: what next? J Obstet Gynaecol India. 2018;68(5):366–8.
52. Snijders RJ, Shawa L, Nicolaides KH. Fetal choroid plexus cysts and trisomy 18: assessment of risk based on ultrasound findings and maternal age. Prenat Diagn. 1994;14(12):1119–27.
53. Leonardi MR, Wolfe HM, Lanouette JM, Landwehr JB, Johnson MP, Evans MI. The apparently isolated choroid plexus cyst: importance of minor abnormalities in predicting the risk for aneuploidy. Fetal Diagn Ther. 1998;13(1):49–52.
54. Prabhu M, Kuller JA, Biggio JR. Society for Maternal-Fetal Medicine Consult Series #57: Evaluation and

management of isolated soft ultrasound markers for aneuploidy in the second trimester: (Replaces Consults #10, Single umbilical artery, October 2010; #16, Isolated echogenic bowel diagnosed on second-trimester ultrasound, August 2011; #17, Evaluation and management of isolated renal pelviectasis on second-trimester ultrasound, December 2011; #25, Isolated fetal choroid plexus cysts, April 2013; #27, Isolated echogenic intracardiac focus, August 2013). Am J Obstet Gynecol. 2021;225(4):B2–B15.
55. Shah PS, Blaser S, Toi A, Fong K, Glanc P, Babul-Hirji R, Rutka J, Chitayat D. Cavum veli interpositi: prenatal diagnosis and postnatal outcome. Prenat Diagn. 2005;25(7):539–42.
56. D'Addario V, Pinto V, Rossi AC, Pintucci A, Di Cagno L. Cavum veli interpositi cyst: prenatal diagnosis and postnatal outcome. Ultrasound Obstet Gynecol. 2009;34(1):52–4.
57. Vergani P, Locatelli A, Piccoli MG, Ceruti P, Patanè L, Paterlini G, Ghidini A. Ultrasonographic differential diagnosis of fetal intracranial interhemispheric cysts. Am J Obstet Gynecol. 1999;180(2 Pt 1):423–8.
58. Sherer DM, Sokolovski M, Dalloul M, Santoso P, Curcio J, Abulafia O. Prenatal diagnosis of dilated cavum septum pellucidum et vergae. Am J Perinatol. 2004;21(5):247–51.
59. Tao G, Lu G, Zhan X, Li J, Cheng L, Lee K, Poon WS. Sonographic appearance of the cavum septum pellucidum et vergae in normal fetuses in the second and third trimesters of pregnancy. J Clin Ultrasound. 2013;41(9):525–31.
60. Schlembach D, Bornemann A, Rupprecht T, Beinder E. Fetal intracranial tumors detected by ultrasound: a report of two cases and review of the literature. Ultrasound Obstet Gynecol. 1999;14(6):407–18.
61. Cornejo P, Feygin T, Vaughn J, Pfeifer CM, Korostyshevska A, Patel M, Bardo DME, Miller J, Goncalves LF. Imaging of fetal brain tumors. Pediatr Radiol. 2020;50(13):1959–73.
62. D'Addario V, Pinto V, Meo F, Resta M. The specificity of ultrasound in the detection of fetal intracranial tumors. J Perinat Med. 1998;26(6):480–5.
63. Sherer DM, Onyeije CI. Prenatal ultrasonographic diagnosis of fetal intracranial tumors: a review. Am J Perinatol. 1998;15(5):319–28.
64. Pilu G, De Palma L, Romero R, Bovicelli L, Hobbins JC. The fetal subarachnoid cisterns: an ultrasound study with report of a case of congenital communicating hydrocephalus. J Ultrasound Med. 1986;5(7):365–72.
65. Anselem O, Mezzetta L, Grangé G, Zerah M, Benard C, Marcou V, Fallet-Bianco C, Adamsbaum C, Tsatsaris V. Fetal tumors of the choroid plexus: is differential diagnosis between papilloma and carcinoma possible? Ultrasound Obstet Gynecol. 2011;38(2):229–32.
66. Isaacs H. Fetal brain tumors: a review of 154 cases. Am J Perinatol. 2009;26(6):453–66.
67. Wakai S, Arai T, Nagai M. Congenital brain tumors. Surg Neurol. 1984;21(6):597–609.
68. Neblett CR, Robertson JW. Symptomatic cysts of the telencephalic choroid plexus. J Neurol Neurosurg Psychiatry. 1971;34(3):324–8.

Neural Tube Defects

Alice D'Amico and Francesco D'Antonio

Abstract

Neural tube defects (NTDs) are among the most common anomalies diagnosed prenatally and occur as a failure of the neural tube to close during the embryonic period. The resulting defect may involve the vertebrae, spinal cord, cranium, and/or brain. NTDs are classified as open or closed depending on the absence or presence of the fetal skin above the defect. Open NTDs are defects commonly covered only by a membrane. The most common NTDs include myelomeningocele (open spina bifida) and anencephaly. Prenatal diagnosis by ultrasound is the mainstay for the detection of these anomalies before birth with reported high diagnostic performance for these anomalies, except that for closed spinal defect.

The aim of the present chapter is to provide an up to date on the pathophysiology, prenatal diagnosis, and prognosis of fetuses with NTDs.

Supplementary Information The online version contains supplementary material available at https://doi.org/10.1007/978-3-031-70192-4_11.

A. D'Amico · F. D'Antonio (✉)
Center for Fetal Care and High-Risk Pregnancies, University of Chieti, Chieti, Italy

Keywords

Neural tube defects · Open spina bifida · Prenatal diagnosis · Myelomeningocele · NTDs screening

1 Introduction

1.1 Definition

Neural tube defects (NTDs) are the most common severely disabling birth defects, with a frequency of approximately 1 of every 2000 births. NTDs include all congenital anomalies that derive from failure of the neural tube to close during the fourth week of embryogenesis. NTDs can occur anywhere along the developing spinal cord, from the brain to the sacrum [1–4].

NTDs include the following anomalies:

- Cranial defects, which includes acrania/exencephaly/anencephaly sequence, and encephalocele.
- Spinal cord dysraphism which include a heterogenous group of anomalies characterized by an aberration in the embryogenesis of the spine and spinal cord.

P. Volpe, T. Ghi (eds.), *Fetal Neurosonography*, Ultrasound in Obstetrics and Gynecology, https://doi.org/10.1007/978-3-031-70192-4_11

1.2 Epidemiology

Neural tube defects are the most common severely disabling birth defects, with a frequency of approximately 1–7 per 1000 livebirth, depending upon ethnic, geographic, and nutritional factors [5, 6].

The recurrence risk in pregnancies with a prior fetus affected by NTD is approximately 20 times higher than that of the general population and has been estimated to be around 2–5% [6, 7].

1.3 Etiology/Pathogenesis

NTDs origin from a failure in the neurulation process, which consists of two phases: primary and secondary neurulation. Primary neurulation is defined as the folding the dorsal part of the neural tube and lengthening of neural plates. Secondary neurulation is characterized by the canalization of neural tubes, forming the distal part of the spinal cord. In the initial stages of its development, the neural tube is open anteriorly and posteriorly through which the lumen of the neural tube connects with the amniotic cavity [8, 9]. The anterior part (anterior neuropore) closes on day 25 while the posterior (posterior neuropore) closes on day 28 after conception. Failure of closure of the anterior neuropore during embryogenesis will lead to absence of the cranial vault and exposition of the brain parenchyma to the amniotic fluid (acrania followed by anencephaly) or, alternatively, to different forms of encephalocele. Conversely, failure of closure of the posterior neuropore during embryogenesis will lead to myelomeningocele [8–10].

The etiology of NTDs is multifactorial, related to genetic, environmental, and autoimmune factors. NTDs may result from an underlying abnormality of one or more of the pathways necessary to achieve neural tube closure or from a genetic variant or environmental insult that disrupts the closure process of the neural tube when the underlying pathway is intact [11–14].

Risk factors include folate deficiency, amniotic bands, genetic factors, and complex structural anomalies, including limb-body wall complex, cloacal exstrophy, and OEIS complex (omphalocele, exstrophy of the cloaca, imperforate anus, and spine abnormalities) [11–14].

1.4 Genetic Background

Although no specific genetic pathway have been reported in association with NDTs, genetic factors have been associated with the development of such anomalies in view of the reported higher risk after a prior defect, concordance in monozygotic twins and recurrence within the same family group [13, 15].

Genetic anomalies associated with NTDs include polymorphisms that affect the efficiency of folate metabolism, DNA methylation/epigenetics, chromosomal abnormalities, and syndromes such as Meckel–Gruber, Roberts, Jarcho-Levin, HARD (hydrocephalus, agyria, and retinal dysplasia), trisomy 13 or 18, and triploidy [16, 17].

2 Acrania-Exencephaly-Anencephaly Sequence

2.1 Definition

Acrania is the most severe type of NDTS resulting from a failure of the anterior neuropore to close at 10–20 post-ovulatory day and characterized by the absence of meninges and calvarium around the fetal brain [18, 19].

2.2 Epidemiology

Acrania was the most common NTDs prior to the era of folic acid supplementation, and its incidence has significantly fallen since the widespread of this practice. It has been reported to occur in approximately 1 per 1000 pregnancies [20].

2.3 Etiology Pathogenesis

The etiology of acrania/exencephaly/anencephaly sequence is multifactorial, including genetic and environmental factors. Folic acid deficiency (serum levels <200 μg/L) represents the major risk factor for this anomaly. Other risk factors include chromosomal and genetic anomalies, teratogens, and maternal chronic conditions (pregestational diabetes, obesity, and hyperthermia among the others) [18].

The generally accepted pathogenetic mechanism of anencephaly is the acrania-exencephaly-anencephaly sequence.

The first stage of the anomaly implies the occurrence of "dysraphia," which occurs as the consequence of the failure of the anterior neuropore to close at 10–20 post-ovulatory dates, resulting in the absence of meninges and calvarium (acrania) which induces the exposition of the normally formed forebrain and a variable amount of brainstem to the amniotic fluid (exencephaly) [18, 19]. Subsequently, the direct exposure of the brain tissue to the amniotic fluid and the trauma exerted by the uterine walls determines the progressive destruction of the initially well-formed and differentiated brain tissue [19] determining anencephaly. Acrania/exencephaly/anencephaly may be sporadically associated with craniorachischisis totalis in which the cranial defect is accompanied by an open defect of the spine [18].

2.4 Sonographic Findings

Prenatal diagnosis of acrania can be accomplished since the early first trimester of pregnancy [21, 22] with high-resolution transvaginal probes. Ultrasound appearance of the anomaly is related to its specific developmental stage. In the early first trimester of pregnancy, there is lack of visualization of the calvarium (acrania) and the direct exposure of the brain parenchyma to the amniotic fluid (exencephaly), which determines an abnormal bilobed brain contour, whose appearance has been named "Mickey Mouse" head [21–24] (Fig. 1). With advancing gestation, the progressive destructive effect of the amniotic fluid determines the loss of a large portion of the forebrain and brainstem (anencephaly) (Fig. 1).

Up to 25–50% percent of the cases during the late-second and the third trimester develops polyhydramnios due to the destruction of the cerebral structures which are responsible for fetal swallowing, and a vast majority of fetuses undergo spontaneous miscarriage [21, 22].

2.5 Differential Diagnosis

Prenatal diagnosis of acrania is relatively straightforward, especially in the first trimester of pregnancy. Lack of cranial vault, exposure of brain tissue within the amniotic cavity and its degeneration with advancing gestation are typical of this condition. Differential diagnosis includes large frontal encephalocele and cranial teratoma. In frontal encephalocele, part of the cranial vault is preserved although in large lesion the exposure of a significant portion of the brain parenchyma may resemble acrania. Cranial teratoma may present with the same ultrasound appearance of exencephaly, although in this case a relatively normal intracranial anatomy is present.

2.6 MRI

Ultrasound is the primary imaging modality in identifying fetuses with acrania/exencephaly/anencephaly sequence, and the use of fetal magnetic resonance imaging has been rarely reported in this anomaly. Several small studies suggest that fetal MRI can be useful in differentiating between acrania and large cranial vault defects [25].

2.7 Prognosis

It is an almost invariably lethal condition and can be reliably detected since the early first trimester of pregnancy. Newborns with acrania/anencephaly die immediately after birth. Recurrence risk of acrania has been estimated to be approximately 2–4% [26].

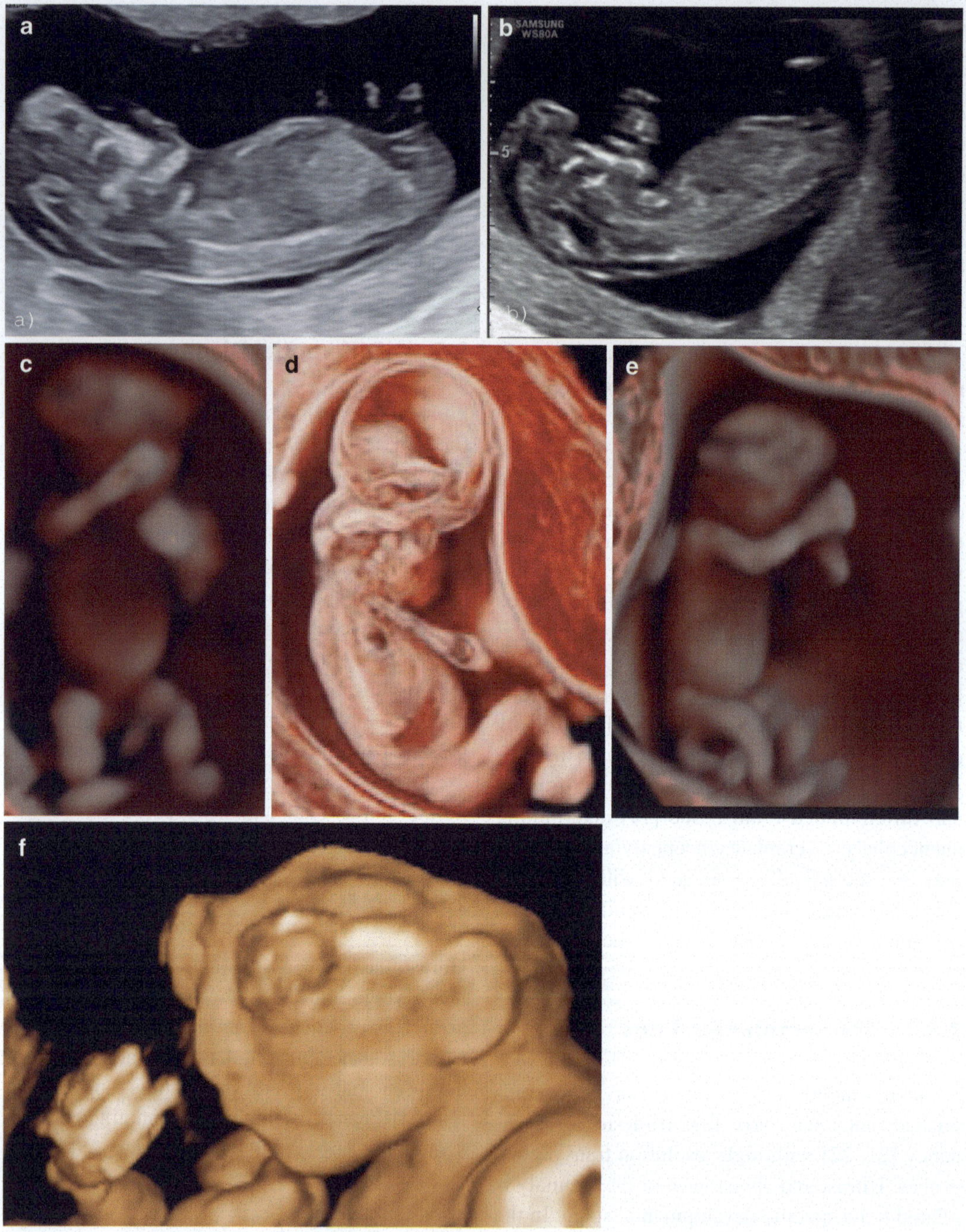

Fig. 1 (**a–f**) Fetuses with acrania/exencephaly/anencephaly. (**a–b**) Sagittal view of a fetus at 11 weeks of gestation, showing absence of cranial vault and direct exposure of the brain tissue to the amniotic fluid. (**d–f**) 3D ultrasound of fetuses with acrania showing exposure of the brain tissue (**d–e**) and anencephaly (**e–f**)

2.8 Option of Treatment

There is no current recognized treatment for acrania, being this anomaly associated with an almost unavoidable risk of in utero or post-natal demise.

2.9 Obstetric Management

Pregnancies affected by fetal acrania/anencephaly do not require a specific prenatal management in view of the unavoidable risk of in utero or post-natal fetal demise. Progressive destruction of the brain stem may impair the ability of the fetus to swallow and lead to polyhydramnios with the subsequent higher risk of post-partum hemorrhage. Cesarean section is not indicated.

2.10 Spinal Dysraphism (Spina Bifida)

Spinal dysraphism (spina bifida) encompasses a heterogenous group of anomalies that result in an abnormal bony formation of the spine and/or the spinal cord caused by a maldevelopment of the ectodermal, mesodermal, and neuroectodermal tissues [9].

According to their clinical appearance, there are two major types of spinal dysraphism:

1. Open spinal dysraphism (spina bifida aperta, which includes meningocele and myelomeningocele), a neural tube defect characterized by a cleft in the vertebral column, with a corresponding defect in the overlying skin so that the meninges and spinal cord are exposed [9].
2. Closed spinal dysraphism ("occult spinal dysraphism" or "spina bifida occulta") characterized by a cleft in the vertebral column, without a corresponding epithelial defect, so that the neural tissue is not exposed [9].

3 Open Spinal Dysraphism (Meningocele and Myelomeningocele)

3.1 Definition

Open spinal dysraphism (or spina bifida) is characterized by a cleft in the spinal column, with herniation of the meninges or meninges and spinal cord through the defect. It is also known as "open spinal dysraphism," as opposed to "closed spinal dysraphism" or "spina bifida occulta" when the cleft in the vertebral column is not associated with a corresponding defect of the overlying skin and the neural tissue is not exposed to the amniotic fluid [1–3].

When the sac contains meninges and cerebrospinal fluid, but the spinal cord and spinal roots are in their normal position, the defect is referred to as a *meningocele*. Conversely, *meningomyelocele* is characterized by protrusion of the spinal cord and meninges through a defect in the vertebral arch, it can occur anywhere along the spinal column but is most common in the lumbar region [1–3].

3.2 Epidemiology

Myelomeningocele is among the most common congenital anomalies identified prenatally with a reported prevalence of around 1–7 per 1000 births [1]. The prevalence of myelomeningocele is dependent upon several factors such as ethnic origin, geographic, and nutritional factors [3–5].

3.3 Genetic Background

Open spinal dysraphism is a multifactorial disease. Polymorphism in maternal folate pattern genes, DNA methylation/epigenetics, chromosomal abnormalities, and genetic syndromes can be associated with the occurrence of this anomaly [16, 17].

3.4 Etiology/Pathogenesis

Myelomeningocele is caused by a failure of primary neurulation. In normal conditions, the central nervous system appears as a plate of thickened ectoderm, the neural plate, whose lateral edges elevate to form the neural folds. Subsequently, these folds fuse to form the neural tube. The fusion begins in the cervical part of the neural tube and proceeds in both the cephalad and caudal direction [9, 10]. The cranial neuropore commonly closes on the 25th day after conception, while the closure of the caudal neuropore is delayed by approximately 2 days in order to allow an open communication between the lumen of the neural tube, neurocele, and the amniotic cavity [27, 28]. However, before the closure of the caudal neuropore, the neurocele closes and this process allows isolation of cranial vesicles, maintains them distended, and prevents drainage of fluids. The neurocele then reopens approximately 2 days after the caudal neuropore has closed, thus preventing the loss of fluid from the cranial vesicles [28]. Myelomeningocele occurs when the neural tube fails to close prior to the reopening of the neurocele, leading to the collapse of the cranial vesicles and to the development of the so-called Chiari II malformation. In this scenario, the reduction of intracranial volume leads to a development of a very small posterior fossa; more importantly, the cerebellum and brainstem are extruded into the spinal canal [29, 30].

3.5 Sonographic Diagnosis

Prenatal diagnosis of spina bifida is commonly accomplished in the second trimester of pregnancy although there is increasing evidence on the role of first trimester ultrasound in identifying fetuses with this anomaly. Midtrimester ultrasound has an excellent diagnostic accuracy for these anomalies with a reported sensitivity of 97–98% [31–34].

Prenatal diagnosis of spina bifida is based upon the presence of direct and indirect signs.

3.5.1 Direct Ultrasound Signs

Prenatal diagnosis of spina bifida mainly relies on the direct visualization of the spinal defect with herniation of meningeal tissue through the bony defect itself in a sagittal view of the fetal spine. In this view, the fetal spine shows irregularities of its bony posterior profile, and a protrusion of a hypoechoic sac lined by a thin hyperechogenic membrane through the fetal vertebral body defect with disruption of the fetal skin contour. The coronal plane of the affected bony segment shows a splaying of the ossification centers replacing the normal parallel lines of the normal vertebral arches, while on the transverse plane, a posterior opening of the ossification centers is documented, resulting in U-shaped vertebrae (Fig. 2) [33, 34] (Video 1).

3.5.2 Non-direct Ultrasound Signs

Myelomeningocele is commonly suspected at ultrasound due to the presence of specific cranial signs related to the presence of the defect. The most common indirect sign of myelomeningocele is due to the Chiari type II malformation, which refers to downward displacement of inferior cerebellar vermis, cerebellar tonsils, and medulla through the foramen magnum into the upper cervical canal, typically in association with a myelomeningocele at the lumbosacral or occasionally at a more cranial level of the spinal cord. Herniation of cerebellar vermis through the foramen magnum is encountered in about 96% of cases (Fig. 2).

Herniation of the hindbrain through the foramen magnum induces profound changes of the supratentorial intracranial anatomy which include:

1. Loss of the convex outward shape of the frontal bones (lemon sign). This sign is present in 90–98% of fetuses with spina bifida and is thought to be the result of the decrease intraspinal pressure which is due to the leakage of the spinal fluid in the amniotic cavity at the level of the defect.

2. Anterior wrapping of the cerebellum around the brainstem (banana sign) with obliteration of the cisterna magna due to downward displacement of the vermis through the foramen magnum. This is caused by the leakage of the CSF fluid in the amniotic cavity at the level of the open spinal defect which produces a reduced intraspinal pressure and concomitant ex vacuo caudal herniation of the hindbrain. In such cases, the transverse cerebellar diameter is reduced.
3. Ventriculomegaly.
4. Small biparietal diameter and head circumference (<5th percentile)

The banana sign has an almost 100% sensitivity and specificity for spina bifida, whereas the lemon sign has excellent sensitivity but can be occasionally seen also in normal fetuses.

Spina bifida can co-exist with cerebral and extra-cerebral anomalies such as complete and partial agenesis of the corpus callosum, callosal dysgenesis, heterotopia, malformations of cortical development, inter-hemispheric cyst, scoliosis, kyphosis, hip deformities, or clubfeet [31–34]. When spina bifida presents with other anomalies, the risk of aneuploidy or genetic disorders is increased, suggesting the need for invasive prenatal diagnosis in order to rule out these anomalies.

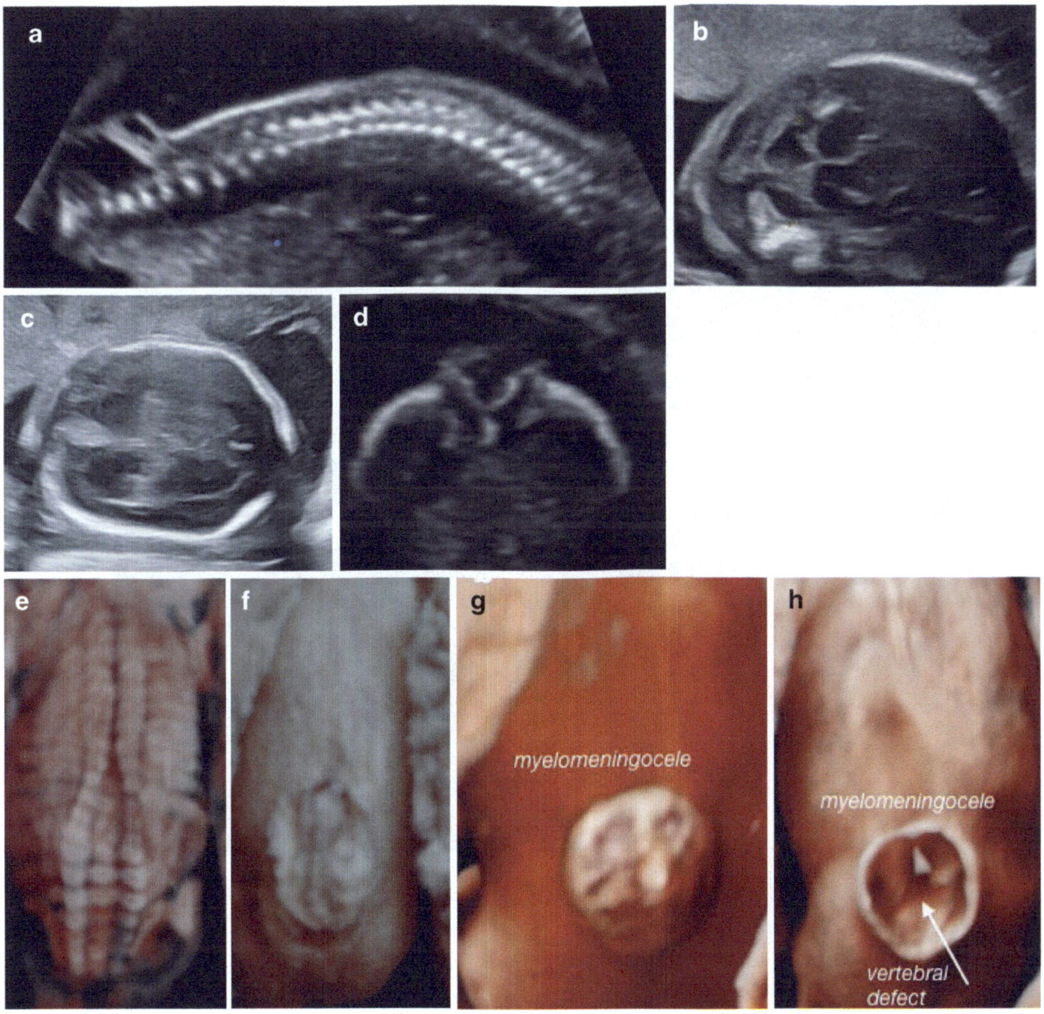

Fig. 2 (**a**) Gray scale ultrasound showing the spinal defect in fetuses with spina bifida. (**b**) Lemon sign, (**c**) banana sign, (**d**) transverse view of the lumbar spine showing the bony defect. (**e–n**) 3D ultrasound of fetuses with spina bifida

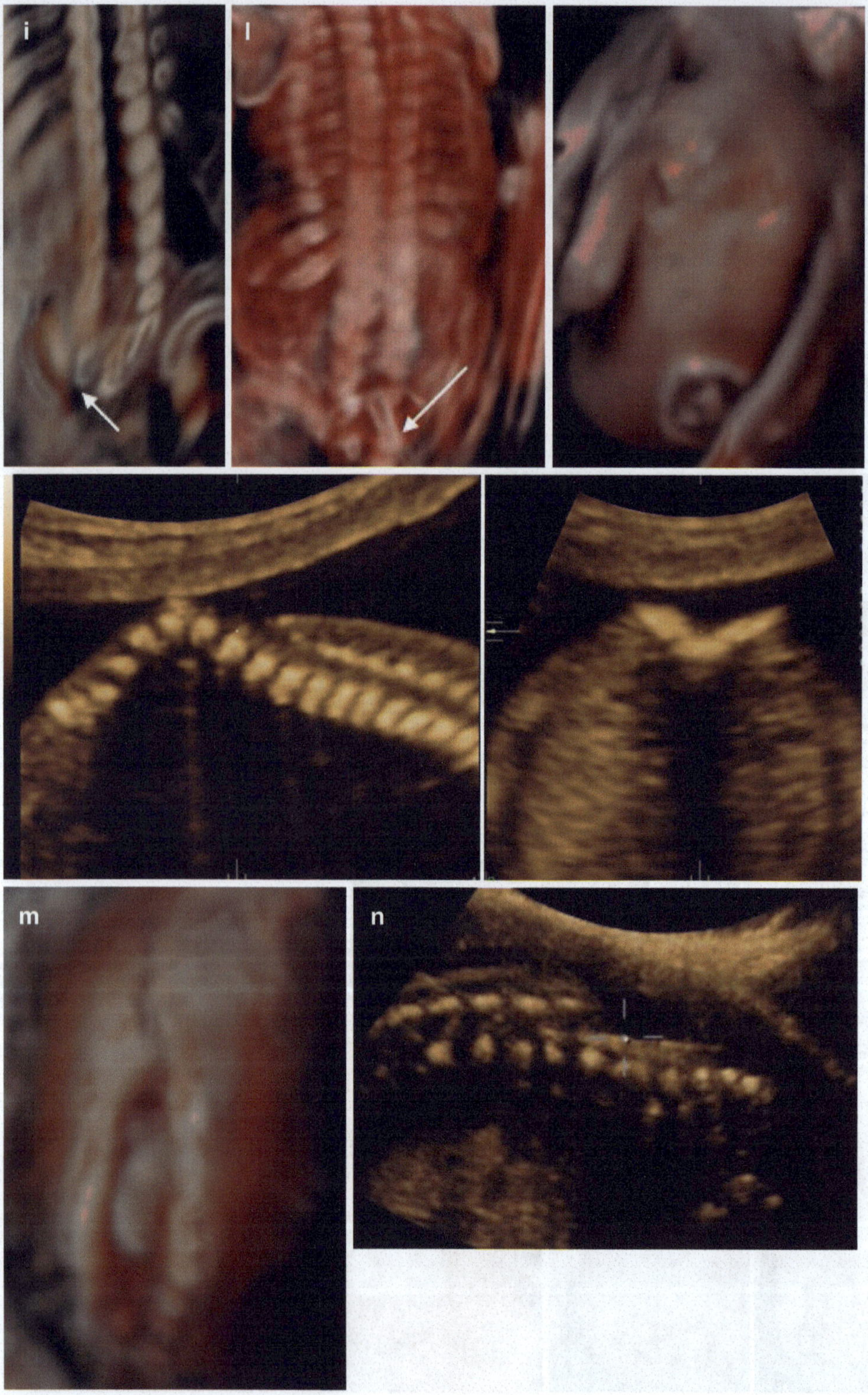

Fig. 2 (continued)

3.5.3 Ultrasound Determinants of Outcome in Fetuses with Spina Bifida

Infants born with open spina bifida are at higher risk of mortality and impaired neurodevelopmental outcome.

The level of the lesion is among the major determinants of post-natal motor and neurological performance in children with spina bifida. According to the lesion level, the newborn can have impaired motor function, sensory deficiency, bladder or anal incontinence, sexual dysfunction, low school performance, and respiratory and cardiac problems in adulthood [8, 35].

Children with cervical, thoracic, and high lumbar lesion level defects suffer of greater disability and have a higher risk of mortality. About 70–99% of children with thoracic or high lumbar lesions may require orthosis for ambulation and a wheelchair for mobility in adulthood; conversely, the large majority (95–100%) of those with low sacral lesions maintain ambulation without support [8, 35].

Therefore, prenatal identification of the level of the lesion is crucial for parental counseling. More importantly, an accurate identification of the level of the lesion is also fundamental when assessing candidacy for prenatal surgical repair of the defect. A recent systematic review [36] exploring the role of prenatal imaging in detecting the exact level of the lesion in fetuses with a prenatal diagnosis of spina bifida reported that that ultrasound has a moderate diagnostic accuracy in correctly identifying the upper level of the lesion in fetuses with open spina bifida. The agreement between ultrasound and post-natal or postmortem assessment was within one vertebral body in 76% and within two in 92% of cases, respectively. Although a direct comparison between the two techniques was not possible, the level of agreement between fetal MRI and post-natal assessment was similar to that reported on ultrasound. Finally, 3D ultrasound was associated with a higher rate of agreement compared to 2D ultrasound although the small number of included cases limited the robustness of the analysis. The detection rate of ultrasound and MRI in detecting the level of the lesion in fetuses with spina bifida is reported in Table 1.

Table 1 Pooled proportions (95% CI) showing the rate of agreement between ultrasound (either 2D or 3D), MRI, and post-natal or postmortem assessment. (Adapted from Di Mascio et al)

	Pooled proportions (95% CI)		Pooled proportions (95% CI)
	Ultrasound		MRI
Same level than post-natal	40.86 (26.9–55.6)	Same level than post-natal	42.50 (35.9–49.2)
US higher than post-natal	31.71 (11.9–55.8)	MRI higher than post-natal	26.41 (20.0–33.3)
US lower than post-natal	25.71 (10.5–44.8)	MRI lower than post-natal	32.37 (25.5–39.7)
Within one level	76.24 (65.0–85.9)	Within one level	76.21 (65.9–85.2)
Within two levels	92.38 (84.3–97.7)	Within two levels	94.18 (90.2–97.2)
One level than post-natal	34.28 (25.2–43.9)	One level than post-natal	40.65 (33.5–48.0)
One level higher than post-natal	16.10 (10.2–23.1)	One level higher than post-natal	24.85 (13.7–38.1)
One level lower than post-natal	17.45 (13.5–21.8)	One level lower than post-natal	20.74 (10.5–33.4)
Two levels than post-natal	20.49 (8.2–36.6)	Two levels than post-natal	13.43 (8.8–19.9)
Two levels higher than post-natal	5.88 (1.2–13.8)	Two levels higher than post-natal	7.84 (2.0–17.1)
Two levels lower than post-natal	8.54 (2.2–18.5)	Two levels lower than post-natal	9.55 (2.9–19.5)
Three levels than post-natal	4.31 (1.4–8.7)	Three levels than post-natal	5.28 (2.5–9.1)
Three levels higher than post-natal	1.72 (0.3–4.4)	Three levels higher than post-natal	0 (0–5.6)
Three levels lower than post-natal	2.61 (0.9–5.2)	Three levels lower than post-natal	3.57 (0.2–10.7)
Four or more levels than post-natal	2.40 (0.03–6.2)	Four or more levels than post-natal	0 (0–19.3)
Four or more levels higher than post-natal	2.68 (0.2–7.7)	Four or more levels higher than post-natal	0 (0–5.6)
Four or more levels lower than post-natal	2.38 (0.01–7.5)	Four or more levels lower than post-natal	0 (0–5.6)

On this basis, prenatal counseling of parents whose fetus is affected by spina bifida should highlight the potential weaknesses of prenatal imaging in correctly identifying the upper level of the defect.

Although the assessment of the level of the lesion on prenatal ultrasound has not been fully standardized yet, many authors use to consider T12 as the insertion of the most caudal rib and the iliac crests as a landmark to locate L5 level. Identifying the level of the conus medullaris might be also helpful during spinal examination, as it usually ends at L4 level between 13 and 18 weeks and then tends to ascend, so it may often be recognized at L3 between 19 and 36 weeks and at L2 after 36 weeks of gestation [37].

Most of children born with myelomeningocele present with Chiari II malformation which predisposes to the development of hydrocephalus and the need for post-natal ventriculoperitoneal shunt placement [38]. Although hydrocephaly per se does not predict the cognitive and neuropsychological outcome in fetuses with spina bifida, shunt complications, including malfunction, infection, and hemorrhage, are associated with a higher risk of adverse neurodevelopmental outcome and even post-natal death [39, 40]. There are few studies exploring the role of the severity of ventriculomegaly in predicting the need for shunt placement in fetuses with spina bifida. A retrospective series including 124 fetuses with isolated spina bifida, of which 48 were born alive, reported that the width of the posterior horn of the lateral ventricle and the ratio between its width and that of the cerebral hemisphere at antenatal diagnosis were higher in cases requiring compared to those not requiring a post-natal shunting, with a detection rate of 68.2% and 86.4%, respectively, and for a false-positive rate of 13%. In this study, all fetuses with a posterior ventricle measuring more than 12 mm or with a ratio of the posterior ventricle width with the cerebral hemisphere >0.6 required post-natal shunt insertion with a positive predictive value of 100% [41].

3.5.4 First Trimester Diagnosis of Spina Bifida

Advances in prenatal imaging techniques and higher probe resolution have made early sonographic diagnosis of spina bifida feasible. Some of the cranial signs described at midtrimester in fetuses with open spina bifida such as downward displacement of the cerebellum, and the brainstem obliteration of the cisterna magna can be sonographically suspected also in the first trimester of pregnancy.

One of the first proposed ultrasound tool for detection of spina bifida in the first trimester was the non-visualization of the fourth ventricle on the midsagittal plane [42]. The fourth ventricle presents as an intracranial translucency parallel to the standard nuchal translucency and is delineated by two echogenic borders: the dorsal part of the brain stem anteriorly and the choroid plexus of the fourth ventricle posteriorly. In the normal fetuses, the fourth ventricle is always visible, while in the fetuses with open spina bifida, this black space may be collapsed due to the caudal displacement of the hindbrain [42]. Other authors have questioned the correspondence between the fourth ventricle and intracranial translucency, reporting a more likely association of this sign with the cisterna magna [43].

A systematic review on the diagnostic accuracy of intracranial translucency to detect fetuses with open spina bifida reported a sensitivity 53.5%, a specificity of 99.7%, a positive likelihood ratio of 62.1, a negative likelihood ratio of 0.55, and diagnostic odds ratio of 223, thus questioning on its role as a primary screening tool for spina bifida in the first trimester of pregnancy [44].

The profound infratentorial reorganization due to the spinal defect may alter the relationship between the occipital bone and the brain stem. Several authors have assessed on the midsagittal plane the ratio between the brain stem (BS) diameter and its distance to the occipital bone (BSOB) (BS/BSOB ratio) as a reliable tool for spina bifida in the first trimester. In a systematic review including 27 cases with open spina bifida, Sirico et al. reported that the BS/BSOB ratio showed a sensitivity of 70% and a specificity of 100% in identifying fetuses with spina bifida with an area under the curve of 0.96 [45].

Fetuses with spina bifida also present with small head size since the second trimester of pregnancy. On this basis, several authors have explored the role of head measurement as a screening test for spina bifida in the first trimester of pregnancy. Khalil et al. reported that the mean size of the biparietal diameter (BPD) at 11–13 weeks' gestation was below the fifth centile in 44.4% of cases of with open spina bifida and that in these fetuses the median BPD MoM values were smaller compared to unaffected cases. More importantly, the authors reported that BPD measured in the first trimester was an independent predictor of spina bifida with a detection rate of 55.6% and a false-positive rate of 11.6% [46].

Cerebrospinal fluid leakage induced by the spinal defect with the secondary expansion of the choroid plexus into the lateral ventricle is responsible for the so-called dry brain effect, which can also be used in the first trimester to identify fetuses with spina bifida. Several authors have reported that the mean choroid plexus length to occipitofrontal diameter ratio is increased in fetuses with open spina bifida. In a study including 24 cases with spina bifida for which first trimester images were available, Kalafat et al. reported that the mean choroid plexus length to occipitofrontal diameter ratio had a high diagnostic accuracy in identifying fetuses with open spina bifida with an area under the curve of 0.921 for and 0.933 for its multiple of the median. Mean choroid plexus length-to-biparietal diameter ratio indicated similar results (area under the curve of 0.928) and for a cut-off point 0.662 yielded a positive predictive value of 90.9% and a negative predictive value of 99.6% [47].

3.6 Differential Diagnosis

The association between indirect and direct ultrasound signs previously described make prenatal identification of open spina bifida very accurate with reported detection rate up to 100%. Differential diagnosis includes mainly sacrococcygeal teratoma. In such case, the fetus present with a lumbar mass of mixed echogenicity but without associated cranial signs.

3.7 MRI

Fetal magnetic resonance imaging (MRI) has been reported to provide valuable prognostic information in fetuses with brain abnormalities not detected by ultrasound and may be considered to confirm the diagnosis, exclude any additional malformations, while it has not been shown to have greater precision in establishing the upper level of the lesion [36, 48, 49]. However, MRI has been reported to potentially identify supratentorial lesion which may commonly co-exist with spina bifida, such as dysgenesis of the corpus callosum or heterotopia. A recent series including 115 fetuses with spina bifida reported that with MRI anomalies of the corpus callosum (either complete or partial agenesis and dysgenesis) were identified in 50.4% and nodular heterotopia in about 4%. In this study, factors independently associated with anomalies of the corpus callosum or heterotopia were non-sacral spina bifida, ventriculomegaly, and abnormal septum pellucidum [49].

Recent studies also proposed MRI assessment as a complimentary prognostic tool in fetuses presenting with spina bifida.

A study including about 40 fetuses affected by spina bifida undergoing prenatal MRI reported that when the upper level of the lesion was between T12 and L2, dysphagia was observed in 50% of cases compared to 13% of cases presenting with a lesion in the lower lumbar or in the sacral tract. Conversely, the absence of a membrane covering the defect was associated with scoliosis and bladder dysfunction [50].

3.8 Prognosis

The short- and long-term outcome of fetuses with myelomeningocele is strictly related to the level of the lesion and to the presence of associated anomalies. Neurological symptoms associated with this anomaly are commonly presenting at birth but may become more evident later especially when specific complications of spinal dysraphism such as hydrocephalus or tethered cord develop [51].

Almost all children with myelomeningocele have Chiari II malformation characterized by downward displacement of the cerebellar tonsils and medulla leading to progressive hydrocephaly. About 60% of children with myelomeningocele require a ventriculoperitoneal shunt [52]. Persistence of hydrocephaly increased the risk of impaired cognitive and motor function, stridor and apnea which are responsible for the increased risk of mortality observed in these children [52]. Most children with myelomeningocele have normal intelligence, although a large majority of them have learning disabilities [53, 54]. Hydrocephaly and infection may increase the risk of abnormal cognitive function.

Almost all children with myelomeningocele present abnormal bladder function (neurogenic bladder), which may lead to progressive deterioration of renal function [52]. Eventually, about 60–70% of these children suffer of bowel incontinence [55].

3.9 Option of Treatment

Although the precise pathogenesis of the neuronal injury in fetuses with open spina bifida has not been fully elucidated yet, it is thought to be the result of a multi-hit insult. First, the primary defect in fetal neurulation is itself cause of neuronal loss or disruption [56]. Subsequently, a secondary damage can occur due to the direct toxic effect of the amniotic fluid on the exposed neural tissue or to the trauma on the sac content [57]. Finally, a third pathogenic hit may occur from internal forces within the myelomeningocele sac that stretch the placode and its derivative nerves [58].

Children with myelomeningocele are commonly operated after birth. However, recent evidence supports the role of prenatal repair of these anomalies.

The rationale behind in utero repair of the spina bifida is to create a complete, water-tight coverage of the defect, with the objective of preventing or limiting the progressive intrauterine injury on the neural tissue due to the amniotic fluid exposure.

The multicenter randomized controlled trial Management of Myelomeningocele Study (MOMS) [59] demonstrated that prenatal repair of open spina bifida by open hysterotomy, compared with post-natal repair, decreases the need for ventriculoperitoneal shunting and increases the chances of independent ambulation. In this study, fetal therapy was offered only to fetuses affected by myelomeningocele with the upper limit of the lesion located between T12 and S1, evidence of hindbrain herniation and gestational age comprised between 19 + 0 and 25 + 6 weeks at the time of the procedure.

However, the surgical approach adopted in the MoM trial implies hysterotomy on the uterine corpus or fundus which can increase the occurrence of preterm birth, oligohydramnios, spontaneous rupture of membranes, placental abruption, pulmonary edema, and uterine dehiscence at the hysterotomy site.

More recently, less invasive approaches using fetoscopy have been proposed. A recent study including 300 fetuses undergoing in utero repair of spina bifida reported that one-third of fetuses undergoing fetoscopic repair had vaginal delivery compared to none of those receiving open fetal surgery [60]. Furthermore, none of the women operated with fetoscopic surgery had signs of scar dehiscence at the time of cesarean section compared to 34 in the group of open fetal surgery. Finally, there was no difference in the need for shunt placement 12 months after birth between the two groups, thus suggesting that fetoscopic repair may represent a safe and effective approach to treat spina bifida in utero [60].

3.10 Obstetric Management

Pregnancies complicated by fetal spina bifida should be referred to tertiary centers with multidisciplinary facilities for the post-natal treatment of these anomalies, including neonatal intensive care unit and pediatric neurosurgery. Indicated preterm delivery is not indicated in these pregnancies and has not been shown to improve the short-term outcome of these children [61].

The presence of spina bifida per se does not represent a primary indication to cesarean section, and based on the evidence coming from observational studies, vaginal delivery can be safely accomplished, unless the fetus is in breech position. A systematic review reporting the outcome of fetuses with spina bifida according to the mode of delivery and including more than 600 cases not subjected to in utero repair reported that the children born vaginally compared to those undergoing cesarean section were less likely to require a shunt or have sac disruption. There was also no difference in the walking ability between the two groups [62]. A more recent retrospective study including nearly 2000 cases of isolated spina bifida did not show a reduced risk of fetal death in pregnancies undergoing prelabor cesarean delivery [63].

However, despite the lack of evidence on the influence of prelabor cesarean delivery in improving the outcome of newborns with spina bifida, decision about the mode of delivery should involve shared decision-making between the woman and the obstetric and pediatric team. Vaginal birth is a reasonable option if the fetal head size is within the normal range, conversely, in case of increased fetal head size, cesarean delivery may be considered.

4 Closed Spinal Dysraphism

4.1 Definition

"Closed spinal dysraphism" is characterized by a cleft in the vertebral column with unexposed neural tissue and intact overlying skin. Closed spinal dysraphism accounts for approximately 10–15% percent of cases of spinal dysraphism. In most cases, closed spinal dysraphism consists of isolated vertebral bony defects although such defect may co-exist with more severe anomalies involving the spinal cord and sacral structures [64].

4.2 Epidemiology

Closed spinal dysraphism occurs in approximately 10–15% percent of cases of spinal dysraphism [65].

4.3 Genetic Background

Closed spinal dysraphism has been anecdotally associated with genetic anomalies, compared to open defect in which chromosomal and genetic anomalies occur in about 2% of cases [13, 16].

4.4 Etiology/Pathogenesis

Closed spinal dysraphism occurs as the result of disruption of secondary neurulation when there is a failure of fusion of the vertebral bodies due to incomplete fusion of the posterior vertebral arches leading to unexposed neural tissue and intact skin overlying the defect. The most common types of closed spinal dysraphism consist of isolated vertebral bony defects although it may present with variable anatomical anomalies, including tethered cord syndrome, terminal diplomyelia, sacrococcygeal teratomas, spinal lipoma, and sacral agenesis [66].

The vertebral defects may occur in association with other more severe anomalies of the spinal cord and sacral structures, such as split spinal cord malformation or various cavitary defects of the spinal cord [66, 67].

Closed spinal dysraphism can be classified into two main groups [67]:

- Those presenting with a subcutaneous mass.
- Those not presenting with a subcutaneous mass. These anomalies can be further classified as simple (such as persistent terminal ven-

tricle) or complex dysraphic (including diastematomyelia and caudal regression syndrome) states.

4.5 Sonographic Findings

Prenatal diagnosis of closed spinal dysraphism has been not extensively reported because affected fetuses do not commonly present with the ultrasound signs typical of open defects, such as lemon or banana sign and the defect is commonly discovered after birth, unless the fetus presents with associated anomalies [68, 69]. The most common ultrasound signs associated with closed spinal dysraphism include vertebral defects with intact skin, anechoic or echogenic cystic mass in the lower spine, and an abnormally low position of the conus medullaris.

Closed spinal dysraphism may be associated with cord tethering which may gradually progress to tethered cord syndrome and which includes symptoms of progressive neurological, urological, and orthopedic dysfunction during the post-natal growth spurt. A classic sign of tethered cord syndrome is the low-lying position of conus medullaris. Assessment of the position of the conus medullaris has been reported to be feasible prenatally with a good level of agreement with prenatal and post-natal MRI. In a study including 14 fetuses with spina bifida occulta and 245 controls, the authors identified all cases with normal insertion of the conus medullaris in unaffected fetuses and an abnormally low insertion in 5/14 of those presenting with closed spina bifida [70]. Assessment of the position of the conus medullaris has been reported to be feasible since the first trimester of pregnancy. In a multicenter study including 143 fetuses undergoing transvaginal ultrasound in the first trimester of pregnancy, the authors assessed the distance between the most caudal part of the CM and the distal end of the coccyx and determined the level of this line in relation to the umbilical cord insertion. The authors reported that the distance between the distal part of the conus medullaris and the coccyx, which was never found below the fetal umbilical cord insertion, increased with gestational age [71].

In another study including 112 cases of NTDs, of which 43% were represented by closed defects, the authors reported an ultrasound staging system for these defected based on the position of the conus medullaris and the presence of associated anomalies [72]:

- Class 1: Isolated low-lying conus (below L3).
- Class 2: Low-lying conus with a lump on the dorsal side (echogenic or cystic lesions).
- Class 3: Caudal regression syndrome or low-lying conus with additional major spinal defects (scoliosis, kyphosis).

Although they did not specifically look at neurological outcome, the authors reported that the live birth rate was 100% in fetuses with class 1, i.e., without other anomalies and 33.3% in the cases with other anomalies. Likewise, pregnancy continuation rate was 50.0% in cases labeled as class 2 without other anomalies and 20.0% in cases with other anomalies [72].

Children with closed spinal dysraphism commonly present with associated cutaneous lesions such as a subcutaneous mass above the spinal defect; in another multicenter series, prenatal diagnosis of closed spinal dysraphism was facilitated by the identification of subcutaneous lipomas or fibrolipoma [73].

Closed spinal dysraphism is commonly associated with other extra-cerebral anomalies, including omphalocele, bladder exstrophy, imperforated anus, vertebral anomalies, anorectal malformations, cardiovascular anomalies, and VACTERL syndrome [74].

4.6 Differential Diagnosis

Differential diagnosis of closed spinal dysraphism includes sacrococcygeal teratomas, isolated subcutaneous lipoma, lymphangiomas, hemivertebra and caudal regression syndrome, diastematomyelia.

4.7 MRI

There are few studies exploring the role of fetal MRI in closed spinal bifida A study including 20 cases of closed spina bifida reported a similar diagnostic accuracy for ultrasound and MRI in detecting closed spina bifida [71]. On the other hand, MRI had a superior capacity in identifying vertebral arch fissures, while the two-techniques had similar agreement in identifying the conus medullaris and scoliosis. MRI may be superior to ultrasound in detecting specific cranial features of fetuses with closed spinal dysraphism, including abnormal clivus–supraocciput angle, presence of cerebellar towering, clival concavity, brainstem compression, and tectal beaking [68].

4.8 Prognosis

The clinical manifestations of closed spinal dysraphism are heterogenous. The large majority of patients are usually asymptomatic or minimally symptomatic, with other experiencing symptoms only in adult life [75]. Sacrococcygeal cutaneous manifestations are among the commonest clinical signs observed in patients with closed spinal dysraphism, mainly in those non-presenting with other clinical symptoms and have been reported in up to 90% of these cases [72]. These lesions include skin tag, areas of hyper or hypopigmentation, and hemangiomas [75].

Other common symptoms include spondylosis, degenerative disc disease, or spinal stenosis, while in some cases, patients can present with more severe manifestations including neurologic, genitourinary, gastrointestinal, or musculoskeletal anomalies. Tethered cord syndrome is among the most common clinical manifestations in symptomatic patients with closed spinal dysraphism. It is caused by a stretch-induced dysfunction of the caudal spinal cord which can lead to a large variety of symptoms including back pain, bladder dysfunction, leg weakness, calf muscle atrophy, diminished or absent deep tendon reflexes, scoliosis, foot deformity, and dermatomal sensory loss [76].

4.9 Obstetric Management

Obstetric management of fetuses presenting closed spinal dysraphism which have been antenatally diagnosed depends upon the presence and severity of associated anomalies which are the main determinants of post-natal outcome of these children. In apparently isolated cases, timing and mode of delivery are not to be influenced by the presence of this anomaly.

5 Cephalocele

5.1 Definition

Cephalocele is defined as the herniation of cranial contents, mainly brain and/or meninges, through the skull [77]. They are commonly classified according to their location:

- Sincipital, including frontoethmoidal, nasofrontal, nasoethmoidal, and naso-orbital lesions.
- Basal, including trans-sphenoidal, trans-ethmoidal, and spheno-orbital lesions.
- Occipital.
- Parietal.

Although it commonly presents as an isolated condition, cephalocele can be potentially associated with cerebral and extra-cerebral anomalies, including ventriculomegaly, microcephaly, microphthalmia, spinal dysraphism, and cardiac and facial defects [78]. Cephalocele is commonly a congenital anomaly although it can rarely present as secondary lesion mainly due to the amniotic band syndrome or to a traumatic event.

5.2 Genetic Background

The risk of chromosomal, mainly Trisomy 18 and 13, or genetic anomalies, such as Meckel–Gruber syndrome, is increased in fetuses with cephalocele, thus supporting the need for genetic testing, including karyotype, microarray and, in case the latter are negative, exome sequencing [78].

5.3 Etiology/Pathogenesis

Although the exact pathogenic mechanism of cephalocele has not been fully elucidated yet, the most severe types of cephalocele involve a defective closure of the anterior neural tube usually prior to 26 days from conception. Nasofrontal lesions are thought to result from defective separation of neural and surface ectoderm at the site of final closure of the rostral neuropore [79, 80]. Anterior cephaloceles are likely to occur as the result of a defective development of the prosencephalic neural crest tissue, while occipital lesions as the consequence of a defective segmentation of the bones of the posterior cranium [81, 82].

5.4 Sonographic Findings

Prenatal diagnosis of cephalocele can be accomplished since the first trimester of pregnancy as a defect in the bony skull with a protruding sac containing a cystic or solid mass which may contain only the meninges (meningocele) or which can also show brain content (encephalocele) (Fig. 3) [83].

Occipital cephalocele is the most common type of these lesions and presents on ultrasound as an anechoic cystic mass protruding through an occipital bony defect [84]. Sincipital encephalocele appears as a cystic anechoic mass located in the midline of the anterior part of the calvarium [85]. Frontoethmoidal lesions appear as midline cysts, projecting anteriorly through a bony defect, from the lower part of the forehead between the orbits and are commonly associated with hypertelorism [86].

5.5 Differential Diagnosis

Posterior lesion can be misdiagnosed with cystic hygroma, cervical teratoma or hemangioma, or epidermal scalp cysts although in such cases the intracranial anatomy appears normal. Differential diagnosis in anterior lesion includes teratomas and epignatus.

5.6 MRI

Ultrasound has a high diagnostic accuracy to identify cephalocele, especially when it presents as an occipital lesion and therefore the usefulness of antenatal MRI to confirm or clarify the sonographic findings is questionable. In a series including 15 cases of occipital cephalocele undergoing fetal MRI, the authors reported that MRI identified displaced brain tissue and abnormal brain stem in almost half of the cases [87]. MRI can be considered in anterior or frontoethmoidal lesions in which differential diagnosis with teratomas is more challenging.

5.7 Prognosis

Prognosis of fetuses with cephalocele is dependent on the size and location of the defect and presence of associated anomalies, but it is commonly associated with a high risk of in utero fetal demise and abnormal neurodevelopmental outcome [88]. Occipital lesions can be associated with cranial nerve anomalies, blindness, seizures, spasticity, and severe developmental delay which can be worsened by the post-natal occurrence of hydro-

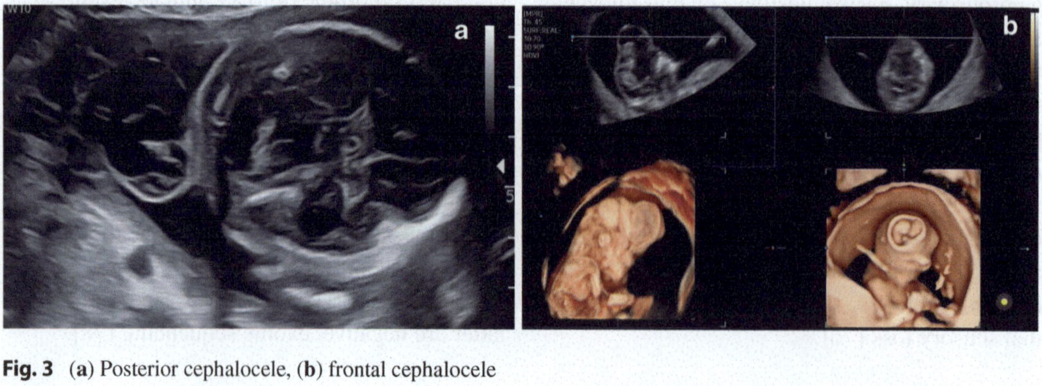

Fig. 3 (**a**) Posterior cephalocele, (**b**) frontal cephalocele

cephaly. Occipital encephalocele may be also associated with hindbrain anomaly (Chiari III malformation) [88]. Conversely, frontoethmoidal cephaloceles may be clinically asymptomatic in case of small lesion or presenting with severe symptoms including hypertelorism, orbital dystopia, and unilateral micro or anophthalmia [80].

5.8 Option for Treatment

Surgical treatment is feasible in the large majority of cases unless the lesion is large or co-exists with associated lethal anomalies. However, the prognosis is strictly related to the size and location of the defect or to the presence of associated anomalies and development of hydrocephaly.

Frontoethmoidal encephalocele has generally a good prognosis after surgery if the lesion is small and a normal intelligence has been reported in a good proportion of cases [80].

Posterior encephalocele has been associated with a mortality rate of about 30%. In those surviving, about half do not present with severe mental or physical disability, 30% show normal intelligence and physical disability while 20% of cases suffer from severe developmental delay [89]. Prognostic factors associated with abnormal neurodevelopmental delay include size of the sac, presence of neural tissue, hydrocephaly, infections, and associated anomalies [89].

5.9 Obstetric Management

Pregnancies complicated by fetal encephalocele should be managed in tertiary referral centers with availability of pediatric neurosurgery. There is no robust data on the preferred mode of delivery in these fetuses, and the decision should be made according to the size, location, and presence of associated anomalies. In case the lesion is small, vaginal birth represents a reasonable option due to the exceedingly low risk of trauma or dystocia. Conversely, cesarean section should be considered in large lesion to avoid dystocia and preserve the mass from trauma.

6 Craniorachischisis

6.1 Definition

Craniorachischisis is the most severe and rare type of NTD and is characterized by the presence of both acrania and spina bifida resulting from the complete failure of the neural tube to close [90]. Craniorachischisis can also present in association with structural anomalies, such as pentalogy of Cantrell and chromosomal and genetic disorders [90].

6.2 Epidemiology

Craniorachischisis is among the less common types of NTD. Its incidence has been estimated to be about 1:10000 pregnancies [5].

6.3 Genetic Background

As for the other NTDs, genetic anomalies associated with NTDs include polymorphisms that affect the efficiency of folate metabolism, DNA methylation/epigenetics, chromosomal abnormalities, and syndromes [16, 17].

6.4 Etiology Pathogenesis

Craniorachischisis is a disorder of the primary neurulation due to the inability of both anterior and caudal neuropore to close [91], and it is thought to occur at the 23 post-ovulatory date, before the neural plate begins to fold.

6.5 Sonographic Findings

Fetuses with craniorachischisis present with both acrania/exencephaly sequence and open spinal defect mainly involving the cervicothoracic part of the spine (Fig. 4) [92, 93].

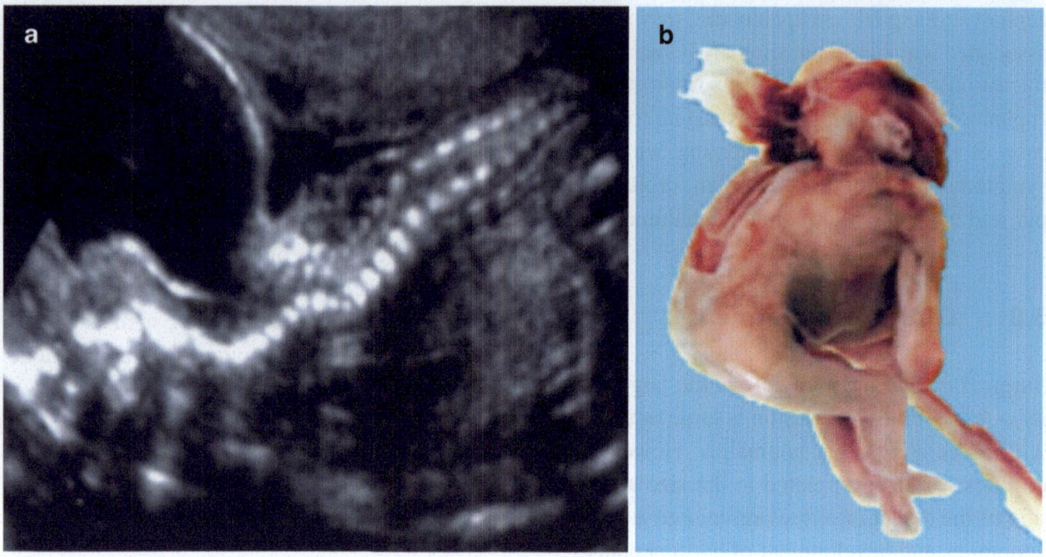

Fig. 4 (**a**) Ultrasound appearance of craniorachischis in the early second trimester of pregnancy. Note the association between acrania and the presence of an open spinal defect starting from the cervical region of the spine. (**b**) Pathological correlation after miscarriage. (Courtesy of Dr. Paolo Volpe)

6.6 Differential Diagnosis

Craniorachischisis can be misdiagnosed with both acrania/exencephaly/anencephaly sequenceor iniencephaly. In acrania/exencephaly/anencephaly, there is absence of cranial vault with exposition of the brain parenchyma into the amniotic fluid while the posterior part of the spine is usually intact. In iniencephaly, there is involvement of the cranial base and cervical vertebrae, but the cranial vault is usually intact.

6.7 MRI

Ultrasound is the primary imaging modality to identify fetuses with craniorachischisis, and the use of fetal MRI to diagnose this condition has only been anecdotally reported and does not seem to improve the diagnostic accuracy for this anomaly [94].

6.8 Prognosis

Craniorachischisis is a universally lethal condition, and no recognized treatment has been reported for this anomaly [90].

6.9 Obstetric Management

Fetuses with craniorachischisis, especially when associated with other structural anomalies genetic or chromosomal disorders are associated, are at high risk of intrauterine death. No specific care is recommended during pregnancy.

7 Iniencephaly

7.1 Definition

Iniencephaly is a complex, and severe form of NTD, characterized by a deficit of the occipital bones, enlarged foramen magnum, partial or total absence of cervical and thoracic vertebrae, shortening of the spinal column due to marked lordosis, hyperextension of the malformed cervicothoracic spine; and an upward-turned face and mandibular skin in direct continuity with that of the chest due to the lack of the neck [95].

7.2 Epidemiology

The incidence of iniencephaly is about 1:1000–2000 births [95].

7.3 Genetic Background

Like other NTDs, iniencephaly can be associated with genetic anomalies including polymorphisms that affect the efficiency of folate metabolism, DNA methylation/epigenetics, chromosomal abnormalities, and syndromes [16, 17].

7.4 Etiology Pathogenesis

Although the pathogenesis of iniencephaly has not been fully elucidated yet, this condition is likely to occur as the consequence of a defect in the closure of the neural tube at the base of the skull, and is featured by the cervical and fixed retroflection of the head [96]. Iniencephaly is associated with cerebral and extra-cerebral anomalies in about 75% of cases, including anencephaly, encephalocele, posterior fossa anomalies, lissencephaly, and holoprosencephaly. Extra-cerebral anomalies, including diaphragmatic hernia, cardiac and gastrointestinal defects are also common [96]. Iniencephaly can be classified into open iniencephalus (iniencephaly with encephalocele) and closed iniencephalus (iniencephaly without encephalocele) [95].

7.5 Sonographic Findings

Prenatal diagnosis of iniencephaly can be accomplished in the early second and first trimester of pregnancy. The most common ultrasound signs observed in this anomaly are the presence of occipital bone defects with enlarged foramen magnum, complete or partial absence of cervical and thoracic vertebrae which appears fused or incompletely closed and fixed, hyperextension of the cervicothoracic spine with upward-turned face (Fig. 5). Iniencephaly can co-exist with encephalocele [97–99].

7.6 Differential Diagnosis

Differential diagnoses included acrania/exencephaly/anencephaly, arthrogryposis, and anterior cervical tumors.

7.7 MRI

Ultrasound is the primary imaging modality to identify fetuses with iniencephaly, and the use of fetal MRI to diagnose this condition has only been rarely reported [100].

7.8 Prognosis

Iniencephaly is a lethal condition, and no recognized treatment has been reported for this anomaly.

However, long survivors with this anomaly have been sporadically reported [101].

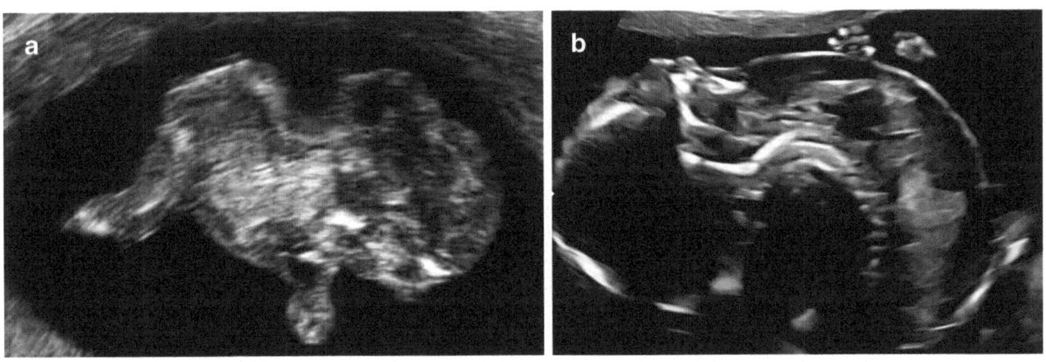

Fig. 5 Iniencephaly in two fetuses at 12 (**a**) and 18 (**b**) weeks of gestation, respectively. Note that open cervical defect, fixed hyperextension of the cervicothoracic spine with upward-turned face spine. (Courtesy of Dr. Paolo Volpe)

7.9 Obstetric Management

Given its almost invariable association with perinatal loss, no specific care is recommended for fetuses with iniencephaly. The fixed hyperextension of the cervical and thoracic spine and head may lead to maternal trauma or dystocia during labor [95].

References

1. Zaganjor I, Sekkarie A, Tsang BL, et al. Describing the prevalence of neural tube defects worldwide: a systematic literature review. PLoS One. 2016;11:e0151586.
2. Northrup H, Volcik KA. Spina bifida and other neural tube defects. Curr Probl Pediatr. 2000;30(10):313–32. https://doi.org/10.1067/mpp.2000.112052.
3. Ceschier N. ACOG Committee on practice bulletins-obstetrics. ACOG practice bulletin. Neural tube defects. Number 44, July 2003. (Replaces committee opinion number 252, March 2001). Int J Gynaecol Obstet. 2003;83(1):123–33. https://doi.org/10.1016/s0020-7292(03)00390-4.
4. Greene ND, Copp AJ. Neural tube defects. Annu Rev Neurosci. 2014;37:221.
5. Frey L, Hauser WA. Epidemiology of neural tube defects. Epilepsia. 2003;44(Suppl 3):4–13. https://doi.org/10.1046/j.1528-1157.44.s3.2.x.
6. Cowchock S, Ainbender E, Prescott G, Crandall B, Lau L, Heller R, Muir WA, Kloza E, Feigelson M, Mennuti M, Cederquist L. The recurrence risk for neural tube defects in the United States: a collaborative study. Am J Med Genet. 1980;5(3):309–14. https://doi.org/10.1002/ajmg.1320050314.
7. Papp C, Adám Z, Tóth-Pál E, Török O, Váradi V, Papp Z. Risk of recurrence of craniospinal anomalies. J Matern Fetal Med. 1997;6(1):53–7. https://doi.org/10.1002/(SICI)1520-6661(199701/02)6:1<53::AID-MFM11>3.0.CO;2-N.
8. Khoshnood B, Loane M, de Walle H, Arriola L, Addor MC, Barisic I, Beres J, Bianchi F, Dias C, Draper E, Garne E, Gatt M, Haeusler M, Klungsoyr K, Latos-Bielenska A, Lynch C, McDonnell B, Nelen V, Neville AJ, O'Mahony MT, Queisser-Luft A, Rankin J, Rissmann A, Ritvanen A, Rounding C, Sipek A, Tucker D, Verellen-Dumoulin C, Wellesley D, Dolk H. Long term trends in prevalence of neural tube defects in Europe: population based study. BMJ. 2015;351:h5949. https://doi.org/10.1136/bmj.h5949. PMID: 26601850; PMCID: PMC4658393
9. Müller F, O'Rahilly R. The primitive streak, the caudal eminence and related structures in staged human embryos. Cells Tissues Organs. 2004;177(1):2–20. https://doi.org/10.1159/000078423.
10. Ybot-Gonzalez P, Copp AJ. Bending of the neural plate during mouse spinal neurulation is independent of actin microfilaments. Dev Dyn. 1999 Jul;215(3):273–83. https://doi.org/10.1002/(SICI)1097-0177(199907)215:3<273::AID-AJA9>3.0.CO;2-H.
11. Atta CA, Fiest KM, Frolkis AD, Jette N, Pringsheim T, St Germaine-Smith C, et al. Global birth prevalence of spina bifida by folic acid fortification status: a systematic review and meta-analysis. Am J Public Health. 2016;106:e24.
12. van der Put NM, van Straaten HW, Trijbels FJ, Blom HJ. Folate, homocysteine and neural tube defects: an overview. Exp Biol Med (Maywood). 2001;226:243.
13. Ross ME, Mason CE, Finnell RH. Genomic approaches to the assessment of human spina bifida risk. Birth Defects Res. 2017;109:120–8. https://doi.org/10.1002/bdra.23592. PMID: 27883265; PMCID: PMC5388593
14. Boyd PA, Devigan C, Khoshnood B, Loane M, Garne E, Dolk H, EUROCAT Working Group. Survey of prenatal screening policies in Europe for structural malformations and chromosome anomalies, and their impact on detection and termination rates for neural tube defects and Down's syndrome. BJOG. 2008;115:689.
15. Windham GC, Bjerkedal T, Sever LE. The association of twinning and neural tube defects: studies in Los Angeles, California, and Norway. Acta Genet Med Gemellol. 1982;31(3–4):165–72. https://doi.org/10.1017/s0001566000008254.
16. Ekin A, Gezer C, Taner CE, Ozeren M, Ozer O, KoçA GNS. Chromosomal and structural anomalies in fetuses with open neural tube defects. J Obstet Gynaecol. 2014;34:156.
17. Kanit H, Özkan AA, Öner SR, Ispahi C, Endrikat JS, Ertan K. Chromosomal abnormalities in fetuses with ultrasonographically detected neural tube defects. Clin Dysmorphol. 2011;20:190.
18. Obeidi N, Russell N, Higgins JR, O'Donoghue K. The natural history of anencephaly. Prenat Diagn. 2010;30:357.
19. Society for Maternal-Fetal Medicine, Monteagudo A. Exencephaly-anencephaly sequence. Am J Obstet Gynecol. 2020;223:B5.
20. Limb CJ, Holmes LB. Anencephaly: changes in prenatal detection and birth status, 1972 through 1990. Am J Obstet Gynecol. 1994;170(5 Pt 1):1333–8. https://doi.org/10.1016/s0002-9378(94)70152-0.
21. Vergani P, Ghidini A, Sirtori M, Roncaglia N. Antenatal diagnosis of fetal acrania. J Ultrasound Med. 1987;6:715.
22. Cox GG, Rosenthal SJ, Holsapple JW. Exencephaly: sonographic findings and radiologic-pathologic correlation. Radiology. 1985;155:755.
23. Practice bulletin no. 187: neural tube defects. Obstet Gynecol. 2017;130(6):e279–90. https://doi.org/10.1097/AOG.0000000000002412.

24. Andonotopo W, Kurjak A, Kosuta MI. Behavior of an anencephalic fetus studied by 4D sonography. J Matern Fetal Neonatal Med. 2005;17:165.
25. Sharif A, Zhou Y. Fetal MRI characteristics of exencephaly: a case report and literature review. Case Rep Radiol. 2016;2016:9801267. https://doi.org/10.1155/2016/9801267. Epub 2016 Feb 3. PMID: 26955498; PMCID: PMC4756176
26. Seller MJ. Recurrence risks for neural tube defects in a genetic counseling clinic population. J Med Genet. 1981;18(4):245–8. https://doi.org/10.1136/jmg.18.4.245. PMID: 7277415; PMCID: PMC1048724
27. Müller F, O'Rahilly R. The development of the human brain, the closure of the caudal neuropore, and the beginning of secondary neurulation at stage 12. Anat Embryol (Berl). 1987;176(4):413–30. https://doi.org/10.1007/BF00310083.
28. Desmond ME, Jacobson AG. Embryonic brain enlargement requires cerebrospinal fluid pressure. Dev Biol. 1977;57(1):188–98. https://doi.org/10.1016/0012-1606(77)90364-5.
29. McLone DG, Dias MS. The Chiari II malformation: cause and impact. Childs Nerv Syst. 2003;19(7–8):540–50. https://doi.org/10.1007/s00381-003-0792-3. Epub 2003 Aug 12
30. McLone DG, Knepper PA. The cause of Chiari II malformation: a unified theory. Pediatr Neurosci. 1989;15(1):1–12. https://doi.org/10.1159/000120432.
31. Douglas Wilson R, Van Mieghem T, Langlois S, Church P. Guideline no. 410: prevention, screening, diagnosis, and pregnancy management for fetal neural tube defects. J Obstet Gynaecol Can. 2021;43:124.
32. Mace P, Mancini J, Gorincour G, Quarello E. Accuracy of qualitative and quantitative cranial ultrasonographic markers in first-trimester screening for open spina bifida and other posterior brain defects: a systematic review and meta-analysis. BJOG. 2021;128:354.
33. Kunpalin Y, Richter J, Mufti N, Bosteels J, Ourselin S, De Coppi P. Cranial findings detected by second-trimester ultrasound in fetuses with myelomeningocele: a systematic review. BJOG. 2021;128:366.
34. Bahlmann F, Reinhard I, Schramm T, Geipel A, Gembruch U, von Kaisenberg CS. Cranial and cerebral signs in the diagnosis of spina bifida between 18 and 22 weeks of gestation: a German multicentre study. Prenat Diagn. 2015;35:228.
35. Avagliano L, Massa V, George TM, Qureshy S, Bulfamante GP, Finnell RH. Overview on neural tube defects: from development to physical characteristics. Birth Defects Res. 2019;111(19):1455–67. https://doi.org/10.1002/bdr2.1380. Epub 2018 Nov 12. PMID: 30421543; PMCID: PMC6511489
36. Di Mascio D, Greco F, Rizzo G, Khalil A, Buca D, Sorrentino F, et al. Diagnostic accuracy of prenatal ultrasound in identifying the level of the lesion in fetuses with open spina bifida: a systematic review and meta-analysis. Acta Obstet Gynecol Scand. 2021;100:210.
37. Oaks W, Gaskill S. Symptomatic Chiari malformations in childhood. In: Park T, editor. Spinal dysraphism. Boston, MA: Blackwell; 1992. p. 104–25.
38. Elgamal EA. Natural history of hydrocephalus in children with spinal open neural tube defect. Surg Neurol Int. 2012;3:112–9.
39. McLone DG. Results of treatment of children born with a myelomeningocele. Clin Neurosurg. 1983;30:407–12.
40. Caldarelli M, Di Rocco C, La Marca F. Shunt complications in the first postoperative year in children with meningomyelocele. Childs Nerv Syst. 1996;12:748–54.
41. Khalil A, Caric V, Papageorghiou A, Bhide A, Akolekar R, Thilaganathan B. Prenatal prediction of need for ventriculoperitoneal shunt in open spina bifida. Ultrasound Obstet Gynecol. 2014;43(2):159–64. https://doi.org/10.1002/uog.13202. Epub 2014 Jan 8
42. Chaoui R, Benoit B, Mitkowska-Wozniak H, Heling KS, Nicolaides KH. Assessment of intracranial translucency (IT) in the detection of spina bifida at the 11-13-week scan. Ultrasound Obstet Gynecol. 2009;34:249.
43. Martinez-Ten P, Illescas T, Adiego B, Estevez M, Bermejo C, Wong AE, Sepulveda W. Non-visualization of choroid plexus of fourth ventricle as first-trimester predictor of posterior fossa anomalies and chromosomal defects. Ultrasound Obstet Gynecol. 2018;51(2):199–207.
44. Maruotti GM, Saccone G, D'Antonio F, Berghella V, Sarno L, Morlando M, Giudicepietro A, Martinelli P. Diagnostic accuracy of intracranial translucency in detecting spina bifida: a systematic review and meta-analysis. Prenat Diagn. 2016;36(11):991–6. https://doi.org/10.1002/pd.4883. Epub 2016 Aug 23
45. Sirico A, Raffone A, Lanzone A, Saccone G, Travaglino A, Sarno L, Rizzo G, Zullo F, Maruotti GM. First trimester detection of fetal open spina bifida using BS/BSOB ratio. Arch Gynecol Obstet. 2020;301(2):333–40. https://doi.org/10.1007/s00404-019-05422-3. Epub 2019 Dec 24
46. Khalil A, Coates A, Papageorghiou A, Bhide A, Thilaganathan B. Biparietal diameter at 11-13 weeks' gestation in fetuses with open spina bifida. Ultrasound Obstet Gynecol. 2013;42(4):409–15. https://doi.org/10.1002/uog.12420. Epub 2013 Aug 22
47. Kalafat E, Ting L, Thilaganathan B, Papageorghiou AT, Khalil A. Diagnostic accuracy of fetal choroid plexus length to head biometry ratio at 11 to 13 weeks for open spina bifida. Am J Obstet Gynecol. 2021;224(3):294.e1–294.e14. https://doi.org/10.1016/j.ajog.2020.08.058. Epub 2020 Aug 22
48. Fidon L, Viola E, Mufti N, David AL, Melbourne A, Demaerel P, Ourselin S, Vercauteren T, Deprest J, Aertsen M. A spatio-temporal atlas of the developing fetal brain with spina bifida aperta. Open Res

Eur. 2022;1:123. https://doi.org/10.12688/openreseurope.13914.2. PMID: 37645096; PMCID: PMC10445840

49. Trigo L, Eixarch E, Bottura I, Dalaqua M, Barbosa AA, De Catte L, Demaerel P, Dymarkowski S, Deprest J, Lapa DA, Aertsen M, Gratacos E. Prevalence of supratentorial anomalies assessed by magnetic resonance imaging in fetuses with open spina bifida. Ultrasound Obstet Gynecol. 2022;59(6):804–12. https://doi.org/10.1002/uog.23761.
50. Chao TT, Dashe JS, Adams RC, Keefover-Hicks A, McIntire DD, Twickler DM. Fetal spine findings on MRI and associated outcomes in children with open neural tube defects. AJR Am J Roentgenol. 2011;197(5):W956–61.
51. Chakraborty A, Crimmins D, Hayward R, Thompson D. Toward reducing shunt placement rates in patients with myelomeningocele. J Neurosurg Pediatr. 2008;1(5):361–5. https://doi.org/10.3171/PED/2008/1/5/361.
52. Matson MA, Mahone EM, Zabel TA. Serial neuropsychological assessment and evidence of shunt malfunction in spina bifida: a longitudinal case study. Child Neuropsychol. 2005;11(4):315–32. https://doi.org/10.1080/09297040490916910.
53. Hampton LE, Fletcher JM, Cirino P, Blaser S, Kramer LA, Dennis M. Neuropsychological profiles of children with aqueductal stenosis and Spina Bifida myelomeningocele. J Int Neuropsychol Soc. 2013;19(2):127–36. https://doi.org/10.1017/S1355617712001117. Epub 2012 Nov 16. PMID: 23153482; PMCID: PMC4076150
54. Burke R. Liptak GS; council on children with disabilities. Providing a primary care medical home for children and youth with spina bifida. Pediatrics. 2011;128(6):e1645–57. https://doi.org/10.1542/peds.2011-2219. Epub 2011 Nov 28
55. Sawin KJ, Liu T, Ward E, Thibadeau J, Schechter MS, Soe MM, Walker W, NSBPR Coordinating Committee. The National Spina Bifida Patient Registry: profile of a large cohort of participants from the first 10 clinics. J Pediatr. 2015;166(2):444–50.e1. https://doi.org/10.1016/j.jpeds.2014.09.039. Epub 2014 Oct 30. PMID: 25444012; PMCID: PMC4535790
56. Ben Miled S, Loeuillet L, Duong Van Huyen JP, Bessières B, Sekour A, Leroy B, Tantau J, Adle-Biassette H, Salhi H, Bonnière-Darcy M, Tessier A, Martinovic J, Causeret F, Bruneau J, Saillour Y, James S, Ville Y, Attie-Bitach T, Encha-Razavi F, Stirnemann J. Severe and progressive neuronal loss in myelomeningocele begins before 16 weeks of pregnancy. Am J Obstet Gynecol. 2020;223(2):256.e1–9. https://doi.org/10.1016/j.ajog.2020.02.052. Epub 2020 Apr 10
57. Heffez DS, Aryanpur J, Hutchins GM, Freeman JM. The paralysis associated with myelomeningocele: clinical and experimental data implicating a preventable spinal cord injury. Neurosurgery. 1990;26(6):987–92.
58. Corroenne R, Sanz Cortes M, Johnson RM, Whitehead WE, Donepudi R, Mehollin-Ray AR, Huisman TAGM, Espinoza J, Nassr AA, Belfort MA, Shamshirsaz AA. Impact of the cystic neural tube defects on fetal motor function in prenatal myelomeningocele repairs: a retrospective cohort study. Prenat Diagn. 2021;41(8):965–71. https://doi.org/10.1002/pd.5992. Epub 2021 Jul 10
59. Adzick NS, Thom EA, Spong CY, Brock JW 3rd, Burrows PK, Johnson MP, et al. A randomized trial of prenatal versus postnatal repair of myelomeningocele. N Engl J Med. 2011;364:993.
60. Sanz Cortes M, Chmait RH, Lapa DA, Belfort MA, Carreras E, Miller JL, Brawura Biskupski Samaha R, Sepulveda Gonzalez G, Gielchinsky Y, Yamamoto M, Persico N, Santorum M, Otaño L, Nicolaou E, Yinon Y, Faig-Leite F, Brandt R, Whitehead W, Maiz N, Baschat A, Kosinski P, Nieto-Sanjuanero A, Chu J, Kershenovich A, Nicolaides KH. Experience of 300 cases of prenatal fetoscopic open spina bifida repair: report of the international fetoscopic neural tube defect repair consortium. Am J Obstet Gynecol. 2021;225(6):678.e1–678.e11. https://doi.org/10.1016/j.ajog.2021.05.044. Epub 2021 Jun 3
61. Ho P, Quigley MA, Tatwavedi D, Britto C, Kurinczuk JJ. Neonatal and infant mortality associated with spina bifida: a systematic review and meta-analysis. PLoS One. 2021;16(5):e0250098. https://doi.org/10.1371/journal.pone.0250098. PMID: 33979363; PMCID: PMC8115829
62. Tolcher MC, Shazly SA, Shamshirsaz AA, Whitehead WE, Espinoza J, Vidaeff AC, et al. Neurological outcomes by mode of delivery for fetuses with open neural tube defects: a systematic review and meta-analysis. BJOG. 2019;126:322.
63. Benjamin RH, Lopez A, Mitchell LE, Sao K, Johnson A, Langlois PH, et al. Mortality by mode of delivery among infants with spina bifida in Texas. Birth Defects Res. 2019;111:1543.
64. Nabizadeh N, Dimar JR. Congenital spine deformities: timing of insult during development of the spine in utero. Spine Deform. 2022;10(1):31–44. https://doi.org/10.1007/s43390-021-00395-3. Epub 2021 Aug 9
65. Saitsu H, Yamada S, Uwabe C, Ishibashi M, Shiota K. Development of the posterior neural tube in human embryos. Anat Embryol (Berl). 2004;209(2):107–17. https://doi.org/10.1007/s00429-004-0421-2. Epub 2004 Oct 14
66. Ikenouchi J, Uwabe C, Nakatsu T, Hirose M, Shiota K. Embryonic hydromyelia: cystic dilatation of the lumbosacral neural tube in human embryos. Acta Neuropathol. 2002;103(3):248–54. https://doi.org/10.1007/s00401-001-0465-9. Epub 2001 Dec 21
67. Trapp B, de Andrade Lourenção Freddi T, de Oliveira Morais Hans M, Fonseca Teixeira Lemos Calixto I, Fujino E, Alves Rojas LC, Burlin S, Cerqueira Costa DM, Carrete H Jr, Abdala N, Tobaru Tibana LA, Takehara ET, Dalul Gomez G. A practical approach to diagnosis of spinal Dysraphism. Radiographics.

2021;41(2):559–75. https://doi.org/10.1148/rg.2021200103. Epub 2021 Jan 15
68. Bedei I, Krispin E, Sanz Cortes M, Lombaard H, Zemet R, Whitehead WE, Belfort MA, Huisman TAGM. Prenatal diagnosis and postnatal outcome of closed spinal dysraphism. Prenat Diagn. 2024;44(4):499–510. https://doi.org/10.1002/pd.6454. Epub 2023 Nov 27
69. Milani HJF, Barreto EQS, Chau H, To NH, Moron AF, Meagher S, Da Silva CF, Araujo JE. Prenatal diagnosis of closed spina bifida: multicenter case series and review of the literature. J Matern Fetal Neonatal Med. 2020;33(5):736–42. https://doi.org/10.1080/14767058.2018.1500543. Epub 2018 Sep 6
70. Lei T, Xie HN, Zheng J, Feng JL, Du L, Wang N. Prenatal evaluation of the conus medullaris position in normal fetuses and fetuses with spina bifida occulta using three-dimensional ultrasonography. Prenat Diagn. 2014;34(6):564–9. https://doi.org/10.1002/pd.4349. Epub 2014 Mar 18
71. Ramirez Zegarra R, Volpe N, Bertelli E, Amorelli GM, Ferraro L, Schera GBL, Cromi A, di Pasquo E, Dall'Asta A, Ghezzi F, Frusca T, Ghi T. Three-dimensional sonographic evaluation of the position of the fetal conus medullaris at first trimester. Fetal Diagn Ther. 2021;48(6):464–71. https://doi.org/10.1159/000516516. Epub 2021 Jun 9
72. Huang YS, Lussier EC, Olisova K, Chang YC, Ko H, Chang TY. Prenatal ultrasound diagnosis of neural tube defects in the era of intrauterine repair—eleven years' experiences. Taiwan J Obstet Gynecol. 2021;60(2):281–9. https://doi.org/10.1016/j.tjog.2021.01.006.
73. Zhang W, Wang J, Wu H, Chen L. Comparison between MRI and the combination of 2D and 3D US in the prenatal diagnosis of closed spina bifida. Pediatr Neurosurg. 2023;58(6):392–400. https://doi.org/10.1159/000533205. Epub 2023 Sep 12
74. Rossi A, Biancheri R, Cama A, Piatelli G, Ravegnani M, Tortori-Donati P. Imaging in spine and spinal cord malformations. Eur J Radiol. 2004;50(2):177–200.
75. Soonawala N, Overweg-Plandsoen WC, Brouwer OF. Early clinical signs and symptoms in occult spinal dysraphism: a retrospective case study of 47 patients. Clin Neurol Neurosurg. 1999;101(1):11–4. https://doi.org/10.1016/s0303-8467(98)00073-0.
76. Michelson DJ, Ashwal S. Tethered cord syndrome in childhood: diagnostic features and relationship to congenital anomalies. Neurol Res. 2004;26(7):745–53. https://doi.org/10.1179/016164104225017974.
77. Society for Maternal-Fetal Medicine, Monteagudo A. Posterior Encephalocele. Am J Obstet Gynecol. 2020;223:B9.
78. Towgifhi J. Cephaloceles. MedLink Neurology 1995 (updated 12/2010). http://www.medlink.com/medlinkcontent.asp. Accessed 15 Nov 2011.
79. Hoving EW. Nasal encephaloceles. Childs Nerv Syst. 2000;16(10–11):702–6. https://doi.org/10.1007/s003810000339.
80. Hoving EW, Vermeij-Keers C. Frontoethmoidal encephaloceles, a study of their pathogenesis. Pediatr Neurosurg. 1997;27(5):246–56. https://doi.org/10.1159/000121262.
81. Francis-West PH, Robson L, Evans DJ. Craniofacial development: the tissue and molecular interactions that control development of the head. Adv Anat Embryol Cell Biol. 2003;169:III–VI, 1–138. https://doi.org/10.1007/978-3-642-55570-1.
82. Tavella S, Bobola N. Expressing Hoxa2 across the entire endochondral skeleton alters the shape of the skeletal template in a spatially restricted fashion. Differentiation. 2010;79(3):194–202. https://doi.org/10.1016/j.diff.2009.11.004. Epub 2010 Jan 14
83. Sepulveda W, Wong AE, Andreeva E, Odegova N, Martinez-Ten P, Meagher S. Sonographic spectrum of first-trimester fetal cephalocele: review of 35 cases. Ultrasound Obstet Gynecol. 2015;46(1):29–33. https://doi.org/10.1002/uog.14661. Epub 2015 Jun 4
84. Weichert J, Hoellen F, Krapp M, Germer U, Axt-Fliedner R, Kempe A, Geipel A, Berg C, Gembruch U. Fetal cephaloceles: prenatal diagnosis and course of pregnancy in 65 consecutive cases. Arch Gynecol Obstet. 2017;296(3):455–63. https://doi.org/10.1007/s00404-017-4424-7. Epub 2017 Jun 20
85. Kehila M, Ghades S, Abouda HS, Masmoudi A, Chanoufi MB. Antenatal diagnosis of a rare neural tube defect: Sincipital Encephalocele. Case Rep Obstet Gynecol. 2015;2015:613985. https://doi.org/10.1155/2015/613985. Epub 2015 Jul 29. PMID: 26294989; PMCID: PMC4532954
86. Biberoglu EH, Kirbas A, Daglar K, Danisman N. Prenatal diagnosis of a case with frontoethmoidal encephalocele and the neonatal outcome. J Clin Diagn Res. 2015;9(7):QD05–7. https://doi.org/10.7860/JCDR/2015/13746.6166. Epub 2015 Jul 1. PMID: 26393172; PMCID: PMC4573004
87. Kasprian GJ, Paldino MJ, Mehollin-Ray AR, Shetty A, Williams JL, Lee W, Cassady CI. Prenatal imaging of occipital encephaloceles. Fetal Diagn Ther. 2015;37(3):241–8. https://doi.org/10.1159/000366159. Epub 2014 Oct 29
88. Siffel C, Wong LY, Olney RS, Correa A. Survival of infants diagnosed with encephalocele in Atlanta, 1979–1998. Paediatr Perinat Epidemiol. 2003 Jan;17(1):40–8. https://doi.org/10.1046/j.1365-3016.2003.00471.x.
89. Kiymaz N, Yilmaz N, Demir I, Keskin S. Prognostic factors in patients with occipital encephalocele. Pediatr Neurosurg. 2010;46(1):6–11. https://doi.org/10.1159/000314051. Epub 2010 May 5
90. French BN. Midline fusion defects and defects of formation. In: Youmans JR, editor. Neurological surgery. Philadelphia, PA: WB Saunders; 1990. p. 1164.
91. Saraga-Babić M, Sapunar D, Stefanović V. Histological features of axial structures during embryonic and fetal stages of human craniorachischisis. Acta Neuropathol. 1993;86:289–94. https://doi.org/10.1007/BF00304144.

92. Coskun A, Kiran G, Ozdemir O. Craniorachischisis totalis: a case report and review of the literature. Fetal Diagn Ther. 2009;25(1):21–5. https://doi.org/10.1159/000188662. Epub 2009 Jan 8
93. Costa P, Fontoura Oliveira A, Baptista VA. Prenatal diagnosis of craniorachischisis totalis. BMJ Case Rep. 2022;15(4):e244682. https://doi.org/10.1136/bcr-2021-244682. PMID: 35470163; PMCID: PMC9039352
94. Jaganmohan D, Subramaniam P, Krishnan N, Mahajan P. Two cases of Craniospinal Rachischisis Totalis: role of magnetic resonance imaging in diagnosis and review of neural tube defects in the Indian context with implications for folate fortification. J Pediatr Neurosci. 2017;12(1):32–5. https://doi.org/10.4103/1817-1745.205632. PMID: 28553376; PMCID: PMC5437784
95. Lewis HL. Iniencephalus. Am J Obstet. 1897;35:11–53.
96. Joó JG, Beke A, Papp C, Szigeti Z, Csaba A, Papp Z. Major diagnostic and pathological features of iniencephaly based on twenty-four cases. Fetal Diagn Ther. 2008;24(1):1–6.
97. Morocz I, Szeifert GT, Molnar P, Toth Z, Csecsei K, Papp Z. Prenatal diagnosis and pathoanatomy of iniencephaly. Clin Genet. 1986;30:81–6.
98. Foderaro AE, Abu-Yousef MM, Benda JA, Williamson RA, Smith WL. Antenatal ultrasound diagnosis of iniencephaly. J Clin Ultrasound. 1987;15:550–4.
99. Meizner I, Bar-Ziv J. Prenatal ultrasonic diagnosis of a rare case of iniencephaly apertus. J Clin Ultrasound. 1987;15:200–3.
100. Gadodia A, Gupta P, Sharma R, Kumar S, Gupta G. Antenatal sonography and MRI of Iniencephaly apertus and clausus. Fetal Diagn Ther. 2010;27(3):178–80. https://doi.org/10.1159/000291472. Epub 2010 Mar 2
101. Agostini L, Massimi L, Tamburrini G, Frassanito P, Bianchi F. Iniencephaly and long-term survival: a possible association-case report and review of the literature. Childs Nerv Syst. 2023;39(8):2027–35. https://doi.org/10.1007/s00381-023-06003-1. Epub 2023 May 26
102. Petrovski S, Aggarwal V, Giordano JL, Stosic M, Wou K, Bier L, et al. Whole-exome sequencing in the evaluation of fetal structural anomalies: a prospective cohort study. Lancet. 2019;393:758.
103. Naidich TP, McLone DG, Fulling KH. The Chiari II malformation: part IV. The hindbrain deformity. Neuroradiology. 1983;25(4):179–97. https://doi.org/10.1007/BF00540232.
104. Bowman RM, Lee JY, Yang J, Kim KH, Wang KC. Myelomeningocele: the evolution of care over the last 50 years. Childs Nerv Syst. 2023;39(10):2829–45. https://doi.org/10.1007/s00381-023-06057-1. Epub 2023 Jul 7
105. Singh AK, Upadhyaya DN. Sincipital encephaloceles. J Craniofac Surg. 2009;20(Suppl 2):1851–5. https://doi.org/10.1097/SCS.0b013e3181b6c49a.

Vascular Lesions of the Brain

Giulia Biancotto and Dario Paladini

Abstract

In this chapter, we describe the sonographic and Doppler features of the major arteriovenous malformations of the brain: vein of Galen aneurysmal malformation (VGAM) and dural sinus thrombosis (DST). VGAM represents a high cardiac output condition characterized by echocardiographic signs of cardiac overload/insufficiency and direct evidence of a primary cerebral arteriovenous malformation at the level of the vein of Galen. Neurosonography should investigate the possible presence of signs of secondary cerebral damage, such as hemorrhagic-ischemic necrosis of the white matter or obstructive hydrocephalus. Only 50–60% of liveborn are treated with embolization procedures with no sequelae, while the remaining develop major and/or minor motor and cognitive dysfunction and/or epilepsy. In the fetus, DST is mostly a benign, self-limiting condition. It is characterized by the formation of thrombus at the level of the torcular Herophili, which is often of aberrant morphology. In cases where extensive dilatation of this structure (lake) is present, the blood flows at low velocity favoring the development of a large thrombus which eventually completely obliterates the structure causing a block in venous brain circulation. Most cases resolve then spontaneously after birth.

Keywords

Fetus · Vein of Galen aneurysm · Arteriovenous fistula · Dural sinus · Ultrasound · Power Doppler · Neurosonography

1 Aneurysm of Galen Vein

1.1 Definition

Initially documented in 1937 by Jaeger et al. [1], the vein of Galen aneurysmal malformation (VGAM) is a rare congenital vascular anomaly of the brain. Despite advancements in diagnostic accuracy and treatment, it continues to be linked to considerable morbidity and mortality [2].

1.2 Epidemiology

VGAM constitutes 1% of all pediatric malformations, with an estimated incidence is 1 out of 25,000 deliveries [3]. Despite its rarity, it represents the most common cerebral arteriovenous malformation in the fetus [4].

G. Biancotto · D. Paladini (✉)
Fetal Medicine and Surgery Unit, Istituto IRCCS G. Gaslini, Genoa, Italy

P. Volpe, T. Ghi (eds.), *Fetal Neurosonography*, Ultrasound in Obstetrics and Gynecology,
https://doi.org/10.1007/978-3-031-70192-4_12

1.3 Etiology/Pathogenesis

VGAM results from the development of an abnormal arteriovenous communication. Specifically, between the 8th and 11th weeks of gestation, during the choroidal stage of embryonic development, an arteriovenous fistula emerges between the primitive choroidal arteries and the embryonic median prosencephalic vein of Markowski (PVM), a precursor of the vein of Galen [5, 6]. In this developmental stage, the choroid vessels provide blood supply to the primitive cerebral vesicles, while the PVM drains blood from the choroid plexus [5]. Normally, by the 11th week of gestation, the anterior part of the PVM undergoes involution, and the vein of Galen originates from its posterior part. In fetuses with VGAM, the abnormal flow through this connection hinders the normal involution of the anterior part of PVM, leading to the enlargement of the vein of Galen, eventually becoming aneurysmatic [6].

Two types of VGAM are distinguished based on the angioarchitecture of the malformation: choroidal and mural [7]. The choroidal type, often associated with severe cardiac decompensation at birth [8], is characterized by a nidus composed by multiple choroidal vessels draining into the aneurysmatic pouch of the PVM. It represents 90% of all VGAMs in neonates and children, and almost all of the VGAMs detected prenatally. Conversely, in the mural VGAM type, the fistula may be single or multiple, opening directly into the dilated PVM.

1.4 Genetic Background

Recently, some genetic causes of VGAM have been identified. Notably, 5–15% of VGAM cases stem from single-gene mutations, specifically involving RASA1 (RASp21 Protein Activator 1) and EPHB4 (Ephrin type-B receptor 4), two key genes for vascular development [9–11]. While EPHB4 genetic variants appear to be more specific to VGAM, RASA1 has been reported also in cases of pial fistulas [9], as well as in cases of capillary malformation-arteriovenous malformation syndrome [12]. Therefore, in instances where a neonate with VGAM presents with hemangiomas or other signs of skin erythema, whole exome sequencing is highly recommended, particularly for the assessment of the risk of recurrence in future pregnancies.

1.5 Sonographic Findings

Although antenatal diagnosis typically occurs during the late second or early third trimester of pregnancy [13], there have been documented cases in the literature of earlier prenatal diagnosis [14–16].

The suspicion of VGAM arises during a routine ultrasound scan when an anechoic, round/oval image is observed on the midline of the axial plane of the fetal brain, extending from the quadrigeminal plate cistern posteriorly toward the occiput. Confirmation of the vascular nature of the malformation is easily achieved through the demonstration of high velocity, turbulent flow using color Doppler [17] (Fig. 1).

Once VGAM is suspected, patient should be referred for fetal neurosonography, echocardiography, and magnetic resonance imaging (MRI), to obtain a comprehensive prenatal evaluation.

The first step in VGAM assessment involves measuring diameters and volume of the vascular ampulla through a 3D grayscale transvaginal neurosonography.

The second step entails searching for other cerebral anomalies. Indeed VGAM, particularly when early-onset, may lead to secondary cerebral damage, which can be already present at the time of malformation diagnosis. Ventriculomegaly (VM), hemorrhage, and ischemic lesions of cerebral parenchyma should be excluded (Fig. 2). Obstructive VM and hydrocephalus are present in 33–46% and 11% of antenatal cases of VGAM, respectively [13, 18]. VM could result from aqueductal obstruction due to compression from a large aneurysm, while high-flow shunt in the nidus leading to venous hypertension could cause hydrocephalus. Spontaneous hemorrhages may contribute to hydrocephalus formation [19], and in some cases lead to necrotic damage of the cortex. Ischemic white matter lesions have been

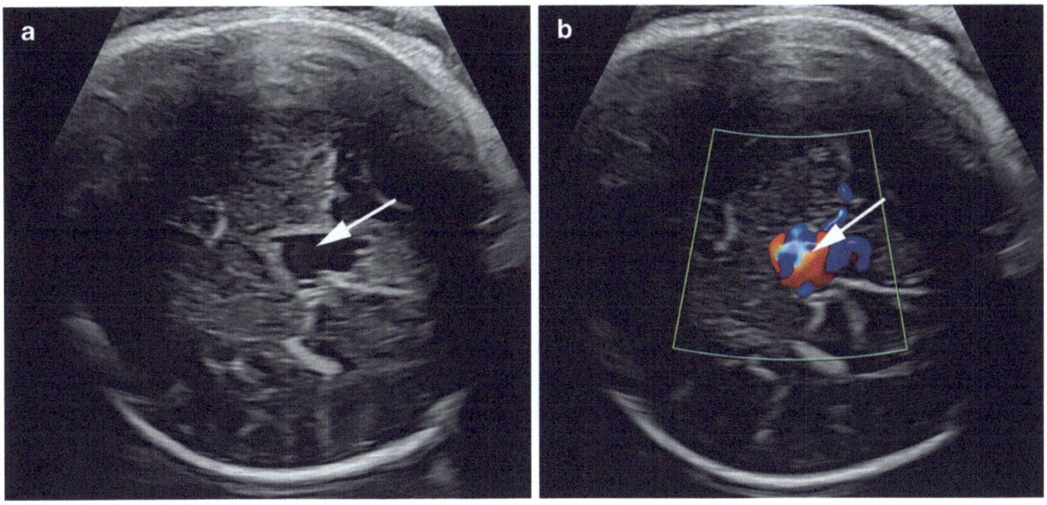

Fig. 1 Vein of Galen Aneurysmal Malformation (VGAM), 36 gestational weeks. (**a**) The suspicion arises on an axial view of the fetal head. An anechoic oval/round structure is visible along the midline, in the central part of the head, slightly toward the posterior part (arrow); (**b**) confirmation that this structure is related to VGAM is achieved switching to color Doppler, which demonstrates high velocity turbulent flow (arrow) at this level

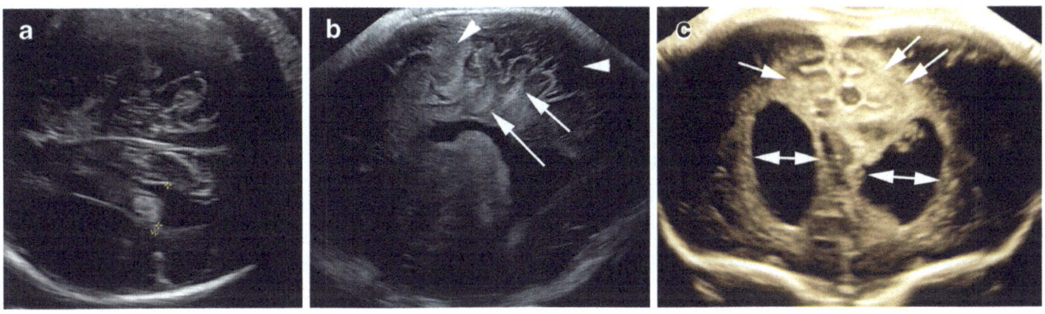

Fig. 2 Secondary lesions observed in fetuses with Vein of Galen Aneurysmal Malformation (VGAM). (**a**) Axial transventricular plane at 37 gestational weeks. Mild ventriculomegaly (11.9 mm), usually from compression of the Sylvian aqueduct, is visible; (**b**) Parasagittal transvaginal plane at 30 gestational weeks. Extensive cortical ischemic lesions, appearing as hyperechogenic at the level of the sulci (arrows), are diagnosed. At the same time, the widening of the subdural spaces (arrowheads) is indicative of cortical atrophic changes; (**c**) at 32 gestational weeks, on the coronal, transcaudate plane hyperechoic, cortical damage (arrows) associated with ventriculomegaly (double-headed arrows) is observed

detected in 22–31% of antenatal VGAM cases [13, 18, 20]. This damage is linked to the "vascular steal" phenomenon, where blood normally directed to cerebral parenchyma is diverted to the low-resistance VGAM, leading to focal hypoxia and ischemic lesions [19]. Cerebral ischemia might present sonographically with a wide range of appearances, from a hyperechoic aspect of the involved cortical layers to periventricular leukomalacia or brain atrophy, depending on severity.

Additionally, a detailed evaluation of the vascular architecture of VGAM is essential, using color/power Doppler and 3D multiplanar approach. The type of VGAM (choroidal or mural), although not always feasible, should be assessed. The numbers and origins of the arterial feeders of the aneurysm (e.g., pericallosal, choroidal, mixed), and its venous drainage should be studied. Venous drainage patterns could be different: in some cases, the vein of Galen drains toward the falcine sinus, a persistence of an embryologic remnant although more commonly it drains to the straight sinus, which could be atresic or even significantly dilated [21]. The size of the falcine/straight sinus has recently been reported to have a prognostic value [2] (Fig. 3).

Fetal echocardiography should be also carried out as the high-flow lesions are associated with a hyperdynamic circulation which might lead to high output cardiac failure [22, 23]. Cardiomegaly, tricuspid regurgitation, pericardial effusion, dilatation of superior vena cava / neck vessels, and reverse blood flow in the aortic isthmus are all signs to search during the fetal echocardiographic exam [24–26] (Fig. 4). Of these signs, cardiomegaly and severe tricuspid regurgitation (≥2 m/s) have been shown to be associated with a poor prognosis [3, 13, 18]. In rare instances, heart failure may progress to hydrops presenting with ascites, pleural effusion, skin edema, and polyhydramnios and representing a high risk of fetal death.

At birth, neonates with VGAM necessitate prompt expert evaluation and treatment as the sudden increase in systemic vascular resistances deviates the blood flow toward the fistula, rapidly deteriorating the neonatal cardiac function and possibly leading to severe pulmonary hypertension and multiorgan failure [4, 17, 20].

1.6 Differential Diagnosis

The use of color/power Doppler confirms the vascular nature of the lesion, helping in the distinction between VGAM and other midline anechoic images associated with cerebral anomalies, such as arachnoid or inter-hemispheric cysts or dilatation of the third ventricle [26].

When considering other vascular cerebral anomalies, it becomes crucial to differentiate VGAM from the pial variants of arteriovenous cerebral malformations (Pial Arteriovenous Shunts—PAVS). Despite the distinct anatomical location (i.e., PAVS in the subpial space and VGAM in the subarachnoid space) [24, 27], prenatal differentiation might be challenging. This distinction is however vital as the postanal treatment approach differs. The involvement of subdural sinuses other than the straight sinus, and the lateral positioning of the aneurysmal venous dilatation or the nidus (not on the midline as VGAM), may provide supportive evidence for the diagnosis of PAVS.

1.7 MRI

MRI is particularly of help in characterizing the vascular architecture of VGAM especially at advanced gestational ages (>36 weeks' gestation) where the ossification of the calvarium signifi-

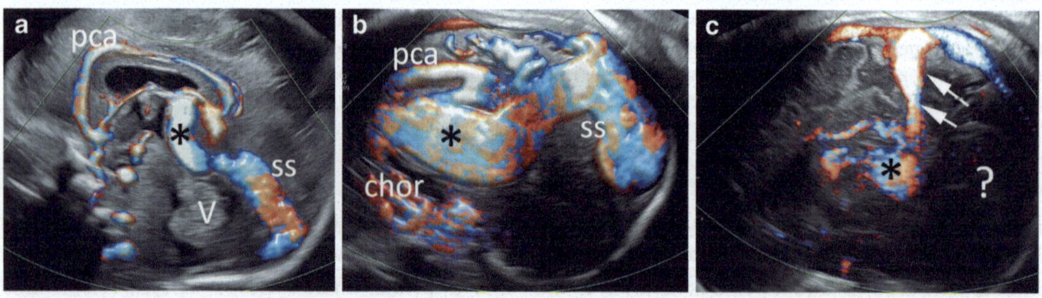

Fig. 3 Venous drainage assessment of the Vein of Galen Aneurysmal Malformation (VGAM). (**a**) in this case, the straight sinus (ss), slightly dilated, represents the only drainage; (**b**) in some more severe cases, the dilatation of the straight sinus is massive. Of note, a significant increase in the arterial feeders is observed compared to figure (**a**); (**c**) rarely, a falcine sinus (arrows) represents the main venous outlet of the malformation, with a very small straight sinus, not evident (?) on this plane. (* VGAM, *chor* choroidal feeders, *pca* pericallosal artery feeders, *V* cerebellar vermis)

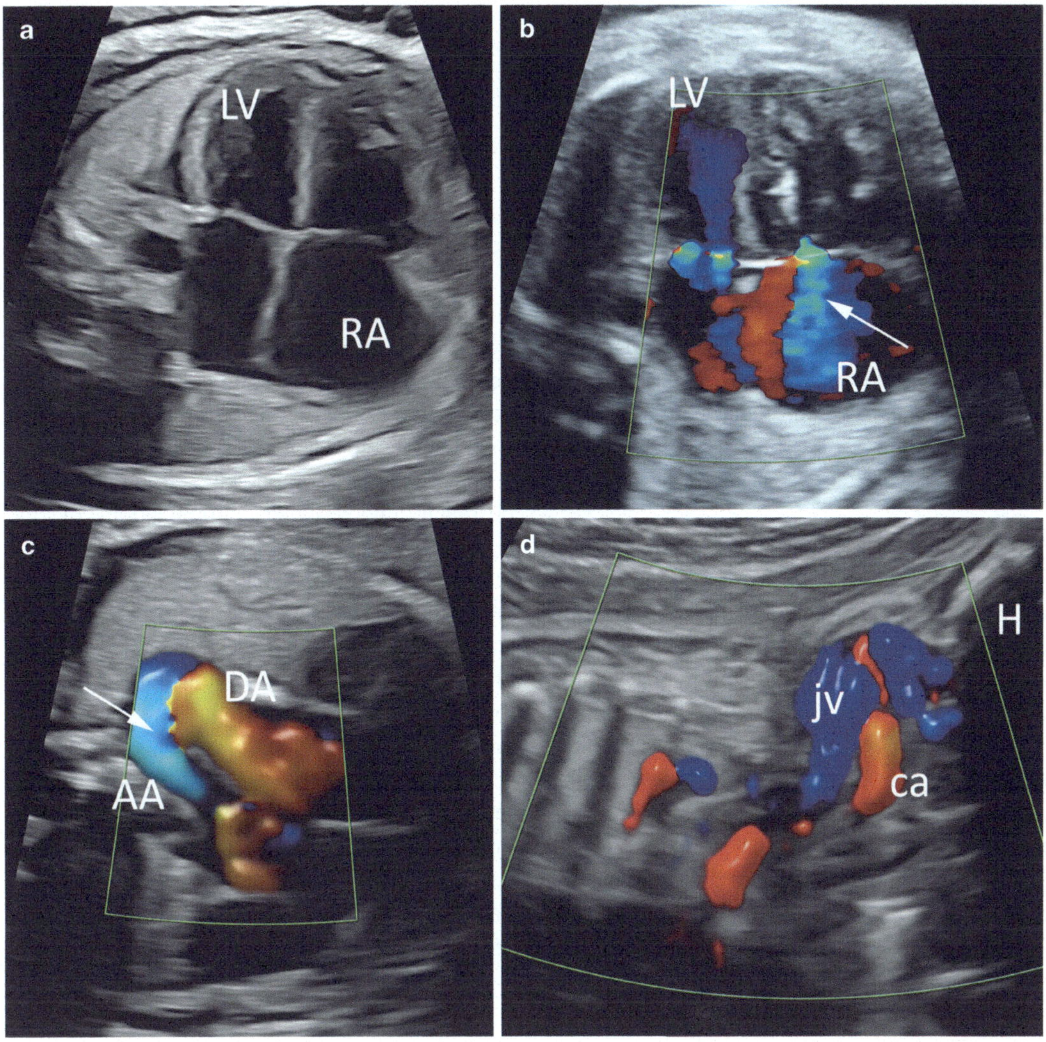

Fig. 4 Fetal echocardiography findings in the Vein of Galen Aneurysmal Malformation. (**a**) Axial, 4-chamber view showing a severe cardiomegaly; (**b**) color Doppler investigation demonstrates severe tricuspid insufficiency (arrow); (**c**) on the three-vessels and trachea view, color Doppler investigation demonstrates reverse blood flow across the aortic arch (arrow); (**d**) severe dilatation of neck vessels (arteries and veins) demonstrates the high output circulation due to the cerebral arteriovenous fistula of the VGAM. *AA* aortic arch, *ca* carotid artery, *DA* ductal arch, *H* fetal head, *JV* jugular vein, *LV* left ventricle, *RA* right atrium

cantly reduces the diagnostic accuracy of transvaginal neurosonography. MRI is nonetheless requested in case of breech presentation as TV neurosonography cannot be performed. Moreover, MRI—particularly in expert hands—represents an effective tool for describing key elements essential for prognostic evaluation. Firstly, it allows for precise measurement of the ampulla's volume, a parameter linked to prognosis [13]. Secondly, it allows the detection (or confirmation) of signs of secondary cerebral damage, such as periventricular calcifications [28] and focal encephalomalacia. Lastly, it facilitates an accurate evaluation of white matter-gray matter differentiation [29].

Fetal MRI proves valuable also in the assessment of the so-called arterial pseudo-feeders, which are challenging to capture through neurosonography due to their position under the skull. These vessels correspond to dilated branches of the middle cerebral artery, visible in the sylvian valley. While they do not supply the VGAM, these vessels irrorate the cerebral parenchyma. There has been a growing interest in detecting these vessels as they appear to be associated with encephalomalacia at birth, as well as with severe heart failure and pulmonary arterial hypertension [29].

Furthermore, the MRI assessment of the medio-lateral diameter of the straight/falcine sinus, measured at its shortest height, has been recently proposed as a prognostic marker, as its dilation appears to be correlated with poor clinical outcomes [2].

1.8 Prognosis

In the pre-embolization era, the mortality rate from VGAM was roughly 100%. Nowadays, the use of endovascular embolization procedures, that represents the gold standard treatment of VGAM, ensures a mortality rate of 14% and a normal/near normal neurological outcome in around 65% of the cases [30, 31]. However, in a recent two-center study of 49 cases of VGAM, 30% of women opted for pregnancy termination (TOP). Of those who opted for pregnancy continuation, feto-neonatal outcomes were the following: neonatal death (32.3%), infant death (2.9%), survived without sequelae (52.9%), and survived with sequelae (8.8%) [13].

Although prenatal prediction of VGAM prognosis remains challenging, several fetal features have been studied to identify prognostic markers. Well-established sonographic indicators of poor outcomes are represented by the presence of secondary lesions (e.g., ischemic cerebral lesions) and of cardiac failure [7, 13, 32]. Of note, when VGAM is detected at 28–30 weeks' gestation, the possibility of progression to irreversible brain damage is about 10% [13].

Other signs have been related to poor prognosis, such as the volume of the VGAM (>20 cm^3 or 20 mL), and the presence of a severe tricuspid regurgitation (≥2 m/s) [13]. As explained before, the medio-lateral diameter of straight/falcine sinus [2] and the presence of perisylvian pseudo-feeders [29], which can be both identified at MRI and even at advanced neurosonography, have been recently proposed.

1.9 Options of Treatment

Isolated VGAM is actually considered a potentially curable condition. In fact, since modern endovascular techniques have been developed and the management of this anomaly has moved toward tertiary referral centers with specialized perinatal intensive care units, several affected patients have been reported to have a normal neurological development [28, 33].

The treatment of choice is represented by postnatal endovascular embolization of the ampulla, supported by medical cardiovascular therapy, if necessary. Thus, prenatal and postnatal imaging, with the assessment of the number, size, and course of the feeders, as well as the type and the number of drainage veins, play a key role to achieve an adequate planning before the procedure.

As for the timing of embolization, it was reported that patients who underwent embolization during neonatal period were less likely to have good neurologic outcomes than those who underwent embolization after 2–3 months of life [31].

Recently, an intra-uterine approach was suggested (and documented in at least 3 cases) in those fetuses showing poor outcome features [34]. The suggested technique consists in puncture of the torcular, allowing ultrasound-guided placement of coils to embolize the malformation. This procedure is considered for fetuses >23 weeks of gestation with medio-lateral diameter of the straight sinus indicating a high risk of neonatal sequelae [2].

1.10 Obstetric Management

Close antenatal surveillance is mandatory, and serial neurosonographic exams should be performed every 2–3 weeks. MRI is recommended at the time of diagnosis and, particularly in early-onset cases of VGAM, it should be repeated at 34–36 weeks of gestation.

Delivery should be planned in a tertiary referral center, even if the fetus does not present signs of cardiac decompensation, because cardio-circulatory conditions may deteriorate suddenly after birth. Although vaginal delivery is not an absolute contraindication, several centers prefer to plan a cesarean delivery to facilitate a prompt management by experts. Most of deliveries are usually planned at ≥37 weeks of pregnancy, but an earlier delivery could be an option as discussed in the following conditions: pseudo-feeders in a fetus with an estimated weight >2000 g [35]; loss of white matter-gray matter differentiation [29]; and more than 40cm^3 of aneurysm volume [13]. However, it is of crucial importance to be aware of the fact that embolization can be performed only after 36 weeks of gestation [31].

2 Dural Sinus Thrombosis

2.1 Definition

Dural sinus thrombosis (DST) in the fetus is a rare condition, since it represents less than 2% of all vascular malformations [36]. DST could affect any of the dural sinuses, but the most common site is the torcular Herophili, which represents the confluence of the superior sagittal sinus, the straight sinus, and the occipital sinus, at the level of the junction between the falx cerebri and the cerebellar tentorium [37]. Lasjaunias et al. described the anatomoclinical characteristics of dural arteriovenous shunts, and they identified a sub-group of cases, "low-flow DAVS," characterized by giant venous lakes, typically involving the posterior dural sinus and the torcular Herophili in neonates and infants, containing blood clots in a high number of cases [38].

2.2 Epidemiology

Although no exact data on the prevalence of this condition during fetal life are available, thrombosis of torcular Herophili is the most frequently diagnosed cerebral thrombotic event during fetal life and affects approximately 0.6 per 100.000 children per year [36, 39–42].

2.3 Etiology/Pathogenesis

The association of DST with thrombophilia, infections, and blood disorders (such as polycythemia and trauma) is well established in childhood and adult life [43]. Conversely, DST etiology in the fetus has not been fully understood; [44] indeed, a link between DST and environmental exposures or thrombophilic conditions has not been proven yet [39–42]. In 40% of cases, DST remains idiopathic [44, 45]. The presence of a vascular anatomical malformation affecting the drainage into the torcular Herophili has been reported as the most common condition associated with DST [37].

2.4 Genetic Background

No correlation with genetic syndromes nor with single-gene disorders is known.

2.5 Sonographic Findings

Depending on the stage of clot evolution, sonographic appearance of DST might be slightly different. Usually, DST presents during the second trimester as a hyperechoic rounded/oval posterior mass—that represents the blood clot—with absence of signals at color Doppler imaging. The mass is surrounded by a hypoechogenic, possibly septate, triangular area, which represents the giant dural lake [46–48]. The clot is usually large and adherent to the wall of the dilated torcular Herophili, above the tentorium (Fig. 5). Over a period of 3–11 weeks, changes in the sonographic aspect of the blood clot might be observed as the clot organizes and retracts [44]. However, in other instances, the size of the clot might increase and fill the whole torcular venous lake and the venous flow becomes as slow as it might become difficult to capture it even with power Doppler and reduced PRF (Fig. 5c).

In many cases, the superior sagittal sinus appears dilated due to the retrograde venous

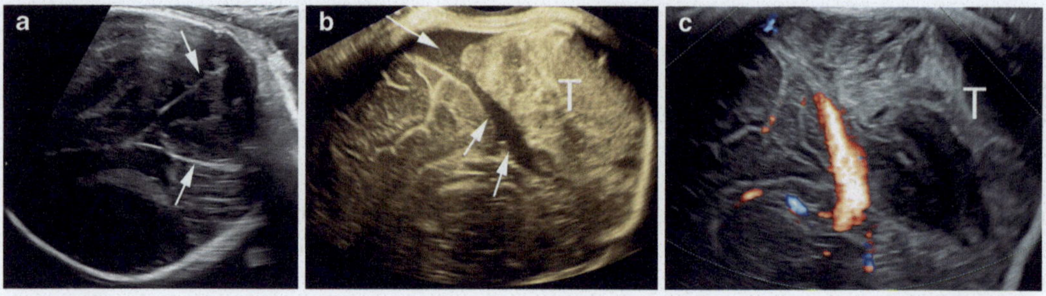

Fig. 5 Dural sinus thrombosis (35 gestational weeks). (**a**) On an axial plane of the fetal head, a large hyperechoic mass confined to the posterior fossa is evident (arrows); (**b**) on transvaginal neurosonography, the midsagittal plane demonstrates a large thrombus protruding from the torcular Herophili into the posterior fossa (arrows). Extremely slow blood flow is visible in front of the thrombus (arrows), within the aneurysmal lake of the dural sinus malformation; (**c**) on power Doppler, blood flow is demonstrated at this level

hypertension, although this finding does not represent a poor prognostic factor [37, 40, 49, 50]. In cases of DST, infratentorial anatomy is normal but it can appear dislocated by the enlargement of the venous lake and thrombus.

2.6 Differential Diagnosis

DST should be distinguished from other cerebral masses, such as intracranial tumors of posterior fossa (e.g., teratoma or lipoma), intracranial bleedings, and arachnoid cysts with intra-cystic hemorrhage.

2.7 MRI

Magnetic Resonance Imaging (MRI) is an effective tool to rule out secondary cerebral damage and associated cerebral malformations [40, 41, 48, 49]. Moreover, it could be helpful in dating the timing of the thrombosis; indeed, during the acute phase (<3 days), the clot is hypointense in T2-weighted MRI sequences due to the presence deoxyhemoglobin, whereas in the subacute phase (<10 days), it might appear hyperintense in T1-weighted MRI sequences for the presence of methemoglobin [44].

2.8 Prognosis

Considering the rarity of this condition, data regarding prognosis are lacking. However, fetal isolated DST seem to be associated with a good prognosis; indeed, the thrombus is often self-limiting and disappears with time [37, 39–42]. Results from a recent systematic review including 78 cases of DST reported regression/reduction in size in 71.2% of the cases and a fetal/neonatal death in 10%. In survivors, good outcomes were reported in 84.6% of patients and abnormal outcomes in 11.5% (including speech delay, developmental delay, autism, and left spastic hemiparesis) [51].

2.9 Options of Treatment

Considering that fetal DST resolves spontaneously in most cases, no treatment is generally required.

2.10 Obstetric Management

Mode and time of delivery are unchanged, with few exceptions.

References

1. Jaeger JR. Bilateral congenital cerebral arteriovenous communication aneurysm. Trans Am Neurol Assoc. 1937;63:173–6.
2. Arko L, Lambrych M, Montaser A, Zurakowski D, Orbach DB. Fetal and neonatal MRI predictors of aggressive early clinical course in vein of Galen malformation. AJNR Am J Neuroradiol. 2020;41(6):1105–11.
3. Gillet de Thorey A, Ozanne A, Melki J, Dumery G, Benachi A, Vivanti AJ. State of the art of antenatal diagnosis and management of vein of Galen aneurysmal malformations. Prenat Diagn. 2022;42(9): 1073–80.
4. Buratti S, Mallamaci M, Tuo G, Severino M, Tortora D, Parodi C, et al. Vein of Galen aneurysmal malformation in newborns: a retrospective study to describe a paradigm of treatment and identify risk factors of adverse outcome in a referral center. Front Pediatr. 2023;11:1193738.
5. Raybaud CA, Strother CM, Hald JK. Aneurysms of the vein of Galen: embryonic considerations and anatomical features relating to the pathogenesis of the malformation. Neuroradiology. 1989;31(2):109–28.
6. Raybaud C. Normal and abnormal embryology and development of the intracranial vascular system. Neurosurg Clin N Am. 2010;21(3):399–426.
7. Lasjaunias PL, Chng SM, Sachet M, Alvarez H, Rodesch G, Garcia-Monaco R. The management of vein of Galen aneurysmal malformations. Neurosurgery. 2006;59(suppl_5):S3-184–94.
8. Ramdani H, Sahri I-E, Elharras Y, Haddad SE, Allali N, Chat L. Vein of Galen aneurysmal malformation presenting as severe heart failure in a neonate. Radiol Case Rep. 2021;16(12):3961–4.
9. Tas B, Starnoni D, Smajda S, Vivanti AJ, Adamsbaum C, Eyries M, et al. Arteriovenous cerebral high flow shunts in children: from genotype to phenotype. Front Pediatr. 2022;10:871565.
10. Vivanti A, Ozanne A, Grondin C, Saliou G, Quevarec L, Maurey H, et al. Loss of function mutations in EPHB4 are responsible for vein of Galen aneurysmal malformation. Brain. 2018;141(4):979–88.
11. Duran D, Karschnia P, Gaillard JR, Karimy JK, Youngblood MW, DiLuna ML, et al. Human genetics and molecular mechanisms of vein of Galen malformation. J Neurosurg Pediatr. 2018;21(4):367–74.
12. Revencu N, Boon LM, Mulliken JB, Enjolras O, Cordisco MR, Burrows PE, et al. Parkes weber syndrome, vein of Galen aneurysmal malformation, and other fast-flow vascular anomalies are caused by RASA1 mutations. Hum Mutat. 2008;29(7): 959–65.
13. Paladini D, Deloison B, Rossi A, Chalouhi GE, Gandolfo C, Sonigo P, et al. Vein of Galen aneurysmal malformation (VGAM) in the fetus: retrospective analysis of perinatal prognostic indicators in a two-center series of 49 cases. Ultrasound ObstetGyne. 2017;50(2):192–9.
14. Ballester MJ, Raga F, Serra-Serra V, Bonilla-Musoles F. Early prenatal diagnosis of an ominous aneurysm of the vein of Galen by color Doppler ultrasound. Acta Obstet Gynecol Scand. 1994;73(7):592–5.
15. Hartung J, Heling KS, Rake A, Zimmer C, Chaoui R. Detection of an aneurysm of the vein of Galen following signs of cardiac overload in a 22-week old fetus. Prenat Diagn. 2003;23(11):901–3.
16. Pires P, Martins L d BA, NMTB P, Werner H, Ferreira AC, Araujo E Jr. Prenatal diagnosis of Galen vein aneurysm using ultrasonography and magnetic resonance imaging and perinatal and long-term neurological outcomes: a case series. Rev Bras Ginecol Obstet. 2017;39(6):309–14.
17. Beucher G, Fossey C, Belloy F, Richter B, Herlicoviez M, Dreyfus M. Antenatal diagnosis and management of vein of Galen aneurysm: review illustrated by a case report. J Gynecol Obstet Biol Reprod (Paris). 2005;34(6):613–9.
18. Deloison B, Chalouhi GE, Sonigo P, Zerah M, Millischer AE, Dumez Y, et al. Hidden mortality of prenatally diagnosed vein of Galen aneurysmal malformation: retrospective study and review of the literature. Ultrasound Obstet Gynecol. 2012;40(6):652–8.
19. Rossitti S. Pathophysiology of increased cerebrospinal fluid pressure associated to brain arteriovenous malformations: the hydraulic hypothesis. Surg Neurol Int. 2013;4:42.
20. Frawley GP, Dargaville PA, Mitchell PJ, Tress BM, Loughnan P. Clinical course and medical management of neonates with severe cardiac failure related to vein of Galen malformation. Arch Dis Child Fetal Neonatal Ed. 2002;87(2):F144–9.
21. Pearl M, Gomez J, Gregg L, Gailloud P. Endovascular management of vein of Galen aneurysmal malformations. Influence of the normal venous drainage on the choice of a treatment strategy. Childs Nerv Syst. 2010;26(10):1367–79.
22. Henrich W, Fuchs I, Bührer C, Van Landeghem FKH, Albig M, Stoever B, et al. Isolated cardiomegaly in the second trimester as an early sign of fetal hydrops due to intracranial arteriovenous malformation. J Clin Ultrasound. 2003;31(8):445–9.
23. Mannaerts D, Muys J, Ramaekers P, Jacquemyn Y. Relapsing fetal bilateral hydrothorax, an isolated expression of a vein of Galen aneurysmal malformation. BMJ Case Rep. 2015;2015:bcr2014208384.
24. Alvarez H, Garcia Monaco R, Rodesch G, Sachet M, Krings T, Lasjaunias P. Vein of galen aneurysmal malformations. Neuroimaging Clin N Am. 2007;17(2):189–206.
25. Chevret L, Durand P, Alvarez H, Lambert V, Caeymax L, Rodesch G, et al. Severe cardiac failure in newborns with VGAM. Prognosis significance of hemodynamic parameters in neonates presenting with severe heart failure owing to vein of Galen arteriovenous malformation. Intensive Care Med. 2002;28(8):1126–30.

26. Sepulveda W, Platt CC, Fisk NM. Prenatal diagnosis of cerebral arteriovenous malformation using color Doppler ultrasonography: case report and review of the literature. Ultrasound Obstet Gyne. 1995;6(4):282–6.
27. Mortazavi MM, Griessenauer CJ, Foreman P, Bavarsad Shahripour R, Shoja MM, Rozzelle CJ, et al. Vein of Galen aneurysmal malformations: critical analysis of the literature with proposal of a new classification system. J Neurosurg Pediatr. 2013;12(3):293–306.
28. Geibprasert S, Krings T, Armstrong D, Terbrugge KG, Raybaud CA. Predicting factors for the follow-up outcome and management decisions in vein of Galen aneurysmal malformations. Childs Nerv Syst. 2010;26(1):35–46.
29. Saliou G, Vraka I, Teglas JP, Senat MV, Durand P, Colmant C, et al. Pseudofeeders on fetal magnetic resonance imaging predict outcome in vein of Galen malformations. Ann Neurol. 2017;81(2):278–86.
30. Yan J, Wen J, Gopaul R, Zhang CY, Xiao S, wen. Outcome and complications of endovascular embolization for vein of Galen malformations: a systematic review and meta-analysis. JNS. 2015;123(4):872–90.
31. Brinjikji W, Krings T, Murad MH, Rouchaud A, Meila D. Endovascular treatment of vein of Galen malformations: a systematic review and meta-analysis. AJNR Am J Neuroradiol. 2017;38(12):2308–14.
32. Rodesch G, Hui F, Alvarez H, Tanaka A, Lasjaunias P. Prognosis of antenatally diagnosed vein of Galen aneurysmal malformations. Childs Nerv Syst. 1994;10(2):79–83.
33. McSweeney N, Brew S, Bhate S, Cox T, Roebuck DJ, Ganesan V. Management and outcome of vein of Galen malformation. Arch Dis Child. 2010;95(11):903–9.
34. See AP, Wilkins-Haug LE, Benson CB, Tworetzky W, Orbach DB. Percutaneous transuterine fetal cerebral embolisation to treat vein of Galen malformations at risk of urgent neonatal decompensation: study protocol for a clinical trial of safety and feasibility. BMJ Open. 2022;12(5):e058147.
35. Taffin H, Maurey H, Ozanne A, Durand P, Husson B, Knebel JF, et al. Long-term outcome of vein of Galen malformation. Dev Med Child Neurol. 2020;62(6):729–34.
36. Barbosa M, Mahadevan J, Weon YC, Yoshida Y, Ozanne A, Rodesch G, et al. Dural sinus malformations (DSM) with Giant Lakes, in neonates and infants. Review of 30 consecutive cases. Interv Neuroradiol. 2003;9(4):407–24.
37. Corral E, Stecher X, Malinger G, Ochoa JH, De Catte L, Sepulveda W. Thrombosis of the torcular herophili in the fetus: a series of eight cases. Prenat Diagn. 2014;34(12):1176–81.
38. Lasjaunias P, Magufis G, Goulao A, Piske R, Suthipongchai S, Rodesch R, et al. Anatomoclinical aspects of dural arteriovenous shunts in children. Review of 29 cases. Interv Neuroradiol. 1996;2(3):179–91.
39. Laurichesse Delmas H, Winer N, Gallot D, Lopes K, Perrotin F, Fluncker S, et al. Prenatal diagnosis of thrombosis of the dural sinuses: report of six cases, review of the literature and suggested management. Ultrasound Obstet Gynecol. 2008;32(2):188–98.
40. Merzoug V, Flunker S, Drissi C, Eurin D, Grangé G, Garel C, et al. Dural sinus malformation (DSM) in fetuses. Diagnostic value of prenatal MRI and follow-up. Eur Radiol. 2008;18(4):692–9.
41. Fanou EM, Reeves MJ, Howe DT, Joy H, Morris S, Russell S, et al. In utero magnetic resonance imaging for diagnosis of dural venous sinus ectasia with thrombosis in the fetus. Pediatr Radiol. 2013;43(12):1591–8.
42. Has R, Esmer AC, Kalelioglu I, Yuksel A, Pata O, Demirbas R. Prenatal diagnosis of torcular herophili thrombosis: report of 2 cases and review of the literature. J Ultrasound Med. 2013;32(12):2205–11.
43. Medlock MD, Olivero WC, Hanigan WC, Wright RM, Winek SJ. Children with cerebral venous thrombosis diagnosed with magnetic resonance imaging and magnetic resonance angiography. Neurosurgery. 1992;31(5):870–6. discussion 876.
44. Sheerin F. The imaging of the cerebral venous sinuses. Semin Ultrasound CT MR. 2009;30(6):525–58.
45. Barron TF, Gusnard DA, Zimmerman RA, Clancy RR. Cerebral venous thrombosis in neonates and children. Pediatr Neurol. 1992;8(2):112–6.
46. Gicquel JM, Potier A, Sitruk S, Girard N. Normal outcome after prenatal diagnosis of thrombosis of the torcular Herophili. Prenat Diagn. 2000;20(10):824–7.
47. Clode N, Gouveia R, Graça LM. Prenatal diagnosis of thrombosis of the dural sinuses. Int J Gynaecol Obstet. 2005;91(2):172–4.
48. Breysem L, Witters I, Spitz B, Moerman P, Smet MH. Fetal magnetic resonance imaging of an intracranial venous thrombosis. Case report. Fetal Diagn Ther. 2006;21(1):13–7.
49. Byrd SE, Abramowicz JS, Kent P, Kimura RE, Elias D, Heydeman PT. Fetal MR imaging of posterior intracranial dural sinus thrombosis: a report of three cases with variable outcomes. Pediatr Radiol. 2012;42(5):536–43.
50. Rayssiguier R, Dumont C, Flunker S, Couture A, Boulot P, Prodhomme O. Thrombosis of torcular herophili: diagnosis, prenatal management, and outcome. Prenat Diagn. 2014;34(12):1168–75.
51. Sacco A, Pannu D, Ushakov F, Dyet L, Pandya P. Fetal dural sinus thrombosis: a systematic review. Prenat Diagn. 2021;41(2):248–57.

First-Trimester Fetal Brain

Nicola Volpe, Andrea Dall'Asta,
Giovanni Morganelli, and Tullio Ghi

Abstract

Detection of congenital malformations of the central nervous system is feasible with expert ultrasound performed between 11 and 13 weeks of gestation. Recent advances in prenatal ultrasound have improved detection rate in the first trimester, nearing 100% for certain brain anomalies characterized by gross distortion of brain anatomy, such as alobar holoprosencephaly, acrania–exencephaly–anencephaly sequence, and cephalocele. The routine fetal brain examination includes the transventricular axial and midsagittal planes to evaluate the main cerebral structures and obtain head biometric measurements. If a brain malformation is suspected during this assessment, prompt referral for early neurosonography is warranted to confirm and characterize the anomaly, ascertain prognosis and establish the most appropriate management. Although the optimal approach for early neurosonography remains uncertain, we recommend a multiplanar examination of the fetal brain, including additional axial (such as transthalamic and transcerebellar planes), coronal (like transfrontal, transcaudate, transthalamic, and occipital planes), and midsagittal planes (including the posterior midsagittal plane). This chapter aims to provide an overview of fetal brain ultrasound examination between 11 and 13 weeks of pregnancy.

Keywords

Anomaly scan · Brain embryology · Fetal central nervous system · Fetal brain · Neurosonography

1 Introduction

The combined screening for major chromosomal anomalies involves an ultrasound assessment of the fetus between 11^{+0} and 13^{+6} weeks of gestation, including the measurement of the nuchal translucency (NT), a key parameter in assessing the risk of fetal chromosomal disorders [1–3]. At the time of the first-trimester screening, the evaluation of fetal anatomy seems to be feasible, allowing the detection of some structural anomalies [4–14]. Despite advancements in detecting major fetal anomalies during first-trimester ultrasound, there remains a lack of standardized methodology for early fetal anatomy ultrasound

N. Volpe (✉) · A. Dall'Asta · G. Morganelli
Department of Medicine and Surgery, Obstetrics and Gynecology Unit, University of Parma, Parma, Italy
e-mail: andrea.dallasta@unipr.it; gmorganelli@ao.pr.it

T. Ghi
Department of Woman and Child Health, Catholic University of Sacred Heart, Fondazione Policlinico Gemelli IRCCS, Rome, Italy
e-mail: tullio.ghi@unicatt.it

P. Volpe, T. Ghi (eds.), *Fetal Neurosonography*, Ultrasound in Obstetrics and Gynecology,
https://doi.org/10.1007/978-3-031-70192-4_13

assessment [15]. Various international societies have thus developed different protocols and guidelines for conducting routine anatomy examinations at 11–13 weeks to address this issue and achieve standardization [15–17].

At first trimester ultrasound the detection rate of fetal central nervous system (CNS) anomalies causing significant distortion of brain anatomy, such as alobar holoprosencephaly, anencephaly, and cephalocele, is close to 100% [4, 14]. Furthermore, other major CNS defects, including cystic anomalies of the posterior fossa [18–20] or open spinal dysraphism with Chiari II malformation [21–26], traditionally considered detectable only at mid-trimester ultrasound, can be suspected as early as 11–13 weeks of gestation when subtle changes in certain fetal brain structures are visible. Achieving high detection rates during routine first-trimester ultrasound requires adherence to a standardized protocol and the visualization of specific brain anatomical landmarks [4].

This chapter provides an overview of fetal brain ultrasound evaluation at 11–13 weeks of pregnancy, focusing particularly on two modalities:

1. Routine examination of the fetal brain, recommended for low-risk pregnancies [27].
2. Targeted early neurosonography, recommended for high-risk pregnancies or those with suspected brain anomalies [28].

2 Routine Examination of the Fetal Brain

2.1 Indication

The basic assessment of the fetal brain is to be performed on axial planes and should be offered to all pregnant women between 11^{+0} and 13^{+6} weeks of gestation as part of routine pregnancy care [17].

2.2 Routine Ultrasound Planes of the Fetal Brain at 11^{+0}–13^{+6} Weeks' Gestation

The routine evaluation of the fetal brain, usually performed using transabdominal ultrasound, relies on the acquisition and assessment of transventricular axial plane, which is defined by specific anatomical landmarks.

2.2.1 Transventricular Axial Plane

The transventricular axial plane of the fetal brain can be obtained by positioning the ultrasound beam transversally to the fetus at the level of the cranial vault and performing a caudal sweep of the probe until the lateral ventricles are visualized (Fig. 1), just above the thalami. This plane is characterized by the following anatomical structures and landmarks:

Transventricular axial plane:

- Fetal calvarium (cranial bone).
- Midline echo representing the interhemispheric fissure.
- Symmetric brain hemispheres.

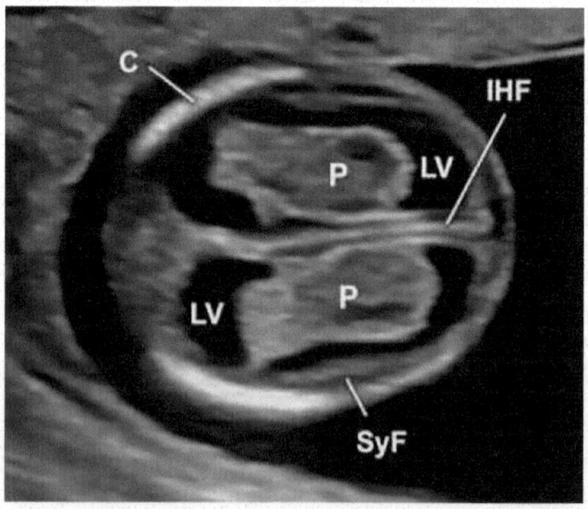

Fig. 1 Axial transventricular plane. The interhemispheric fissure (IHF) and both lateral ventricles (LV) are depicted on this view. *C* calvarium, *P* choroid plexus, *SyF* future Sylvian fissure

- Lateral ventricles on either side of the midline echo, filled with the choroid plexuses.

The ***fetal calvarium*** (skull) appears as a uniformly hyperechoic bony structure with an uninterrupted oval shape. Any bulging or protrusion of the intracranial structures or irregularities in the skull shape should raise suspicion of brain abnormalities, such as cephalocele, acrania–exencephaly–anencephaly sequence, or other neural tube defect [29, 30].

The ***interhemispheric fissure*** appears as a straight, uninterrupted hyperechoic midline echo dividing the fetal brain in two equal-sized hemispheres. Disruption of the continuity of the interhemispheric line is a clue finding of alobar holoprosencephaly [31], characterized by the appearance of an abnormal communication between lateral ventricles across the midline.

The ***lateral ventricles*** are two oval-shaped, fluid-filled structures located on either side of the midline echo. Either lateral ventricle contains the hyperechoic choroid plexus, occupying about half or more of the ventricle length/area [25, 32]. The normal appearance of the choroid plexuses on the axial plane is commonly referred to as the "butterfly sign." A smaller choroid plexus size may indicate an abnormally increased amount of ventricular fluid, as seen in ventriculomegaly [32, 33], whereas a choroid plexus filling most of the ventricular area may suggest fluid reduction, as seen in open spina bifida [25, 34].

The external brain surface is lined with a ***rudimentary cortex***, appearing as a thin smooth layer surrounding the ventricles and the external brain surface with two small recesses on the lateral surface of either brain hemisphere, representing the future Sylvian fissures. No other sulci or gyri are visible at this stage.

2.3 Biometric Measurements of the Fetal Brain

The primary aim of fetal biometry in the first trimester of pregnancy is to estimate gestational age [17]. The crown-rump length (CRL) is considered the most accurate parameter for pregnancy dating [35–37]. Alternatively, the biparietal diameter (BPD) and head circumference (HC) (Fig. 2) can be measured on the axial plane of the fetal head and used to estimate accurately gestational age. Moreover, the routine measurement of BPD has been found to be useful in early screening for open spinal dysraphism [38–41], as smaller values of BPD, i.e. below the fifth percentile, may indicate a cerebrospinal fluid leakage, typically observed in those neural tube defects.

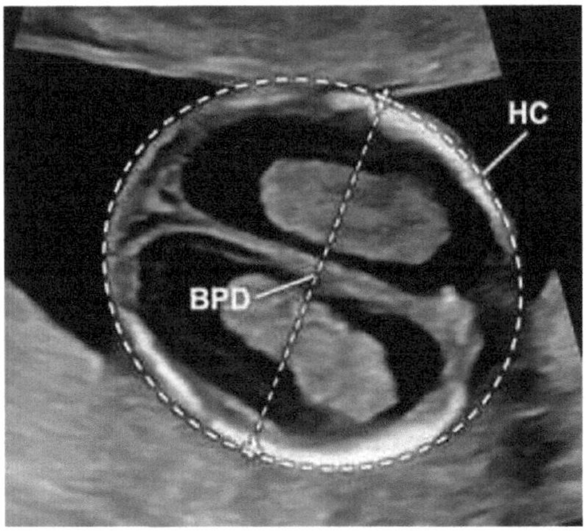

Fig. 2 Biometric measurements of the fetal brain. Measurement of the biparietal diameter (BPD) and head circumference (HC) on the transventricular axial plane

The BPD can be measured using either an outer-to-outer (calipers on the external edges of the parietal bones) or an outer-to-inner technique (calipers on the leading edges of the parietal bones), depending on the reference charts that one uses [42].

2.4 Management of Abnormal Findings

In case of suspected brain abnormality during the first-trimester routine ultrasound, it is important to refer the patient for an early neurosonography. This is an advanced examination including a multiplanar fetal brain assessment, usually conducted in a specialized center for fetal medicine.

3 Advanced Evaluation of the Fetal Brain (Early Fetal Neurosonography)

3.1 Indication

Suspected brain malformation identified during the first-trimester ultrasound screening examination.

3.2 Ultrasound Planes for Advanced Evaluation of the Fetal Brain

The optimal approach for early fetal neurosonography is yet to be established; however, a multiplanar approach not dissimilar from that of second and third trimester neurosonology [43] may be considered [28]. A multiplanar approach including axial, coronal, and sagittal planes of the fetal head allows for a comprehensive evaluation of fetal brain anatomy. While a transabdominal approach suffices in most cases, the vaginal approach may be considered for its potential in offering better resolution images due to the probe characteristics (higher frequency) and the shorter distance to the anatomical structures. Profound knowledge of the fetal CNS embryogenesis and anatomy is required for adequate interpretation of fetal brain findings during first-trimester neurosonography. Detailed neurosonography planes, beyond those necessary for routine examination, are described in the subsequent section.

The *axial planes* to be obtained in addition to the transventricular plane are as follows:

- Transthalamic plane.
- Transcerebellar plane.

Transthalamic plane: The following brain structures are to be visualized and assessed in sequential order from anterior to posterior:

- The frontal portion of the lateral ventricles.
- The anterior part of the interhemispheric fissure.
- The third ventricle.
- The thalami.
- The Sylvian aqueduct, surrounded by the midbrain tectum.

Starting from the transventricular plane, the **transthalamic plane** (Fig. 3) is obtained by a slight caudal movement of the ultrasound probe, angling it toward the cranial posterior fossa. On this plane, the anterior segment of the ***interhemispheric fissure*** is visible between the frontal portion of the ***lateral ventricles***, eventu-

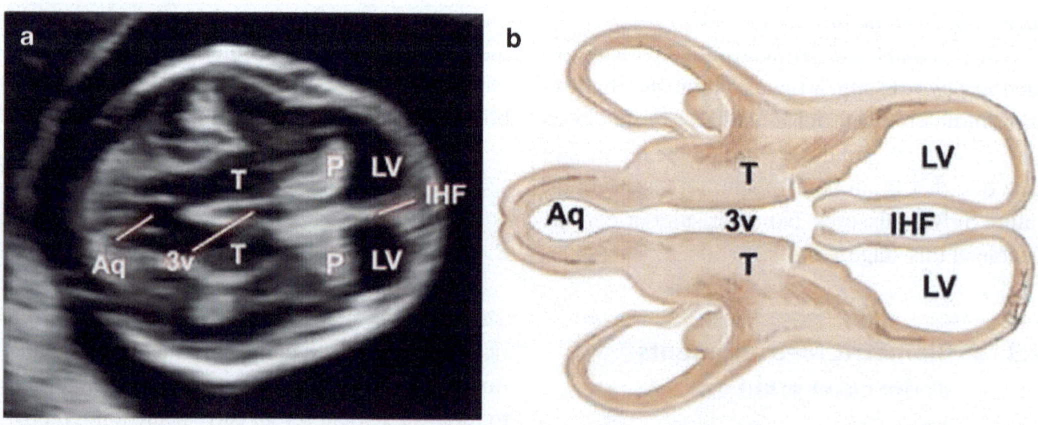

Fig. 3 Axial transthalamic plane. Ultrasound image of the transthalamic plane (**a**) and corresponding anatomic illustration (**b**). The frontal portion of the lateral ventricles (LV), corresponding choroid plexuses (P) and interhemispheric fissure (IHF) are depicted. The third ventricle (3v) between the thalami (T), and more posteriorly the Sylvian aqueduct (Aq) are also visible

ally developing into the frontal horns, filled with the corresponding ***choroid plexus***. The interhemispheric fissure appears to be interrupted by the ***third ventricle***, presenting as a thin, anechoic space at the level of the thalami. The ***thalami*** are visible as two separate, symmetrical, anechoic ovoid structures on each side of the midline, encircling the third ventricle. Posterior to the thalami, the ***Sylvian aqueduct*** lies along the midline, presenting as an anechoic, rectangular cavity surrounded by the midbrain tectum.

Transcerebellar plane: The following brain structures are to be visualized and assessed in sequential order from anterior to posterior:

- The anterior part of the lateral ventricles.
- The anterior part of the interhemispheric fissure.
- The third ventricle.
- The thalami and the midbrain tegmentum.
- The rudimentary cerebellum.
- The cisterna magna.

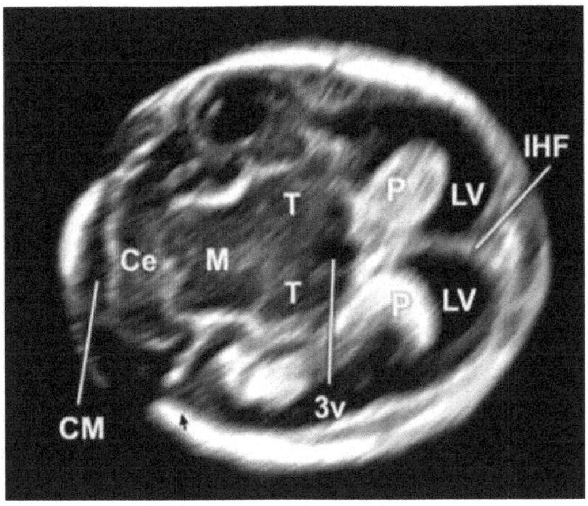

Fig. 4 Axial transcerebellar plane. The frontal portion of the lateral ventricles (LV), corresponding choroid plexuses (P) and interhemispheric fissure (IHF) are depicted. The third ventricle (3v) and the thalami (T) are also visible. The midbrain tegmentum (M), the cerebellum (Ce), and the cisterna magna (CM) are seen in sequence posterior to the thalami

The **transcerebellar plane** (Fig. 4) is obtained by gently angling the probe posteriorly toward the posterior fossa, creating an oblique plane. On this plane, the main ***supratentorial brain structures*** (including frontal portion of the lateral ventricles, interhemispheric fissure, third ventricle, and thalami) are visualized similarly to the transthalamic plane. Posterior to the thalami, the ***midbrain tegmentum***, a region corresponding to the curvature of the midbrain, can be observed just below the Sylvian aqueduct. At this stage, the ***fetal cerebellar hemispheres*** and ***vermis*** are still developing and may not be distinctly visible. The ***cerebellum*** might appear posterior to the thalami and midbrain as an arch-shaped structure. Behind the cerebellum, the ***cisterna magna*** is identifiable as a thin, fluid-filled space, with a central area sometimes appearing darker, representing the lower and posterior portion of the fourth ventricle, referred to as the Blake pouch.

The main *coronal planes* are as follows:

- Transfrontal coronal plane.
- Transcaudate coronal plane.
- Transthalamic coronal plane.
- Occipital coronal planes.

These planes are sequentially acquired by aligning the ultrasound beam perpendicular to the sagittal suture and sweeping the probe from the frontal to the occipital pole of the fetal head (Fig. 5). Each coronal plane is characterized by specific anatomic landmarks, as follows:

Transfrontal coronal plane:
- Interhemispheric fissure.
- Frontal portions of the lateral ventricles with choroid plexus.
- Orbital process of the frontal bone.
- Orbits and lenses.

The **transfrontal coronal plane** (Fig. 6) is the most anterior coronal plane, obtained through the anterior fontanelle. The frontal portions of the ***lateral ventricles*** are partially filled with their corresponding choroid plexuses, appearing symmetrical and lying on either side of the uninterrupted, straight midline echo which represents the ***interhemispheric fissure***. Additionally, the ***orbital processes*** of the frontal bones are visible along with the fetal ***orbits*** and ***lenses*** below.

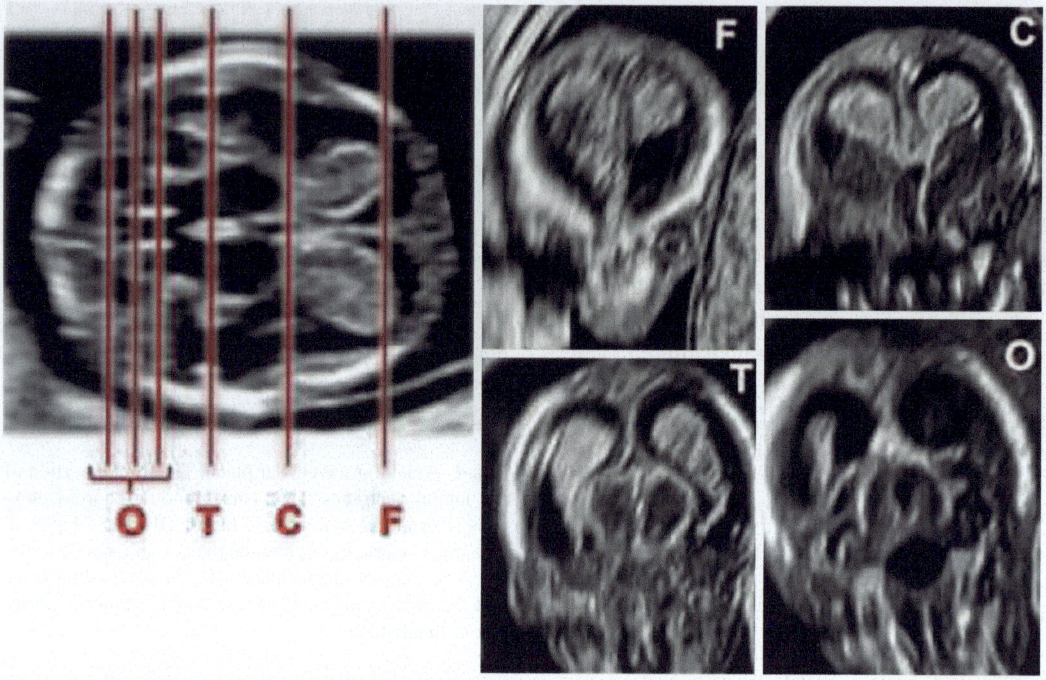

Fig. 5 Coronal planes—overview. Transfrontal (F), transcaudate (C), transthalamic (T), and occipital (O) coronal views. Adapted from Volpe N. et al., 2021 [28]

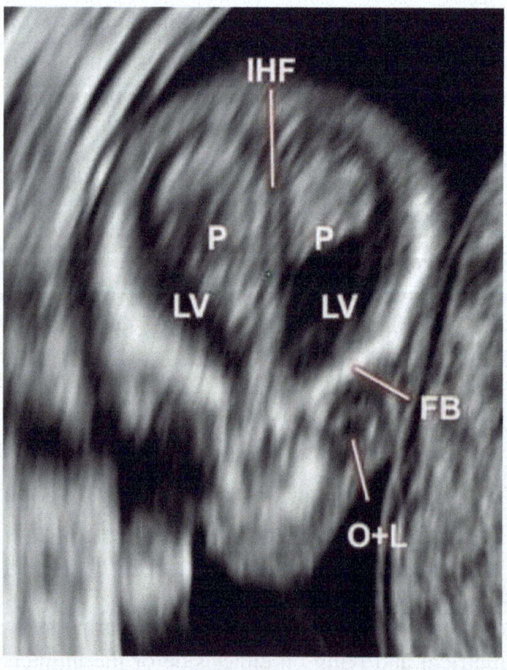

Fig. 6 Transfrontal coronal plane. The lateral ventricles (LV) and choroid plexuses (P) are visible on either side of the interhemispheric fissure (IHF). The orbital processes of the frontal bones (FB), with corresponding eye orbits and lenses (O + L) are also visible. Adapted from Volpe N. et al., 2021 [28]

Transcaudate coronal plane:

- Frontal portion of the lateral ventricles with choroid plexuses.
- Interhemispheric fissure interrupted by the foramina of Monro.
- Third ventricle.
- Ganglionic eminences.
- Basal ganglia.

The **transcaudate coronal plane** (Fig. 7), slightly posterior to the transfrontal plane, is also obtained through the anterior fontanelle. The ***lateral ventricles*** are displayed on either side of the midline, filled by their corresponding ***choroid plexuses***, which are converging downwards and joining at the level of the ***foramina of Monro***, also known as interventricular foramina. The interhemispheric ***fissure*** is interrupted at this junction, whereas the frontal portion of the ***third ventricle*** may be depicted just inferiorly, on the midline, as a thin fluid-filled cavity. The ***ganglionic eminences*** are placed laterally and inferiorly to the frontal portion of each lateral ventricle, in the subventricular zone, appearing as a

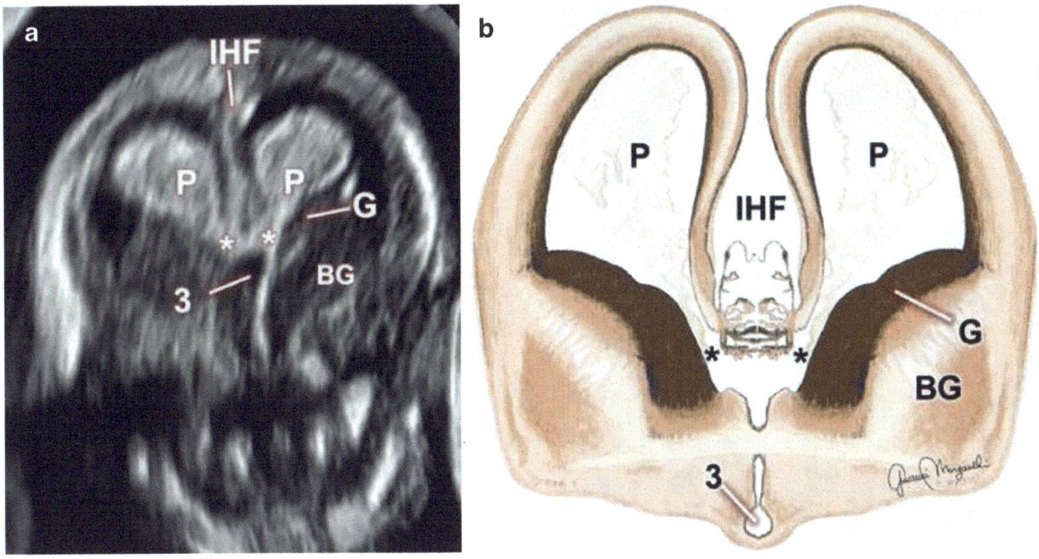

Fig. 7 Transcaudate coronal plane. Ultrasound image of the transcaudate coronal plane (**a**) and corresponding anatomic illustration (**b**). The lateral ventricle choroid plexuses are joining on the midline at the level of the foramina of Monro (*). Below the ventricles, ganglionic eminences (G) and basal ganglia (BG) are also visible. (IHF) interhemispheric fissure; [3] third ventricle

hypoechoic thickening. The ***basal ganglia***, including the caudate nucleus, are also visible, sitting below the ganglionic eminences, on either side of the third ventricle.

Transthalamic coronal plane:

- Interhemispheric fissure.
- Temporal portions of the lateral ventricles with choroid plexus.
- Thalami.
- Third ventricle.

The **transthalamic coronal plane** (Fig. 8) is obtained by gently sweeping the probe further posteriorly. The ***interhemispheric fissure*** has similar appearance to that observed on the previous planes, yet it is interrupted inferiorly by the ***thalami***, appearing as hypoechoic, round, and symmetrical structures. The ***temporal portions of the lateral ventricles*** with their corresponding choroid plexuses are visualized on either side of thalami. Between the thalami, the caudal portion of the ***third ventricle*** can be depicted.

Occipital coronal planes:

- Occipital portions of the lateral ventricles.
- Brainstem (midbrain, pons and medulla oblongata).
- Sylvian aqueduct.
- Cerebellar hemispheres.
- Fourth ventricle with choroid plexus.

The **occipital planes** (Fig. 9) represent the most posterior coronal planes, comprising three distinct sub-planes defined by the position of the ultrasound beam in relation to the fourth ventricle: OC_1 is located anteriorly to the fourth ventricle; OC_2 includes the fourth ventricle; and OC_3 is posterior to the fourth ventricle.

On the ***OC_1*** (Fig. 9a), the ***occipital portions of the lateral ventricles*** are displayed on the upper part of the image. The ***Sylvian aqueduct*** lies on the midline, lined by the ***midbrain tectum*** laterally and superiorly, while the ***midbrain tegmentum*** is just below it. The midbrain represents the most cranial part of the ***brainstem***, which includes also the ***pons*** and ***medulla oblongata***,

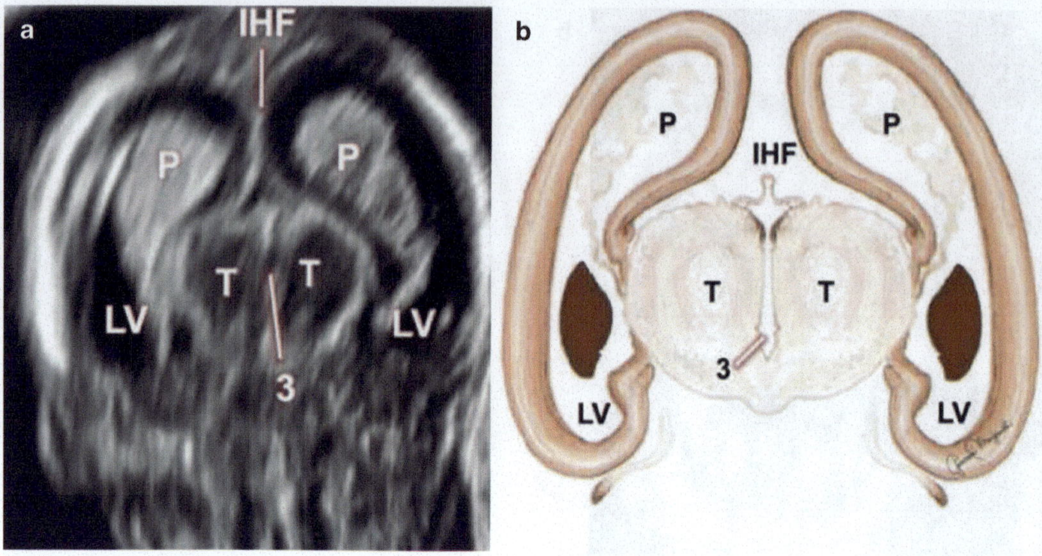

Fig. 8 Transthalamic coronal plane. Ultrasound image of the transthalamic coronal plane (**a**) and corresponding anatomic illustration (**b**). The temporal portions of the lateral ventricles (LV) with their corresponding choroid plexuses (P) are visualized on either side of thalami (T). (IHF) interhemispheric fissure; [3] third ventricle

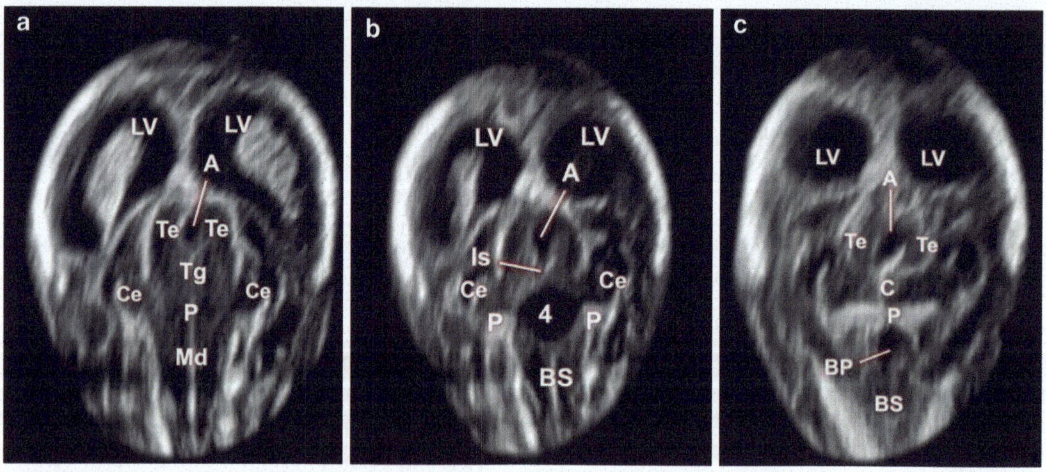

Fig. 9 Occipital coronal planes. On the anterior occipital coronal plane (**a**), the midbrain tectum (Te) is above and aside the aqueduct of Sylvius (A), and the midbrain tegmentum (Tg) is just below it, in continuity with the pons (P) and medulla oblongata (Md). On the transventricular occipital coronal plane (**b**), the fourth ventricle [4] is visible, appearing connected to the aqueduct of Sylvius (A) by the isthmus (Is). The lateral portions of its choroid plexus (P) and the rudimentary cerebellar hemispheres (Ce) are visible on either side of the fourth ventricle. Behind the fourth ventricle, the posterior occipital coronal plane (**c**) allows the visualization of the rudimentary cerebellum (Ce) and the fourth ventricle choroid plexus (P). On the midline, below the plexus, the Blake pouch (BP) is also visible as the lowest posterior part of the fourth ventricle. *LV* lateral ventricle, *BS* brainstem

following the midbrain caudally. On either side of the pons, the rudimentary ***cerebellar hemispheres*** are depicted.

On the ***OC***$_2$ (Fig. 9b), the ***occipital portions of the lateral ventricles***, the ***Sylvian aqueduct,*** and the ***midbrain tectum*** are depicted similarly to OC$_1$. In this view, the Sylvian aqueduct is followed caudally by the ***isthmus***, which connects the aqueduct to the ***fourth ventricle***, appearing as a typically rhombic-shaped structure. At this level, the two lateral portions of the ***choroid plexus*** appear as hyperechoic structures on the two lateral walls of the cavity, just below the rudimentary ***cerebellar hemispheres***. Below the fourth ventricle, the most inferior segment of the brainstem, the ***medulla oblongata***, is visualized.

The ***OC$_3$*** (Fig. 9c), mainly displays the structures of the cranial posterior fossa behind the fourth ventricle. The most posterior part of the ***Sylvian aqueduct***, along with the adjacent ***midbrain tectum*** can be seen on this plane. Below these structures lies the rudimentary ***cerebellum*** and the ***choroid plexus*** of the fourth ventricle, appearing as a hyperechoic thick elongated structure on the lower surface of the cerebellum. Slightly inferior to the choroid plexus, the lowest posterior part of the fourth ventricle, the ***Blake pouch***, appears as an anechoic, round-shaped structure sitting on the midline.

The *sagittal planes* are as follows:

- Anterior midsagittal plane.
- Posterior midsagittal plane.

Anterior midsagittal plane:

- Fetal profile depicting the forehead, nose (bone, skin, and tip), and chin.
- Rectangularly-shaped hard palate.
- Round-shaped anechoic diencephalon.
- Sylvian aqueduct.
- Brainstem, fourth ventricle (with choroid plexus), and cisterna magna appearing as three anechoic spaces in the posterior fossa.

The **midsagittal plane** is obtained with the ultrasound beam aligned longitudinally with the fetal profile and sagittal suture, over the anterior fontanelle, parallel to the midline of the fetal brain (Fig. 10). It is the reference plane for the measurement of the NT and allows the evaluation of the following structures:

The ***diencephalon*** appears as a hypoechoic, round structure in the middle of the fetal brain, including the thalami and the third ventricle. In approximately half of cases when using a transvaginal probe, allowing higher resolution imaging, the *cavum veli interpositi* can be visualized just above the roof of the diencephalon as an anechoic elongated structure [44] (Fig. 10b). Posterior and caudal to the diencephalon, three parallel anechoic spaces of similar size are visible between the sphenoid and occipital bones [45]. From anterior to posterior, these spaces represent the ***brainstem*** (including the mesencephalon, pons, and medulla oblongata), the ***fourth ventricle*** (i.e., "intracranial translucency"), and the ***cisterna magna*** (Fig. 10a). Under normal circumstances, the ratio between the brainstem thickness and the distance between the brain stem and the occipital bone (also called BS/

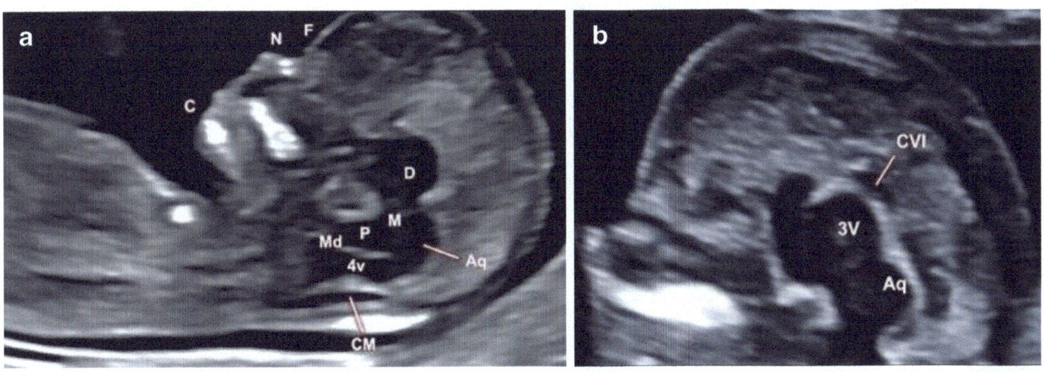

Fig. 10 Midsagittal plane, anterior approach. (**a**) The diencephalon (D) is clearly depicted in the middle of the brain, and the Sylvian aqueduct (Aq) can be also visualized posterior to it. The detailed anatomy of the cranial posterior fossa is also depicted, including the brainstem (M, mesencephalon, P, pons and Md, medulla oblongata), the fourth ventricle (4v), and the cisterna magna (CM). (**b**) Using higher resolution probes, the third ventricle (3v), the cavum veli interpositi (CVI), and the Sylvian aqueduct (Aq) could be visualized. *F* forehead, *N* nose, *C* chin

BSOB) ranges from 0.5 to 1.0 [21, 22]. Posterior to the diencephalon and superior to the mesencephalon and fourth ventricle, the ***Sylvian aqueduct*** could be visualized as an elongated fluid-filled cavity (Fig. 10a, b). Abnormal appearance of the anatomic structures of the posterior fossa should raise suspicion of major CNS anomalies, such as open spinal dysraphism or cystic anomaly of posterior fossa. In case of open spina bifida, the obliteration of the cisterna magna and posterior displacement of the brain structures may cause an increased BS/BSOB ratio [21, 22], whereas a cystic anomaly of the posterior fossa would lead to an enlargement of the spaces behind the brainstem (i.e., fourth ventricle and cisterna magna) with a decreased BS/BSOB ratio [18, 20, 24]. More details on the abnormal ultrasound findings in the first trimester related to posterior fossa malformations are described in the dedicated chapter.

Posterior midsagittal plane:

- Brainstem (midbrain, pons, and medulla oblongata).
- Mesencephalic and pontine flexures.
- Sylvian aqueduct.
- Fourth ventricle and choroid plexus.
- Anterior and posterior membranous area.
- Cerebellar vermis.
- Cisterna magna.

The **posterior midsagittal plane** (Fig. 11) is acquired through the posterior fontanelle and allows a detailed visualization of the infratentorial region of the brain, also referred to as the posterior fossa [46–48].

The most anterior structure within the posterior fossa is the ***brainstem***, comprising ***midbrain***, ***pons***, and ***medulla oblongata***. The brainstem displays a characteristic "S" shape, due to the ***mesencephalic*** and ***pontine flexures***, the latter representing the floor of the ***fourth ventricle***, which appears as an anechoic fluid-filled space lying dorsally to the brainstem. Above the fourth ventricle, another fluid-filled cavity could be depicted, the ***Sylvian aqueduct***, similar in size and connected with the former by a thin ***isthmus*** at the level of the mesencephalic flexure. The Sylvian aqueduct sits above and posterior to the ***midbrain tegmentum***, whereas its posterior wall and roof are covered by the ***midbrain tectum***.

In the first trimester, the ***cerebellar vermis*** develops from a thickening of the most cranial part of the roof of the fourth ventricle, consisting

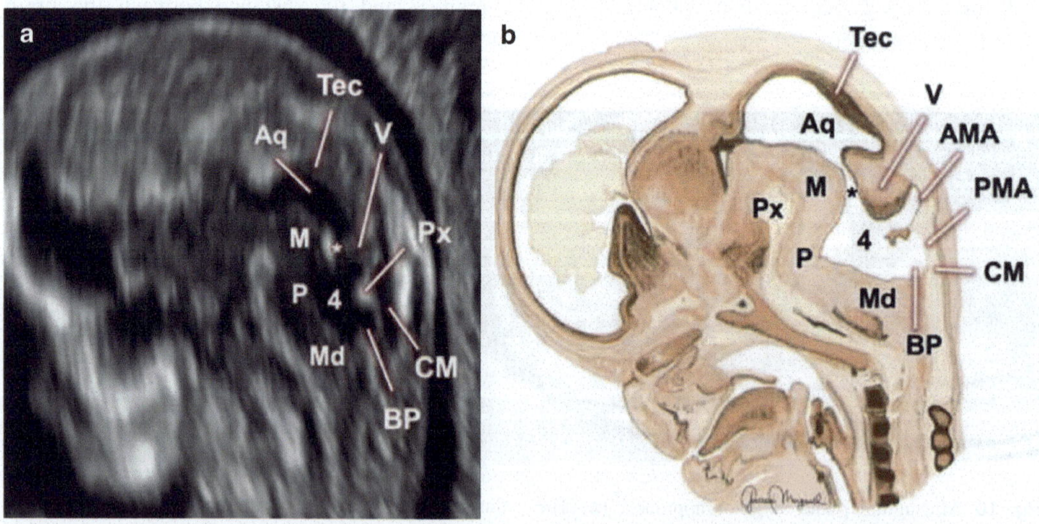

Fig. 11 Midsagittal plane, posterior approach. Ultrasound image of the midsagittal plane (**a**) and corresponding anatomic illustration (**b**). *Aq* aqueduct of Sylvius, *M* mesencephalon, *P* pons, *Md* medulla, * isthmus, *4* fourth ventricle, *CM* Cisterna Magna, *Tec* tectum, *AMA* anterior membranous area, *PMA* posterior membranous area, *Px* plexus of the fourth ventricle, *V* cerebellar vermis, *BP* Blake's pouch

of a medullary velum and divided into ***anterior*** and ***posterior membranous areas*** by the protruding ***choroid plexus***. The anterior membranous area gradually decreases in size as the cerebellar vermis develops caudally toward the choroid plexus. The posterior membranous area protrudes into the developing cisterna magna, forming a finger-shaped structure known as Blake's pouch [48, 49].

As mentioned above, some CNS malformations, such as open spinal bifida and cystic anomalies of the posterior fossa, usually induce specific anatomic alterations of the cranial posterior fossa structures. Consequently, the knowledge of the normal anatomy and embryology of the posterior fossa is a prerequisite for the identification and classification of such conditions. Furthermore, variations in the position or size of some posterior fossa structures— such as the anterior membranous area, choroid plexus of the fourth ventricle, and cerebellar vermis—can potentially serve as sonographic markers for the differential diagnosis of cystic anomalies [19, 49, 50].

References

1. Nicolaides KH. Screening for fetal aneuploidies at 11 to 13 weeks. Prenat Diagn. 2011;31(1):7–15.
2. Pandya PP, Altman DG, Brizot ML, Pettersen H, Nicolaides KH. Repeatability of measurement of fetal nuchal translucency thickness. Ultrasound Obstet Gynecol. 1995;5(5):334–7.
3. Santorum M, Wright D, Syngelaki A, Karagioti N, Nicolaides KH. Accuracy of first-trimester combined test in screening for trisomies 21, 18 and 13. Ultrasound Obstet Gynecol. 2017;49(6):714–20.
4. Syngelaki A, Hammami A, Bower S, Zidere V, Akolekar R, Nicolaides KH. Diagnosis of fetal non-chromosomal abnormalities on routine ultrasound examination at 11–13 weeks' gestation. Ultrasound Obstet Gynecol. 2019;54(4):468–76.
5. Vayna AM, Veduta A, Duta S, Panaitescu AM, Stoica S, Buinoiu N, et al. Diagnosis of fetalstructural anomalies at 11 to 14weeks. J Ultrasound Med. 2018;37(8):2063–73.
6. Bardi F, Smith E, Kuilman M, Snijders RJM, Bilardo CM. Early detection of structural anomalies in a primary care setting in The Netherlands. Fetal Diagn Ther. 2019;46(1):12–9.
7. Rayburn WF, Jolley JA, Simpson LL. Advances in ultrasound imaging for congenital malformations during early gestation. Birth Defects Res Part Clin Mol Teratol. 2015;103(4):260–8.
8. Rossi AC, Prefumo F. Accuracy of ultrasonography at 11-14 weeks of gestation for detection of fetal structural anomalies: a systematic review. Obstet Gynecol. 2013;122(6):1160–7.
9. Grande M, Arigita M, Borobio V, Jimenez JM, Fernandez S, Borrell A. First-trimester detection of structural abnormalities and the role of aneuploidy markers. Ultrasound Obstet Gynecol. 2012;39(2):157–63.
10. Anderson N, Boswell O, Duff G. Prenatal sonography for the detection of fetal anomalies: results of a prospective study and comparison with prior series. Am J Roentgenol. 1995;165:943–50.
11. Iliescu D, Tudorache S, Comanescu A, Antsaklis P, Cotarcea S, Novac L, et al. Improved detection rate of structural abnormalities in the first trimester using an extended examination protocol. Ultrasound Obstet Gynecol. 2013;42(3):300–9.
12. Syngelaki A, Chelemen T, Dagklis T, Allan L, Nicolaides KH. Challenges in the diagnosis of fetal non-chromosomal abnormalities at 11-13 weeks. Prenat Diagn. 2011;31:90–102.
13. Kenkhuis MJA, Bakker M, Bardi F, Fontanella F, Bakker MK, Fleurke-Rozema JH, et al. Effectiveness of 12–13-week scan for early diagnosis of fetal congenital anomalies in the cell-free DNA era. Ultrasound Obstet Gynecol. 2018;51:463.
14. Liao Y, Wen H, Ouyang S, Yuan Y, Bi J, Guan Y, et al. Routine first-trimester ultrasound screening using a standardized anatomical protocol. Am J Obstet Gynecol. 2021;224(4):396.e1–396.e15.
15. Karim JN, Roberts NW, Salomon LJ, Papageorghiou AT. Systematic review of first-trimester ultrasound screening for detection of fetal structural anomalies and factors that affect screening performance. Ultrasound Obstet Gynecol. 2017;50(4):429–41.
16. Volpe N, Sen C, Turan S, Sepulveda W, Khalil A, Rolnik DL, et al. First trimester examination of fetal anatomy: clinical practice guideline by the World Association of Perinatal Medicine (WAPM) and the Perinatal Medicine Foundation (PMF). J Perinat Med. 2022;50(7):863–77.
17. International Society of Ultrasound in Obstetrics and Gynecology, Bilardo CM, Chaoui R, Hyett JA, Kagan KO, Karim JN, et al. ISUOG practice guidelines (updated): performance of 11–14-week ultrasound scan. Ultrasound Obstet Gynecol. 2023;61(1):127–43.
18. Volpe P, Contro E, Fanelli T, Muto B, Pilu G, Gentile M. Appearance of fetal posterior fossa at 11-14 weeks in fetuses with Dandy-Walker malformation or chromosomal anomalies. Ultrasound Obstet Gynecol. 2016;47:720–5.
19. Volpe P, Persico N, Fanelli T, Robertis VD, D'Alessandro J, Boito S, et al. Prospective detection and differential diagnosis of cystic posterior fossa anomalies by assessing posterior brain at 11–14 weeks. Am J Obstet Gynecol MFM. 2019;1(2):173–81.

20. Lachmann R, Sinkovskaya E, Abuhamad A. Posterior brain in fetuses with Dandy-Walker malformation with complete agenesis of the cerebellar vermis at 11-13weeks: A pilot study. Prenat Diagn. 2012;32(8):765–9.
21. Lachmann R, Chaoui R, Moratalla J, Picciarelli G, Nicolaides KH. Posterior brain in fetuses with open spina bifida at 11 to 13 weeks. Prenat Diagn. 2011;31:103–6.
22. Wertaschnigg D, Ramkrishna J, Ganesan S, Tse C, Scheier M, Volpe N, et al. Cranial sonographic markers of fetal open spina bifida at 11 to 13 weeks of gestation. Prenat Diagn. 2020;40(3):365–72.
23. Chaoui R, Nicolaides KH. Detecting open spina bifida at the 11-13-week scan by assessing intracranial translucency and the posterior brain region: mid-sagittal or axial plane? Ultrasound Obstet Gynecol. 2011;38(6):609–12.
24. Volpe P, Muto B, Passamonti U, Rembouskos G, Robertis VD, Campobasso G, et al. Abnormal sonographic appearance of posterior brain at 11-14weeks and fetal outcome. Prenat Diagn. 2015;35:717–23.
25. Loureiro T, Ushakov F, Montenegro N, Gielchinsky Y, Nicolaides KH. Cerebral ventricular system in fetuses with open spina bifida at 11-13 weeks' gestation. Ultrasound Obstet Gynecol. 2012;39(6):620–4.
26. Ushakov F, Sacco A, Andreeva E, Tudorache S, Everett T, David AL, et al. Crash sign: new first-trimester sonographic marker of spina bifida. Ultrasound Obstet Gynecol. 2019;54:740–5.
27. Malinger G, Paladini D, Haratz KK, Monteagudo A, Pilu GL, Timor-Tritsch IE. ISUOG practice guidelines (updated): sonographic examination of the fetal central nervous system. Part 1: performance of screening examination and indications for targeted neurosonography. Ultrasound Obstet Gynecol. 2020;56(3):476–84.
28. Volpe N, Dall'Asta A, Di Pasquo E, Frusca T, Ghi T. First-trimester fetal neurosonography: technique and diagnostic potential. Ultrasound Obstet Gynecol. 2021;57(2):204–14.
29. Sepulveda W, Wong AE, Andreeva E, Odegova N, Martinez-Ten P, Meagher S. Sonographic spectrum of first-trimester fetal cephalocele: review of 35 cases. Ultrasound Obstet Gynecol. 2015;46(1):29–33.
30. Cheng C-C, Lee F-K, Lin H-W, Shih J-C, Tsai M-S. Diagnosis of fetal acrania during the first trimester nuchal translucency screening for down syndrome. Int J Gynecol Obstet. 2003;80(2):139–44.
31. Sepulveda W, Wong AE. First trimester screening for holoprosencephaly with choroid plexus morphology ('butterfly' sign) and biparietal diameter. Prenat Diagn. 2013;33(13):1233–7.
32. Manegold-Brauer G, Oseledchyk A, Floeck A, Berg C, Gembruch U, Geipel A. Approach to the sonographic evaluation of fetal ventriculomegaly at 11 to 14 weeks gestation. BMC Pregnancy Childbirth. 2016;16(1):3.
33. Labrosse KB, Buechel J, Guelmez H, Butenschoen A, Schoenberger H, Visca E, et al. Presentation of ventriculomegaly at 11–14 weeks of gestation: an analysis of longitudinal data. Prenat Diagn. 2023;43(7):910–8.
34. Chaoui R, Benoit B, Entezami M, Frenzel W, Heling KS, Ladendorf B, et al. Ratio of fetal choroid plexus to head size: simple sonographic marker of open spina bifida at 11–13 weeks' gestation. Ultrasound Obstet Gynecol. 2020;55(1):81–6.
35. Salomon LJ, Bernard JP, Duyme M, Dorion A, Ville Y. Revisiting first-trimester fetal biometry. Ultrasound Obstet Gynecol. 2003;22(1):63–6.
36. Salomon LJ, Pizzi C, Gasparrini A, Bernard JP, Ville Y. Prediction of the date of delivery based on first trimester ultrasound measurements: an independent method from estimated date of conception. J Matern Fetal Neonatal Med. 2010;23(1):1–9.
37. Chalouhi GE, Bernard JP, Benoist G, Nasr B, Ville Y, Salomon LJ. A comparison of first trimester measurements for prediction of delivery date. J Matern Fetal Neonatal Med. 2011;24(1):51–7.
38. Suresh S, Sudarshan S, Rangaraj A, Indrani S, Cuckle H. Spina bifida screening in the first trimester using ultrasound biparietal diameter measurement adjusted for crown-rump length or abdominal circumference. Prenat Diagn. 2019;39(4):314–8.
39. Simon EG, Arthuis CJ, Haddad G, Bertrand P, Perrotin F. Biparietal/transverse abdominal diameter ratio ≤ 1: potential marker for open spina bifida at 11–13-week scan. Ultrasound Obstet Gynecol. 2015;45(3):267–72.
40. Bernard JP, Cuckle HS, Bernard MA, Brochet C, Salomon LJ, Ville Y. Combined screening for open spina bifida at 11-13 weeks using fetal biparietal diameter and maternal serum markers. Am J Obstet Gynecol. 2013;209(3):223.e1–5.
41. Karl K, Benoit B, Entezami M, Heling KS, Chaoui R. Small biparietal diameter in fetuses with spina bifida on 11–13-week and mid-gestation ultrasound. Ultrasound Obstet Gynecol. 2012;40(2):140–4.
42. Loughna P, Chitty L, Evans T, Chudleigh T. Fetal size and dating: charts recommended for clinical obstetric practice. Ultrasound. 2009;17(3):160–6.
43. Paladini D, Malinger G, Birnbaum R, Monteagudo A, Pilu G, Salomon LJ, et al. ISUOG practice guidelines (updated): sonographic examination of the fetal central nervous system. Part 2: performance of targeted neurosonography. Ultrasound Obstet Gynecol. 2021;57(4):661–71.
44. Altmann R, Scharnreitner I, Auer C, Hirtler L, Springer C, Falschlehner S, et al. Visualization of the third ventricle, the future cavum Septi Pellucidi, and the Cavum Veli Interpositi at 11+3 to 13+6 gestational weeks on 3D transvaginal ultrasound including normative data. Ultraschall Med - Eur J Ultrasound. 2023;44(01):e72–82.
45. Chaoui R, Benoit B, Mitkowska-Wozniak H, Heling KS, Nicolaides KH. Assessment of intracranial translucency (IT) in the detection of spina bifida at the 11–13-week scan. Ultrasound Obstet Gynecol. 2009;34(3):249–52.

46. Bayer SA, Altman J. The human brain during the late first trimester [internet]. 0th ed. CRC Press; 2006. [cited 2024 Feb 16]. https://www.taylorfrancis.com/books/9781420003277
47. Robinson AJ. Inferior vermian hypoplasia—preconception, misconception. Ultrasound Obstet Gynecol. 2014;43(2):123–36.
48. Altmann R, Scharnreitner I, Scheier T, Mayer R, Arzt W, Scheier M. Sonoembryology of the fetal posterior fossa at 11 + 3 to 13 + 6 gestational weeks on three-dimensional transvaginal ultrasound: Sonoembryology of the fetal posterior fossa at the first trimester scan. Prenat Diagn. 2016;36(8):731–7.
49. Paladini D, Donarini G, Parodi S, Chaoui R. Differentiating features of posterior fossa at 12–13 weeks' gestation in fetuses with Dandy–Walker malformation and Blake's pouch cyst. Ultrasound Obstet Gynecol. 2019;53(6):850–2.
50. Volpe P, Robertis VD, Volpe G, Boito S, Fanelli T, Olivieri C, et al. Position of the choroid plexus of the fourth ventricle in first- and second-trimester fetuses: a novel approach to early diagnosis of cystic posterior fossa anomalies. Ultrasound Obstet Gynecol. 2021;58(4):568.

Prenatal MR Imaging of Brain Malformations

Nevena Fileva, Irina Stavarache, Andrea Righini, and Andrea Rossi

Abstract

While ultrasound remains the cornerstone of prenatal imaging and can recognize and characterize the majority of congenital and acquired brain abnormalities, MR imaging has the potential of refining the diagnosis and can reveal additional findings in cases when ultrasound is unrevealing. MR imaging is typically feasible from 19 to 20 gestational weeks onward. This chapter focuses on the role of MR imaging in fetuses harboring brain malformations; the fundamental bases of prenatal MR imaging diagnoses in these conditions are discussed.

Nevena Fileva and Irina Stavarache contributed equally with all other contributors.

Keywords

Magnetic resonance imaging · Prenatal · Brain malformations · Diagnosis

1 Introduction

The first and pivotal imaging method to explore the fetal brain is ultrasound (US), while magnetic resonance (MR) imaging is applied to further investigate unclear or more complex conditions. In the last two decades, a large body of literature has addressed the issue regarding the indications to perform fetal MR neuroimaging.

The current chapter will focus especially on those conditions where MR imaging is likely to provide a more detailed characterization of anomalies suspected during ultrasound examination. The indication for fetal MR is especially relevant at early gestational ages, especially in the second trimester, since in several countries

N. Fileva
Neuroradiology Unit, Istituto Giannina Gaslini, Genoa, Italy

Department of Diagnostic Imaging, Medical University Sofia, Sofia, Bulgaria

I. Stavarache
Donna Medical Center, Bucharest, Romania

A. Righini
Pediatric Radiology and Neuroradiology Department, Children's Hospital V. Buzzi, Milan, Italy
e-mail: andrea.righini@asst-fbf-sacco.it

A. Rossi (✉)
Neuroradiology Unit, Istituto Giannina Gaslini, Genoa, Italy

Department of Health Sciences (DISSAL), University of Genoa, Genoa, Italy
e-mail: andrearossi@gaslini.org

P. Volpe, T. Ghi (eds.), *Fetal Neurosonography*, Ultrasound in Obstetrics and Gynecology,
https://doi.org/10.1007/978-3-031-70192-4_14

there are stringent limitations concerning the legal limits for pregnancy termination. Indeed, fetal MRI could provide additional information that might be key to formulate a more accurate counseling regarding the prognosis of the suspected condition for guiding patients' choice regarding pregnancy management.

The role of fetal MR neuroimaging depends also on the level of expertise of prenatal ultrasound specialists, since highly specialized professionals might less frequently seek for MRI complementary information to make a definite diagnosis; however, the improvements in expert neurosonography have permitted the identification of very subtle, unusual, and scarcely definable sonographic signs which might also be looked for correlation at MRI imaging. In this sense, the two imaging techniques help each other in a mutual assistance in the diagnostic prenatal neuroimaging workup.

2 Chiari Malformations

2.1 Chiari I Malformation

Chiari I malformation (CMI) represents the caudal descent of the cerebellar tonsils below the foramen magnum due to a smaller than normal posterior fossa. CMI is defined by most authors as caudal tonsil displacement of 5 mm below the McRae line (from basion to opisthion), while others consider that diagnosis is made when, irrespective of the degree of displacement, the tonsils' shape is abnormal, such as "peg-like" or pointed, and they fill the foramen magnum, obstructing the cerebrospinal fluid spaces [1, 2].

Prenatal diagnosis of CMI is rare [3, 4]; it is reported in the literature that the role of fetal MRI is more about understanding the pathogenesis rather than directing the clinical management [3].

Features of CMI, such as tonsillar descent, are not so obvious in utero as on postnatal MR scans, so qualitative prenatal estimation is not predictive. This is because the cerebellum has yet to complete its development prenatally, so the posterior fossa can still accommodate the developing cerebellum before tonsillar descent becomes evident postnatally. Some parameters, however, can be predictive of CMI such as wider basal and clivo-supraoccipital angles, the reduced posterior cranial fossa (PCF) width, posterior cranial fossa height, and the ratio between PCF width (PCFw) and height, and the reduced PCFw/BPDb ratio may indicate an eventually small of PCF and predict postnatal development of CMI [5].

2.2 Chiari II Malformation

Chiari II malformation (CMII) is defined as hindbrain descent through the foramen magnum with herniation of the cerebellar vermis, brainstem, and fourth ventricle, occurring in the context of open spinal dysraphisms such as myelomeningocele. It is also associated with other cranial features such as ventriculomegaly, cerebellar hypoplasia, tentorium hypoplasia, tectal beaking, enlarged interthalamic adhesion, corpus callosum dysgenesis, aqueductal stenosis, and periventricular nodular heterotopia [6, 7].

Cranial anomalies as well as spinal defects of CMII are usually identify at ultrasound imaging. Fetal MRI allows, however, a better evaluation of detailed features such as the morphology of the cerebellum or brain stem, brain parenchyma signal changes, and whether the spinal dysraphism is open or closed (Fig. 1) [3].

Fetal MRI is also usually performed in centers where intrauterine surgery can be offered. In adequate settings, prenatal myelomeningocele surgery can reduce the need for subsequent shunting and improve motor function compared to postnatal surgery [8]. Evidence in the literature showed that there was no change in the severity of cerebellar ectopia/Chiari grade in fetuses with CMII who did not undergo prenatal surgery, while improvement of cerebellar ectopia occurred in those fetuses who underwent prenatal surgery [9].

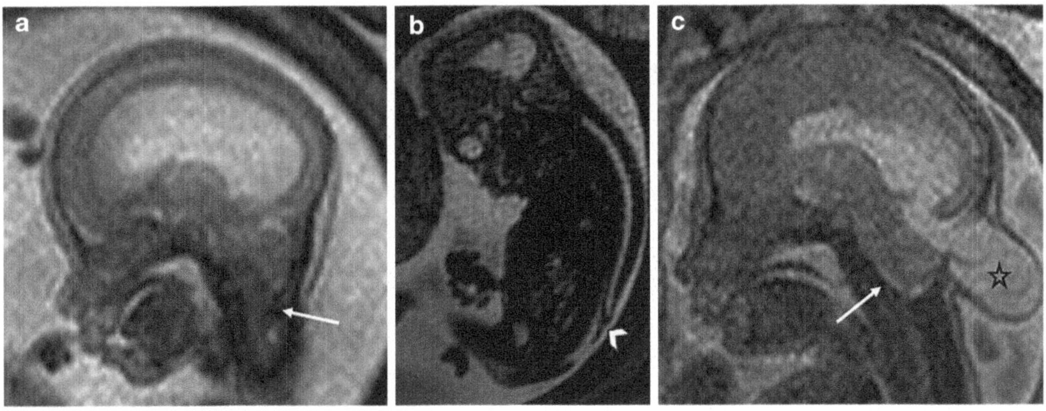

Fig. 1 Chiari II: (**a**, **b**) Herniation of the cerebellar vermis, brainstem, and fourth ventricle through the foramen magnum (arrow, **a**), combined with sacral myelocele (arrowhead, **b**) at 20 GW; (**c**) Chiari II signs (arrow), combined with occipital meningocele (star) at 24 GW; this association has classically been termed as "Chiari III malformation"

3 Posterior Fossa Malformations

3.1 Blake's Pouch Cyst

Under normal circumstances, the process of outpouching and permeabilization of the inferior portion of the fourth ventricular roof (the so-called posterior membranous area) is already completed at 20 gestational weeks, resulting in an acute fastigium and a small foramen of Magendie. MR studies have proven that the primary fissure (between anterior and posterior vermian lobes) and the fastigial point should be visible at 21 weeks' gestation. In addition, it has been reported that after 22 weeks' gestation, seven vermian lobules can usually be reliably detected [10].

In cases of delay or interruption of the normal permeabilization process of the pouch, a remnant structure of the posterior membranous area can be found below the vermis, which is called Blake's pouch cyst (BPC). Typically, no enlargement of the posterior fossa is seen in these cases. The vermis can be completely developed but displaced posteriorly with a widening of the tegmento-vermian angle [11]. Any cystic lesion identified during the routine US examination should be carefully evaluated and eventually sent for MR to aid in the differential diagnosis between pathological cases and anatomical variants; in fact, regression of the pouch can sometimes occur later during the second trimester, thereby leading to a complete vermian rotation only around 28–30 weeks. In fetuses before or at 26 weeks' gestation, the presence of ≥2 factors [(i) a tegmento-vermian angle ≥23°; (ii) width of the cisterna magna ≥9 mm; and (iii) presence of the "cerebellar tail sign"] has been shown to have a sensitivity of 84.21% (95% CI, 60.4–96.6%) and specificity of 80.8% (95% CI, 60.6–93.4%) in identifying cases of postnatal persistence of vermian rotation [12, 13].

In addition, the location of the choroid plexus and tenia-tela choroidea along the anterosuperior aspect of the cyst, inferior to the vermis, can be used as a marker suggestive of the presence of BPC [14]. Mild to moderate ventriculomegaly is commonly reported in utero and can resolve over time, either pre- or postnatally (Fig. 2) [15].

3.2 Vermian Hypoplasia

Vermian hypoplasia (VH) is a malformation characterized by reduced size of the vermis, without posterior fossa enlargement. The different vermian lobules develop from different parts of the mesial primordium. A definition of caudal or inferior vermian hypoplasia can be misleading because the abnormal vermian portion can be dif-

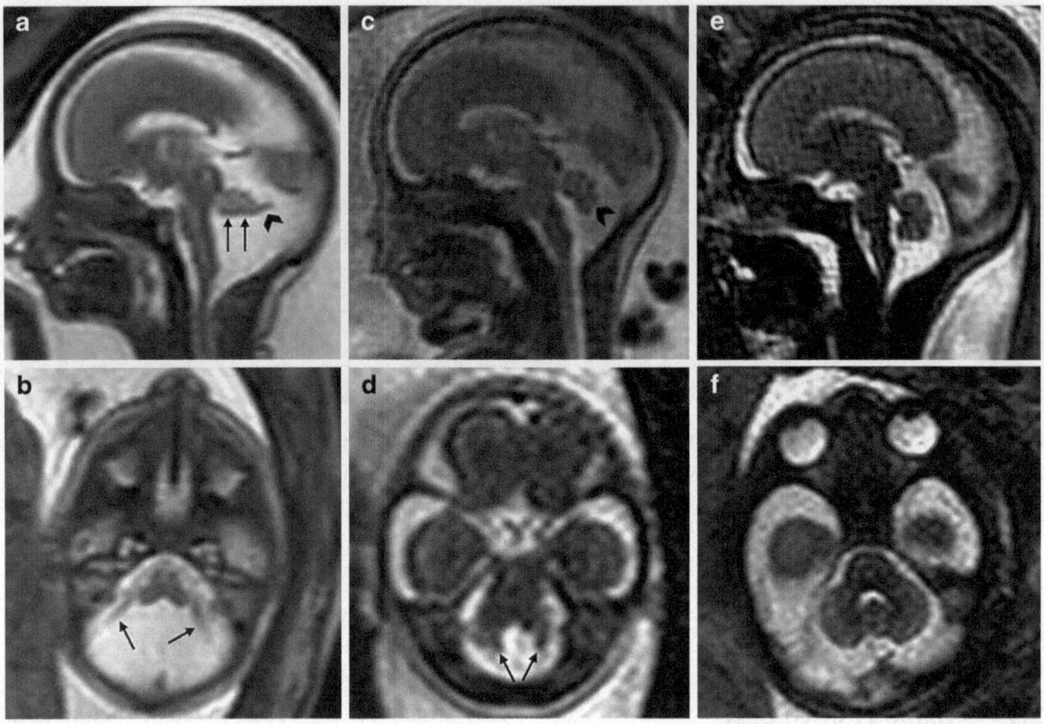

Fig. 2 Posterior fossa malformations: (**a**, **b**) Dandy–Walker malformation at 21 GW, demonstrating the incomplete rotation of the vermis with a flat fastigium (arrows, **a**) and presence of a caudal lobule (arrowhead, **a**) with a wide communication between the fourth ventricle and the cisterna magna (**a**); the taenia–tela choroidea complex spreads out deviating from the midline and the vermis (arrows, **b**); (**c–d**) Blake's pouch cyst at 21 GW with rotated vermis (arrowhead, **c**) and median location of taenia–tela choroidea complex that tends to connect to the inferior vermis (arrows, **d**); normal appearance of the same fetus at 28 GW (**e**, **f**)

ferent in each case depending on the nature and the timing of the triggering factor leading to similar morphological changes, especially during fetal examination [16]. The size of the vermis should be assessed in the midsagittal view by measuring the largest height and the anterior-posterior diameter, which are to be compared with previously published reference values [17, 18]. Due to the already explained mechanism of progressive disappearance of the inferior portion of the fourth ventricular roof (i.e., the posterior membranous area), the vermian displacement, which might happen during normal development, can be falsely interpreted as a partial or caudal hypoplasia. Vermian malrotation can be associated with upward rotation but without enlargement of the posterior fossa or torcular-lambdoid inversion [15]. The MR morphology of the vermis must be carefully evaluated regardless of the tegmento-vermian angle (Fig. 2) [14].

The MR features of VH include reduced size with posterior-to-anterior vermis ratio less than 2:1, normal or slightly enlarged fourth ventricle, preserved size of the posterior fossa without occipital scalloping, and no hydrocephalus. In addition, a major fetal MR study comparing the differentiable vermian lobules reported that patients with VH had four or five lobules (six or more in the normal brain controls). The authors found a correlation between having three or fewer lobules and worse postnatal development [15].

3.3 Dandy–Walker Malformation

Dandy–Walker malformation (DWM) has been variably defined in the literature. According to recent criteria, the phenotype includes the dilatation of the fourth ventricle combined with counter-clockwise rotated hypoplastic vermis,

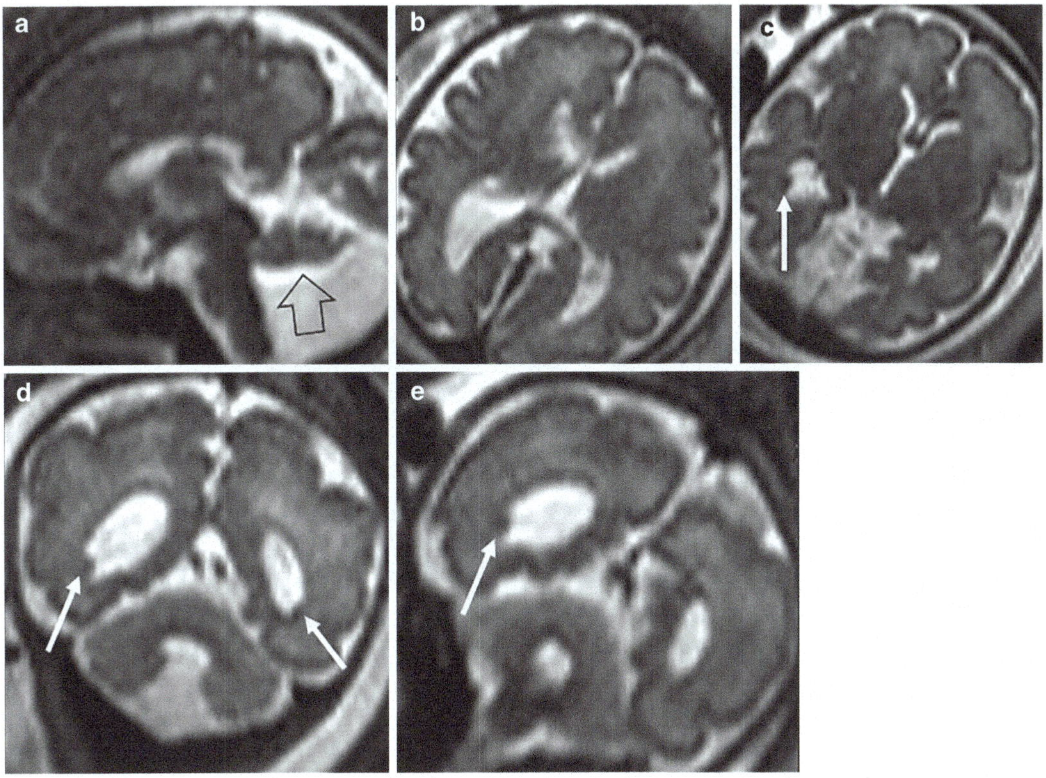

Fig. 3 In this 31 GW fetus with a Dandy–Walker malformation (arrow, **a**), nodular irregularities of the ventricular wall are seen along the ventricular walls, compatible with periventricular nodular heterotopia (arrows, **c–e**)

inferolateral displacement of the tela choroidea/choroid plexus (mandatory when visible), an unpaired caudal lobule or "cerebellar tail," an enlarged tegmento-vermian angle, and an obtuse fastigial recess. Recent research reported that posterior fossa size and torcular elevation (once considered to be cardinal features) are not decisive for the final diagnosis [19].

US provides an excellent characterization of the posterior fossa membranous structures. Fetal MR assists in identifying the exact location of the taenia–tela choroidea complex and choroid plexus along the wall of the fourth ventricle, displaced distantly from the vermis. The cerebellar hemispheres can be hypoplastic and displaced anterolaterally. Hydrocephalus is present in most cases (70–90% of literature). Often, additional commissural or cortical malformation can be found in patients with DWM (Figs. 2 and 3) [20].

3.4 Rhombencephalosynapsis

Rhombencephalosynapsis (RES) is a rare hindbrain malformation characterized by a vermian agenesis or hypogenesis with midline fusion of the cerebellar hemispheres and dentate nuclei. It can be complete or partial, isolated, or part of complex malformation syndromes. The clinical presentation can range from mild ataxia and normal cognitive abilities to severe cerebral palsy and intellectual disability. Often, RES is associated with stenosis or atresia of the aqueduct with or without brainstem malformations, leading to hydrocephalus [21]. In this context, mesencephalosynapsis is frequently associated, and it can range from a fusion of the colliculi to a mass-like stenotic midbrain with aqueductal atresia. The accompanying ventriculomegaly can be the first sign visualized during the routine US exam at early gestational stages, before 20 weeks' gesta-

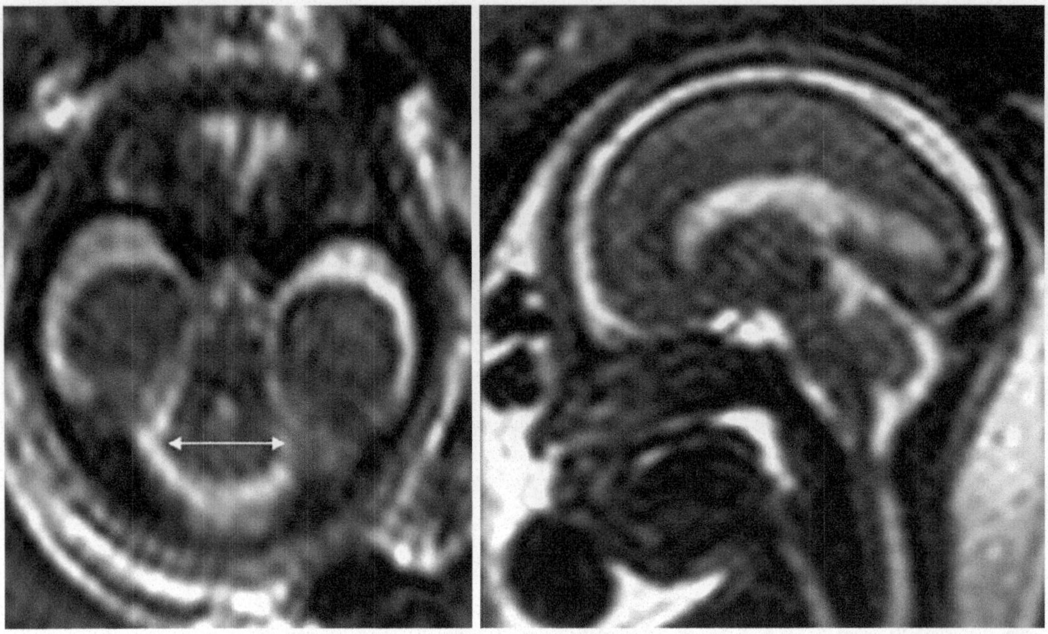

Fig. 4 Rhombencephalosynapsis at 22 GW: Hypoplastic bell-shaped cerebellum with decreased transverse diameter and "keyhole" appearance of the fourth ventricle; no vermis is visualized in sagittal plane (notice absent primary fissure)

tion [22]. Indeed, the possibility of RES should be evaluated in all cases of ventriculomegaly.

The classical form of RES has specific features visible at both US and MR exam: the flattening or absence of the vallecula leading to a usual bell-like (or round) shape of the single-lobed cerebellum, a small transverse cerebellar diameter on the axial views, a continuous foliation in coronal views, and a keyhole-shaped fourth ventricle [21]. On the axial plane, an abrupt angulation between the lateral and posterior profiles of the single-lobed cerebellum is characteristic; on the other hand, sagittal images may be less striking, with absent visibility of the primary fissure and a small, inferiorly displaced fourth ventricle.

Fetal MRI shows a high level of accuracy in the diagnosis of RES, especially in the rare cases of partial RES, and it can be adopted to exclude other brain anomalies. Lack of the midline cleft and cranial cerebellum with a visible vermian cleft in its caudal portion is reported to be observed even at 21 weeks' gestation (Fig. 4). Other associated cerebral anomalies include diencephalic-mesencephalic junction dysplasia, holoprosencephaly, corpus callosum dysgenesis, and agenesis of the septum pellucidum. RES is also included in some syndromes, such as VACTERL-H syndrome (vertebral anomalies, anal atresia, cardiac defects, tracheoesophageal fistula, esophageal atresia, renal anomalies, hydrocephalus) and Gómez–López–Hernández syndrome (parietal alopecia, trigeminal anesthesia, and craniofacial dysmorphism) [13, 23].

4 Brainstem Malformations

4.1 Z-Shaped Brainstem Deformities

A kinked or "z-shaped" brainstem represents a rare anomaly of the brainstem, strongly associated with an array of conditions such as α-dystroglycanopathies (Walker-Warburg phenotype in particular), X-linked hydrocephalus (L1CAM mutation), and tubulinopathies (TUBA1A, TUBB2B, TUBB3 mutations) [24, 25]. Usually, the associated brain derangement is severe and fetal MRI is requested to detect the imaging aspects of kinked brainstem and other signs of associated intracranial malformations.

A kinked brainstem is characterized by exaggerated flexures, resembling the immature embry-

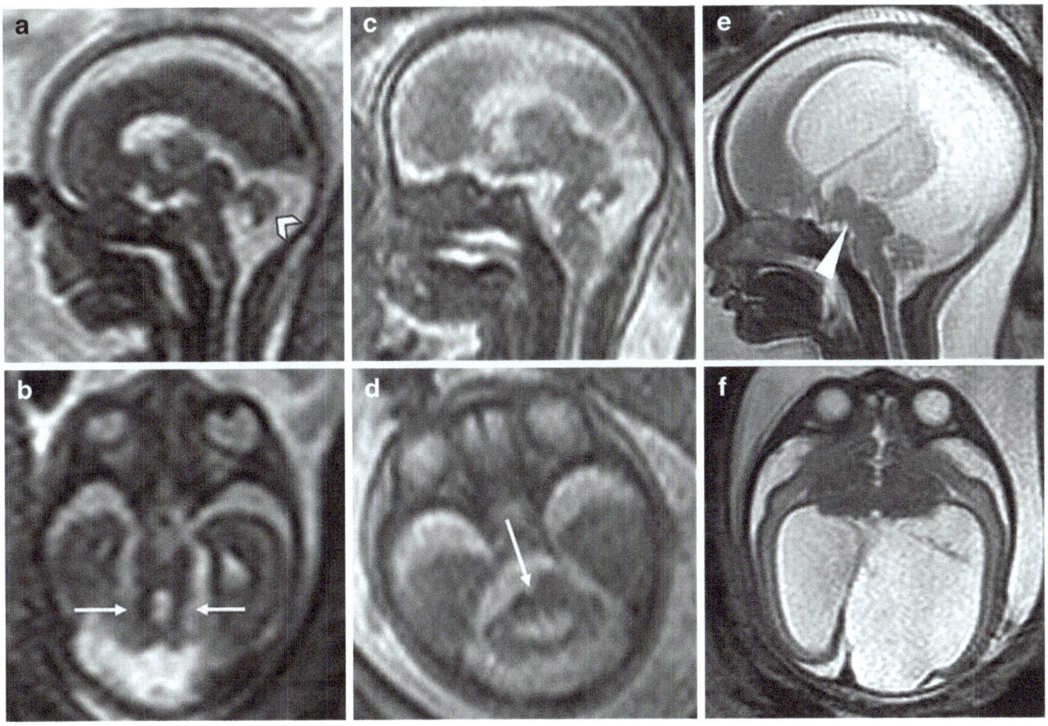

Fig. 5 Brainstem malformations: Molar tooth sign at 20 GW: dysmorphic, hypoplastic vermis (arrowhead, **a**) and the typical "molar tooth" appearance (arrows) (**b**); Z-shaped malformation at 21 GW (**c**) with pontine clefting and asymmetry on axial view (arrow, **d**); Diencephalic-mesencephalic junction dysplasia type B at 26 + 4 GW—lack of separation between the massa intermedia of the thalamus and the upper aspect of the midbrain in sagittal plane (arrowhead, **e**) with extreme asymmetrical ventriculomegaly (**f**)

onal morphology of the brainstem, associated with the inhibition of the normal development of posterior fossa structures. The brainstem can be dislocated posteriorly or anteriorly, thickened or thinned. Cerebellar hypoplasia is frequently associated [26, 27]. Obstructive hydrocephalus is present, and other associated abnormalities can guide the prenatal diagnosis such as dysplastic basal ganglia in tubulinopathies or ocular anomalies in α-dystroglycanopathies (Fig. 5) [25]. Z-shaped brainstem aberrations are, on the other hand, extremely rare in isolation.

4.2 Molar Tooth Sign

Primary nonmotile ciliopathies are a group of complex cerebellar and brainstem malformations associated with the involvement of multiple extracranial organs and structures such as the kidneys, retina, liver, pancreas, and skeletal system. The most common entity is the Joubert syndrome, characterized by the pathognomonic appearance of the superior cerebellar peduncles in the midbrain which are elongated, thickened, and horizontally oriented, surrounding an abnormally deep interpeduncular fossa and resulting in the typical "molar tooth sign," associated with a variable degree of vermian hypoplasia and dysgenesis (Fig. 5) [28].

Oral-facial-digital syndrome type VI (OFD VI) or Varadi-Papp syndrome is a rare phenotypic subtype of Joubert syndrome with polydactyly, oral findings, intellectual disability, and absence of the cerebellar vermis. While US can raise the suspicion of the malformation, MR examination is needed to confirm the suspect and differentiate any additional features. Additional MR findings used as criteria for the diagnosis of OFD VI are the presence of tongue hamartoma, additional frenula, and upper lip notch (oral abnormalities), mesoaxial polydactyly, and hypothalamic hamartoma [29].

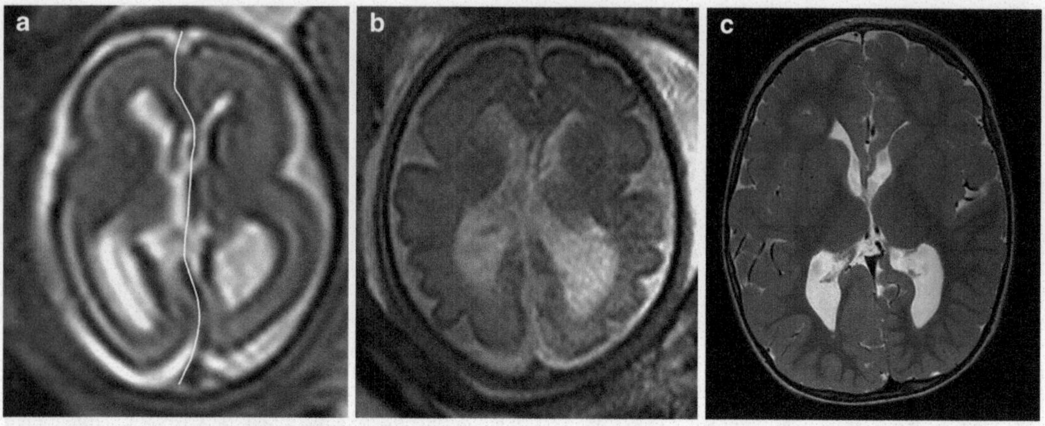

Fig. 6 Confirmed tubulinopathy: typical midline distortion is observed during the fetal MRs performed at 23 GW and 31 GW (**a**, **b**) and confirmed in the postnatal imaging (**c**). Also notice profound asymmetry of sulcation consistent with dysgyria

4.3 Diencephalic-Mesencephalic Junction Dysplasia

Diencephalic-mesencephalic junction dysplasia (DMJD) is a rare malformation characterized by an ill-defined junction between the diencephalon and the midbrain. Based on the Severino classification, DMJD is categorized into two groups [30]. Type A is recognized in the axial plane with enlarged dorsoventral size of the brainstem and abnormal midbrain contour in the axial plane, with or without ventral cleft corresponding to the "butterfly sign" (lack of separation between the thalamus and the midbrain). Type B can be defined in the sagittal plane by the lack of separation between the massa intermedia of the thalamus and the upper aspect of the midbrain (Fig. 5). Often, the first suggestive sign during early developmental stages is ventriculomegaly. In the literature, the butterfly sign is reported to be recognizable at 20–21 gestational weeks at fetal MRI. DMJD usually is observed to be associated with other brain anomalies or as part of complex conditions, such as L1 and L1-like syndromes [30, 31].

4.4 Tubulinopathies

Tubulinopathies are a group of neurodevelopmental disorders associated with a variety of cortical malformations caused by mutations in tubulin genes (including TUBA1A, TUBA8, TUBB3, TUBB5, and TUBG1). The fusion between lenticular nuclei and the head of the caudate nuclei with a lack of anterior limb of the internal capsule is a frequent feature, but it can be more easily described only at postnatal examinations. Two main imaging phenotypes are described in the fetal stage. The first one (severe form) is characterized by microlissencephaly, brainstem anomalies, and enlargement of the germinal matrices (ganglionic eminence) with dysmorphic basal ganglia. The milder form can have a combination of a wide range of malformations such as corpus callosum dysgenesis, reduced Sylvian fissure opercularization, and dysgenesis of the brainstem and cerebellum. Major diagnostic flags suggestive of tubulinopathy are the presence of asymmetry of the ventricular system including distortion of the cavum septi pellucidi and abnormal sulcation of the cerebellum and the cerebral hemispheres. Minor findings include a smaller pontine anteroposterior diameter (≤5th centile), asymmetry or absence of the olfactory sulci, and brainstem asymmetry with abnormal bulge of the pons (Fig. 6). In cases of detection of any major or minor criteria, a genetic test should be performed. MRI shows higher diagnostic rates compared to the US, especially in the visualization of the minor signs [24, 32–34].

5 Ganglionic Eminence Anomalies

The ganglionic eminences (GE) are one of the main areas where progenitor cells are located during early brain development. They can be visualized with transvaginal US as early as 10–13 weeks' gestation as thickenings of the lateral wall and floor of the third and lateral ventricles, but pathological changes are rare observed at this early stage [35]. They become most prominent at 18–22 weeks' gestation, which is followed by a progressive reduction and eventually disappearance of GE around the 30th week [36]. Anomalies affecting the GE are rare and divided into two groups depending on the main presentations: with cavitations or with increased volume. Often, they are associated with other brain malformations such as cortical abnormalities, corpus callosum dysgenesis, vermian hypoplasia, and syndromes such as tuberous sclerosis, tubulinopathies, and Walker-Warburg syndrome. A connection with TUBA1A and MTOR-PIK3CA (PROS) AKT pathway mutations was found [37]. MRI provides an optimal characterization, description of associated features, and differentiation from the more common ischemia or hemorrhages that can occur in those areas [38].

MR findings include disorganized and nodular appearance of the ganglionic eminences. Changes are often bilateral, predominantly with cavitations, but cases combining enlargement and cystic components are also reported (Fig. 7). Diffusion restriction with low ADC values reflects increased cellular density. The differential diagnosis is with germinal matrix hemorrhage that has abnormal T1-weighted hyperintense areas with irregular and shape signal drop on T2*/SWI sequences [37, 38].

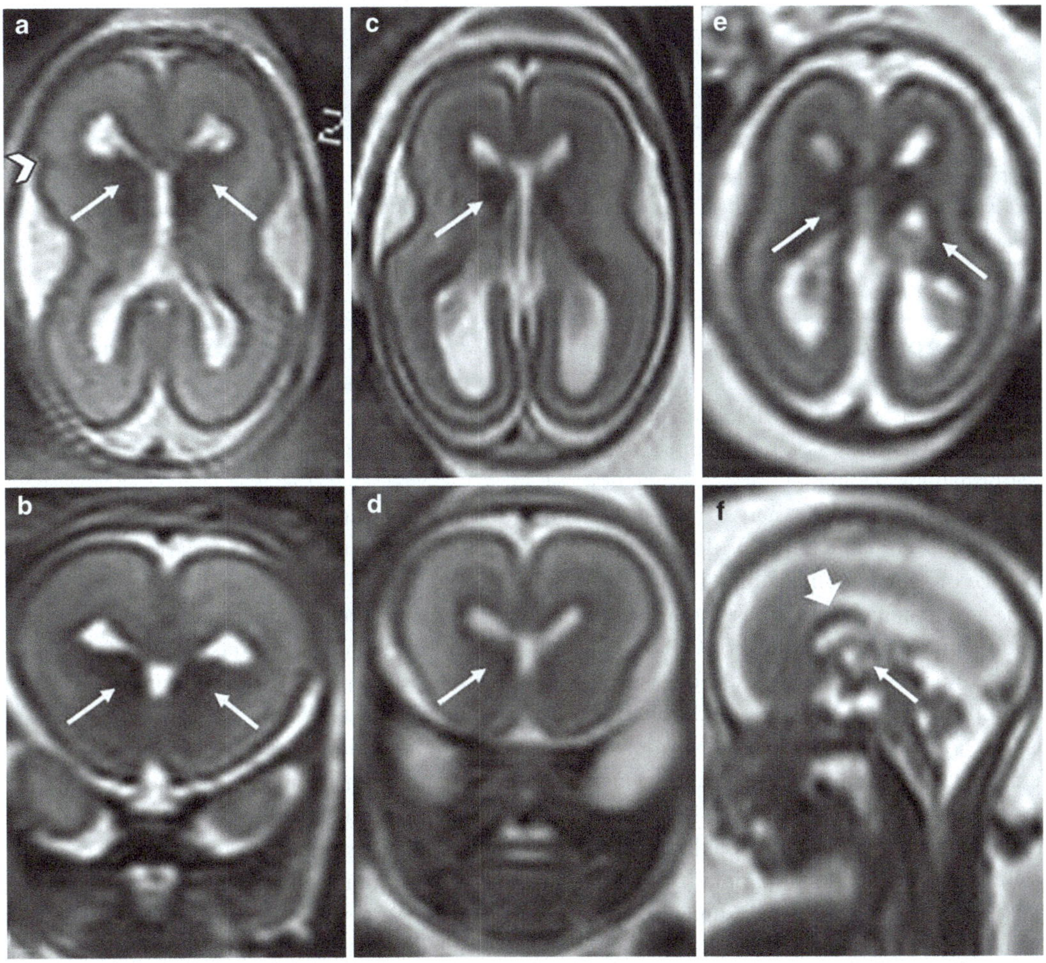

Fig. 7 Ganglionic eminence pathologies at 22 GW: (**a**, **b**) macrocephaly with bilateral enlargement of the ganglionic eminences (arrows) and right-sided polymicrogyria (arrowhead); (**c**, **d**) unilateral right sided enlargement of the ganglionic eminence (arrow); (**e**, **f**) bilateral cavitations (arrows); notice corpus callosum dysgenesis (thick arrow, **f**)

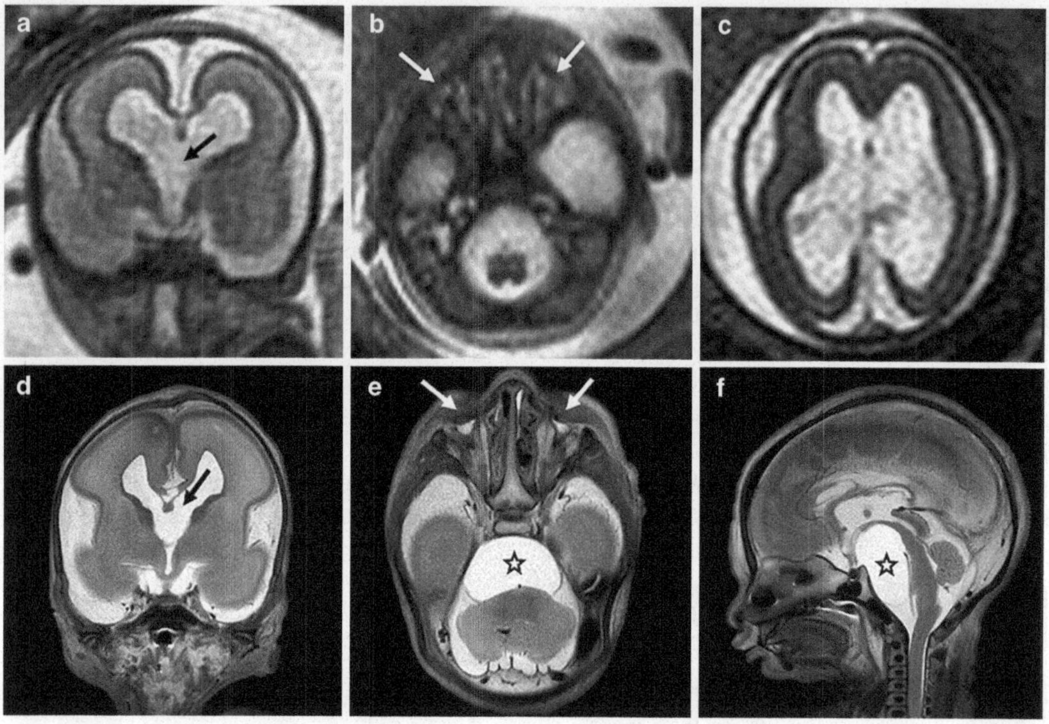

Fig. 8 Septo-optic dysplasia (SOD): MR was performed in 21 GW (**a–c**) and postmortem (**d–f**). It confirmed the agenesis of the anterior septum pellucidum with communication of the lateral ventricles at the level of the frontal horns (black arrows) and additionally bilateral anophthalmia (white arrows). Arachnoid cyst compressing the ventral profile of the pons and midbrain (star, **e**, **f**) and corpus callosum hypoplasia (**f**) were visualized

6 Septo-Optic Dysplasia

Septo-optic dysplasia (SOD), or so-called de Morsier's syndrome, is a rare complex of brain malformations including any combination of hypoplasia of the optic nerve, pituitary gland hypoplasia, corpus callosum dysgenesis, and absence of septum pellucidum (ASP). The latter is the most common suspicious finding of SOD at routine ultrasound. The isolated ASP has a good postnatal prognosis, but the possible association with other anomalies requires additional examinations to exclude SOD. The evaluation of the fetal optic nerves, chiasm, and pituitary gland can be challenging. In such cases, the MRI is used to assist in excluding nerve hypoplasia, pituitary stalk absence, and frontal-parietal polymicrogyria (Fig. 8). The typical MR imaging findings include septal remnants, forniceal fusion, squared anterior horns, and dysplastic temporal with variable thinning of the corpus callosum [39, 40].

7 Malformations of the Corpus Callosum

7.1 Corpus Callosum Agenesis

Corpus callosum agenesis represents a complex malformation and is one of the most frequent brain congenital anomalies. The corpus callosum is the main cerebral commissure that connects the cerebral hemispheres. It is divided, from anterior to posterior, into rostrum, genu, body, and splenium [41]. It develops from the dorsal part of the lamina terminalis between 12 and 20 weeks of gestation, but its maturation and growth continue in the postnatal period, especially the thickening due to myelination of its fibers. Complete corpus callosum agenesis results from a prenatal abnormal process that takes place before the initial induction at 8 weeks of gestation, and it is frequently associated with other central nervous system malformations [42].

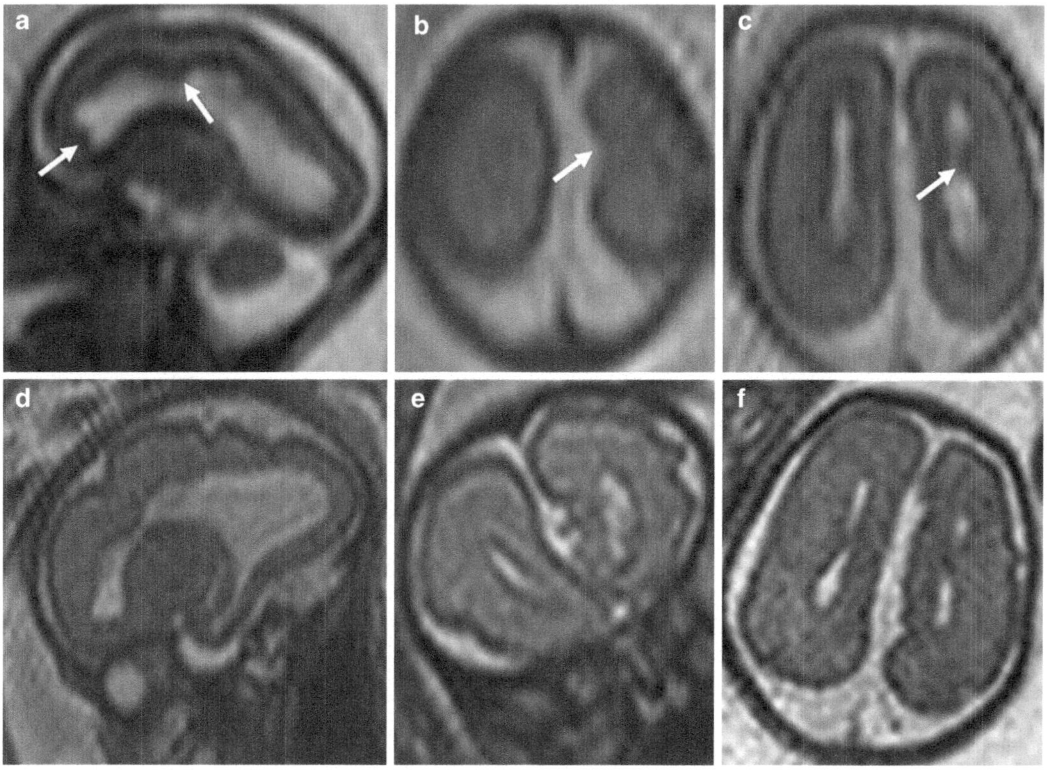

Fig. 9 Corpus callosum agenesis in a fetus at 20 GW. Irregularities of frontal cortical profile and ventricular margins are noted (arrows, **a–c**). (**d–f**) At 26 GW corpus callosum, agenesis is confirmed at MRI which also shows an increase in the irregularities of frontal cortical profile as well as the presence small nodularities consistent with subependymal heterotopia

Ultrasound prenatal diagnosis of corpus callosum agenesis is usually sufficient for the diagnosis, and it is fundamentally suspected when the cavum septum pellucidum is not visualized [41].

MRI offers a detailed characterization of the malformation and confirms whether agenesis is isolated or associated with other anomalies, an important indicator of a more careful neurological prognosis [43]. The characteristic finding of corpus callosum agenesis is represented by the absence of commissural fibers that cross the midline [44]. Anomalies that can be frequently identified on fetal MRI include cortical malformations and posterior fossa malformations [42, 45, 46]. A strong association with corpus callosum agenesis has been reported in males with unilateral cortical malformations and in females with Aicardi syndrome [45, 46]. MRI should be performed between 20 and 34 weeks of gestation, when the basic structure of the corpus callosum is expected to be fully developed, and not before 20 weeks of gestation when the corpus callosum is not yet fully formed [43].

Cortical malformations associated with complete agenesis of the corpus callosum are seen more frequently in male fetuses, especially in frontal or parietal lobes. These cortical malformations have been described as irregular cortical surface ("wart-like"), and irregular invaginations of cortical profile (multiple tiny excessive or few major ones) (Fig. 9). Eventually the postnatal findings in these cases are typically polymicrogyria [46].

In Aicardi syndrome, MR imaging can identify, at an early gestational age (before 24 weeks) anomalies such as cortical malformations (a frontal dysgyria cortical pattern is characteristic), interhemispheric single or multiple cysts, coloboma, posterior fossa malformations, or dysmorphism of the basal ganglia. The prenatal Aicardi

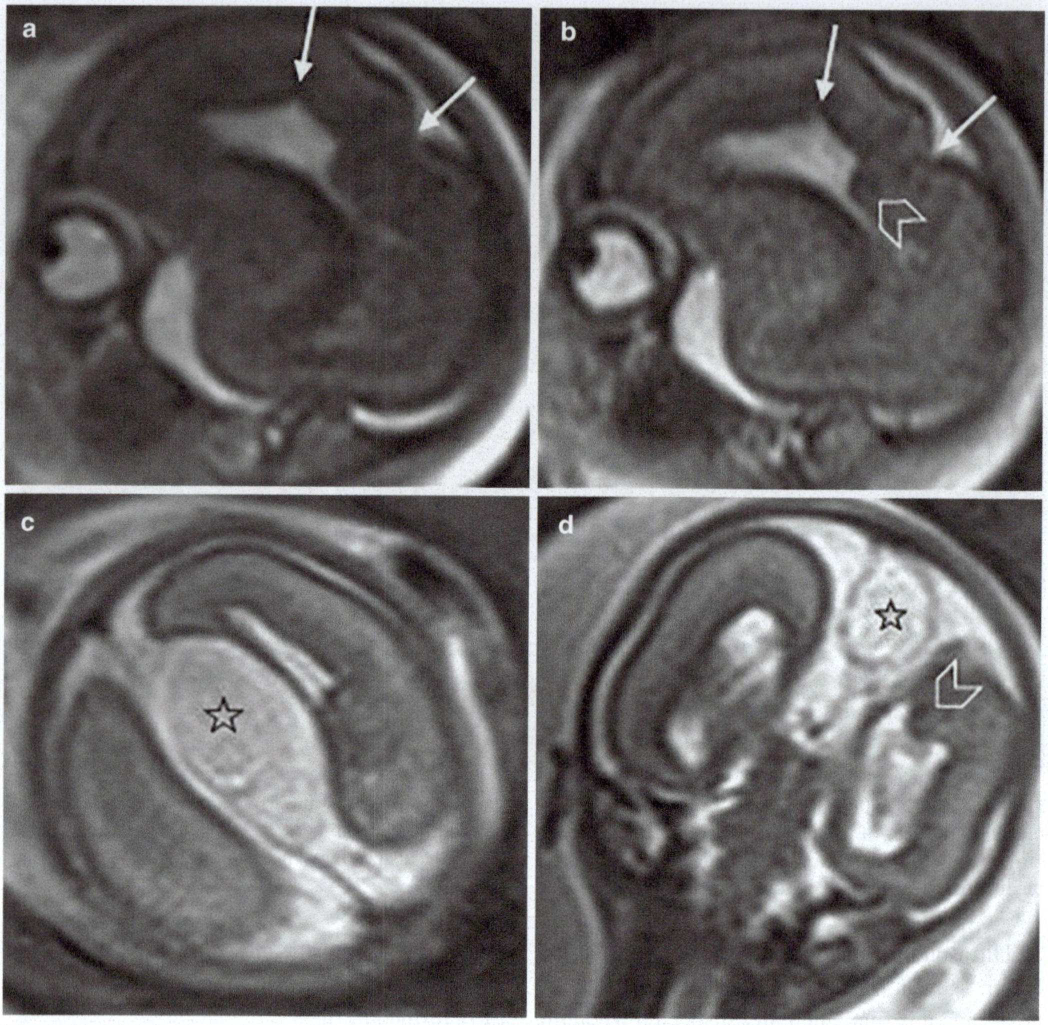

Fig. 10 Aicardi syndrome. Fetal MRI at 21 GW demonstrates agenesis of the corpus callosum, interhemispheric cyst (star, **c**, **d**), and focal cortical formation anomaly (arrows, **a**, **b**) on the frontal lobe with heterotopia (arrowhead, **b**, **d**)

triad consists of corpus callosum agenesis, interhemispheric cysts, and modification of interhemispheric fissure (Fig. 10) [47]. Postnatally, the typical dysgyric cortical pattern can be identified as polymicrogyria [45].

7.2 Corpus Callosum Dysgenesis

Dysgenesis of the corpus callosum can be divided into partial agenesis, hypoplasia, and abnormally thick corpus callosum. Partial agenesis represents missing parts of the corpus callosum. It can be associated with interhemispheric cysts or pericallosal lipoma. Hypoplasia appears when the corpus callosum is apparently fully formed, but it is shorter and thin [45, 48].

Length and thickness should be compared to reference biometric parameters according to the gestational age. The length of the corpus callosum should be measured on the sagittal T2-weighted image from genu to splenium, while the thickness can be more difficult to be reliably determined especially at earlier gestational ages.

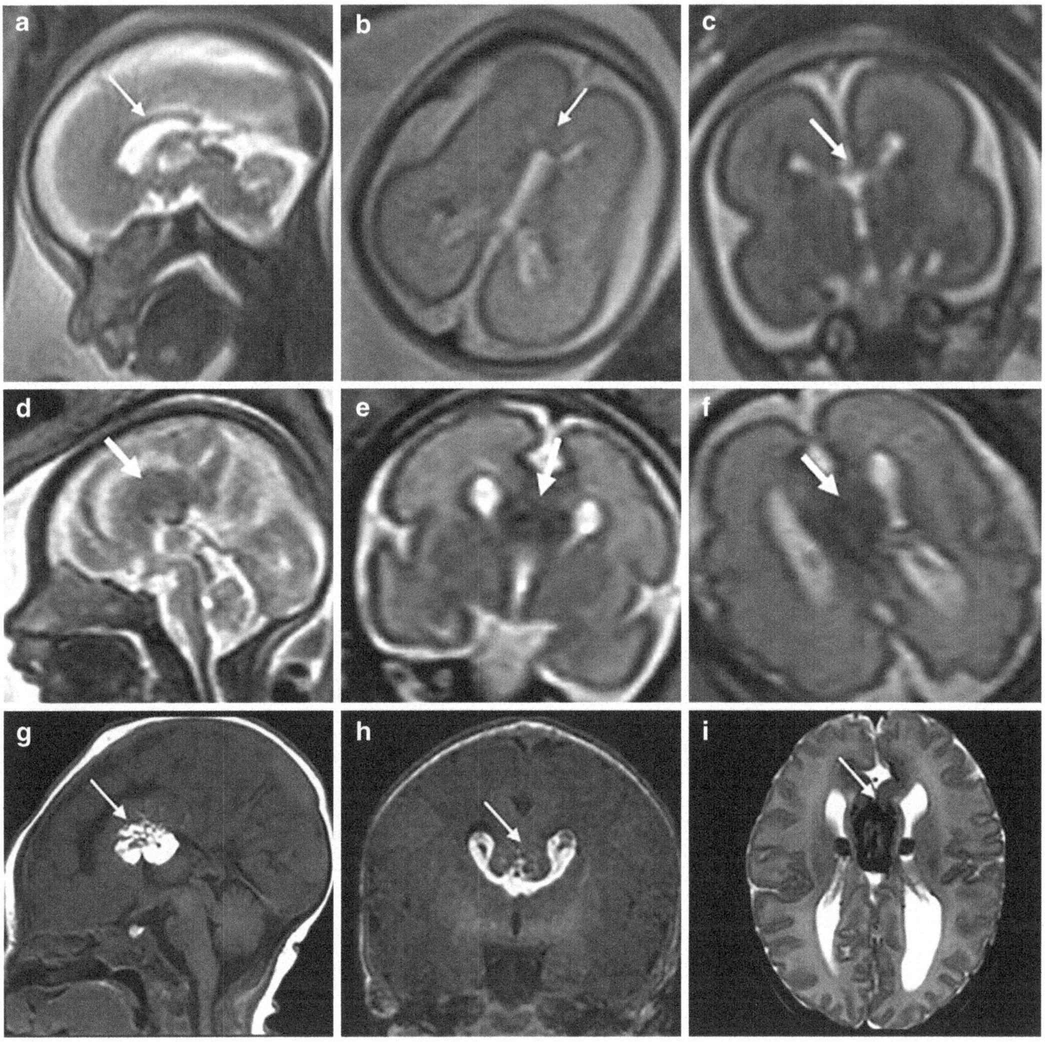

Fig. 11 Corpus callosum malformation. (**a–c**) Corpus callosum thinning-dysgenesis (arrow) associated with a malrotated hippocampus at 23 weeks' gestations. (**d–f**) Dysgenesis of corpus callosum and lipoma can be suspected at 30 GW due to the hypointense signal on T2-weighted images (arrow). Postnatal images (**g–i**) confirmed the lipoma and corpus callosum malformation

A thick corpus callosum can be an isolated finding or associated with complex malformations such as megalencephaly or polymicrogyria. Fetal MRI is strictly needed in these cases, in addition to ultrasound, to detect brain anomalies associated with dysgenesis of the corpus callosum (Fig. 11) [48]. DTI/tractography can be a useful tool to conventional fetal MRI to identify supracallosal bundles, which can also be associated with dysgenesis of the corpus callosum and later in the postnatal period, with neurodevelopmental delay [49].

8 Malformations of Cortical Development

Malformations of cortical development (MCDs) are secondary to abnormal corticogenesis like abnormal cell proliferation, incomplete neuronal migration, neuronal overmigration, or postmigrational cortical organization [50]. MCDs are among the most difficult malformations to detect on prenatal ultrasound, and fetal MRI has the potential to significantly improve the prenatal imaging diagnosis [51].

8.1 Polymicrogyria

Polymicrogyria (PMG) is classically defined as an abnormal cortical gyration pattern with multiple excessive small gyri. PMG is not a single entity; indeed, it can be defined as a generic "umbrella" term that gathers various focal and diffuse cortical abnormalities. PMG is secondary to an abnormal postmigration cortical event, and it can be focal or diffuse, symmetric or asymmetric, unilateral or bilateral [47, 50, 52].

MRI provides important additional information in cases of minor focal PMG, especially in fetuses at less than 24 weeks' gestation, since the anomaly often cannot be accurately detected at prenatal ultrasound [52]. Evidence in the literature shows that at early gestational ages, when the brain is normally lissencephalic (smooth), PMG can be detected in the presence of four main patterns such as "wart-like," "sawtooth," abnormal invaginating sulcus, and "focal bump" (single or multiple) (Fig. 12). These cortical anomalies can also be associated with thinning and blurring of the subplate and intermediate zone. "Sawtooth" anomalies are mainly bilateral and related to clastic insults, while abnormal invaginating sulcus and "wart-like" anomalies are mainly unilateral [53]. An in depth understanding of the processes of brain lamination, sulcation, and gyration is key to formulate the correct diagnosis of a specific cortical anomaly [52]. Of note, at more advanced gestational ages, fetal MRI signs are similar to those seen in postnatal patients [50].

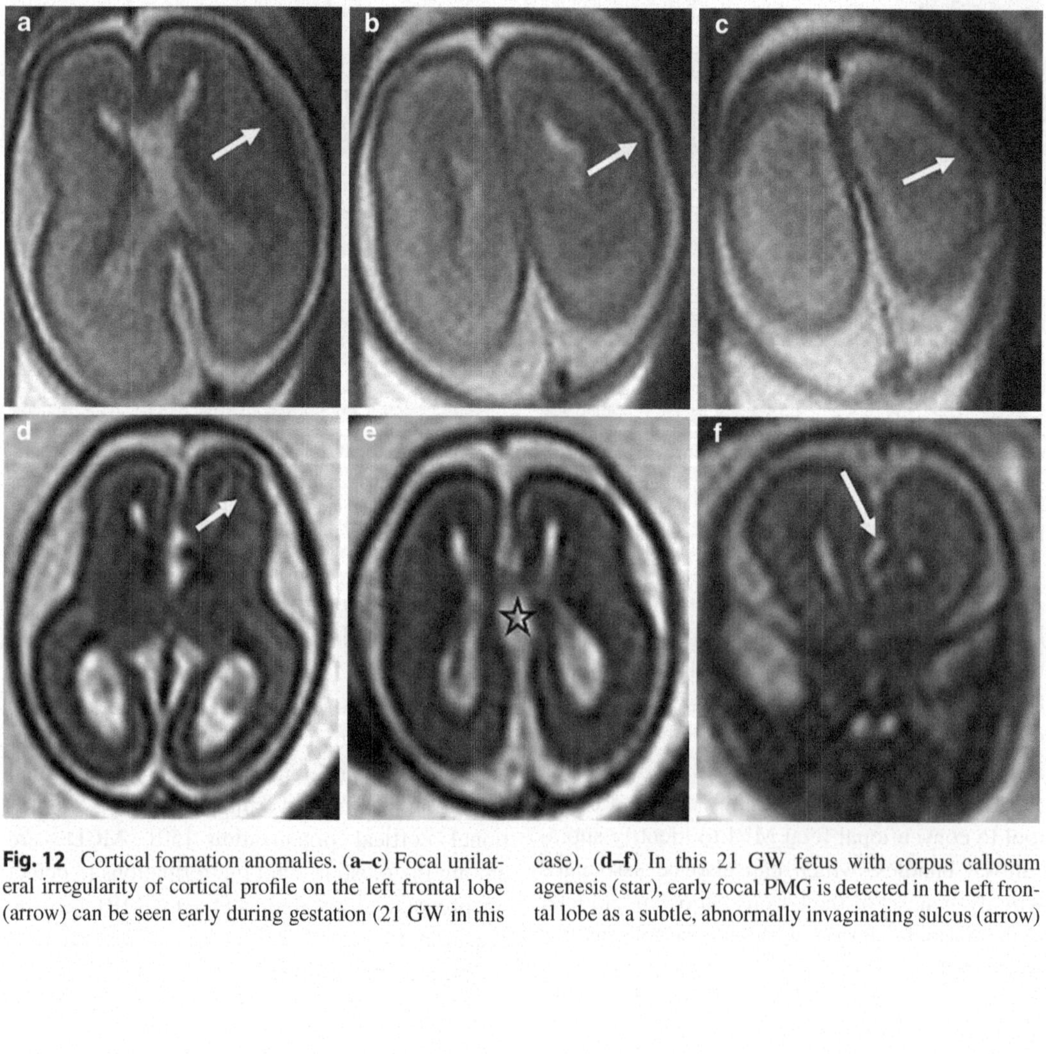

Fig. 12 Cortical formation anomalies. (**a–c**) Focal unilateral irregularity of cortical profile on the left frontal lobe (arrow) can be seen early during gestation (21 GW in this case). (**d–f**) In this 21 GW fetus with corpus callosum agenesis (star), early focal PMG is detected in the left frontal lobe as a subtle, abnormally invaginating sulcus (arrow)

8.2 Lissencephaly

Lissencephaly represents a rare brain malformation mainly due to an interference in the neuroglial migration. The brain appears abnormally "smooth" due to a reduction or absence of sulci and gyri. The prognosis is usually poor because the abnormal corticogenesis takes place before 20 weeks of gestation [54].

Prenatal ultrasound diagnosis is challenging, and it has been reported in the literature that lissencephaly is more easily diagnosed in the third trimester while the sensitivity of US at earlier gestational ages is not as high [55]. Indeed, published data suggest that most of postnatal diagnosis of lissencephaly were missed at prenatal ultrasound [56].

Fetal MRI is an important tool to provide additional information on cerebral gyri and sulci, compared to ultrasound. Although it is easier to detect lissencephaly at advanced gestational ages, earlier diagnosis, between 20 and 24 weeks, is possible [56]. Some early MRI signs such as reduced/absent Sylvian fissure opercularization, parieto-occipital sulcus absence, and shape of frontal lobes should be indeed carefully evaluated.

Patterns of opercularization, best seen in axial and coronal planes, are described according to gestational age, and the presence of an abnormal Sylvian fissure morphology can be a first sign of lissencephaly. Opercularization patterns are based on how much the temporal lobe covers the insula and on the angulation between the insula and the temporal and parietal opercular borders, which typically exhibits an acute angle after 24.5 gestational weeks [57].

The parieto-occipital fissure is seen best on the axial and sagittal plane, appearing as a deep cleft on the brain medial surface; its absence can be a sign of lissencephaly, especially when a coexistent ventriculomegaly is not present and cannot therefore explain the parieto-occipital sulcus absence [58].

The shape of the frontal lobes should be evaluated, with flattening of the frontal lobes representing a significant sign of lissencephaly [13].

8.3 Schizencephaly

Schizencephaly represents a rare cortical development malformation, and it appears as a fluid-filled defect (lined by gray matter), which communicates with the lateral ventricle or subarachnoid space. Two types are recognized: the "closed-lip" type, when the clefts are in contact and "open-lip" type, when the clefts are separated. Prenatal diagnosis by ultrasound or fetal MRI is rare, and most of the cases are diagnosed after 28 weeks of gestation [59]. Most cases are considered to result from an early acquired insult to the entire extent of the brain mantle, probably of ischemic nature.

On fetal MR, "open-lip" is defined as the continuity of cerebrospinal fluid spaces from the lateral ventricle to the subarachnoid space, while "closed-lip" appears when there is a complete apposition of the clefts or if the clefts are detached only by vessels (seen in the three spatial planes). "Open-lip" types are easily detected on prenatal MRI, while "closed-lip" forms are more difficult to be detected on prenatal fetal MRI and are more commonly diagnosed postnatally (Fig. 13). A rigorous check-up of the gray matter lining is compulsory for the correct diagnosis, and analysis of multiple planes is required [60].

8.4 Gray Matter Heterotopia

Gray matter heterotopia is caused by incomplete neuronal migration between 7 and 16 weeks of gestation. Heterotopias can be classified as subependymal, subcortical, or band heterotopia [61]. Compared to other MCDs such as PMG or lissencephaly, the sensitivity of fetal MRI in the diagnosis of heterotopia is lower (it has been reported in the literature to be around 44% before 24 weeks of gestation and 73% after) [51]. Periventricular nodular heterotopia can be diagnosed as a focal thickening or irregularity of the ventricular wall, but its detection might be not straightforward (Fig. 9) [13].

In fetuses with Chiari II malformation and associated hydrocephalus, gray matter heteroto-

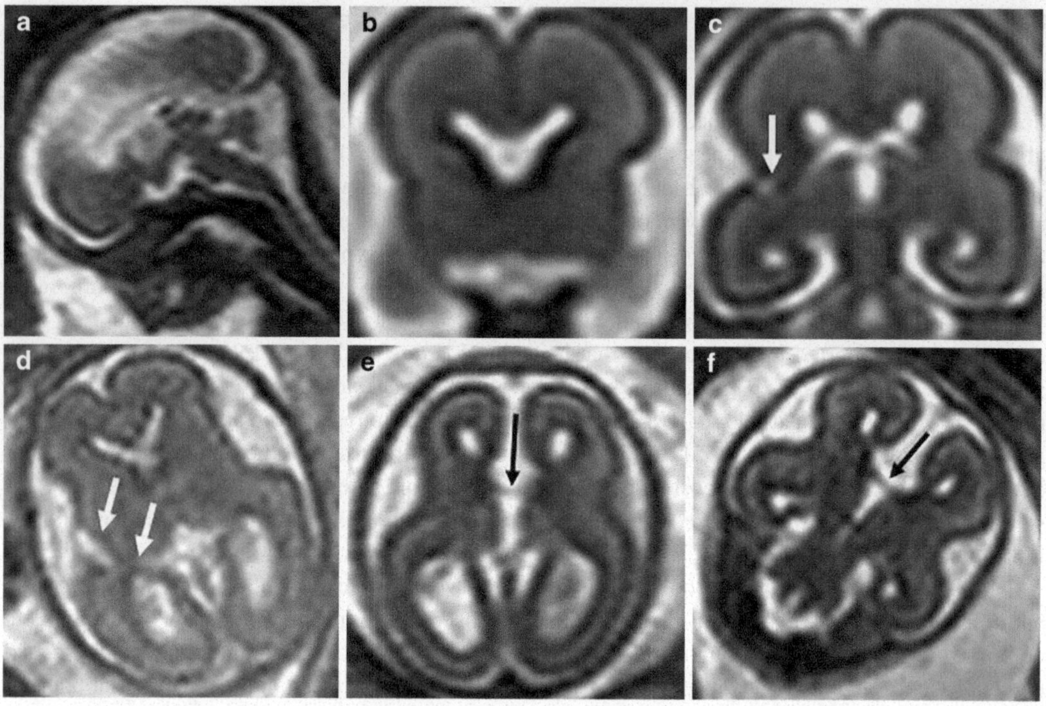

Fig. 13 Schizencephaly. Fetal MRI at 21 GW demonstrates unilateral right closed-lip schizencephaly (arrows, **c**, **d**) and absence of septum pellucidum (**b**) and corpus callosum. Hippocampal commissure has a thin tubular shape (arrows, **e**, **f**)

pia can be observed as the hydrocephalus can lead to a loss of the germinal matrix with a consequent abnormal neuroblast migration [62].

8.5 Megalencephaly

Megalencephaly represents an increase in cerebral structures volume due to anomalies in neuronal cell proliferation, differentiation, or migration. It can be unilateral or bilateral, focal or diffuse. Macrocephaly or macrocrania is defined as an increase in the head circumference above two standard deviations for gestational age and sex-related dimensions, and it is usually due to malformations of the skeletal structures, familial forms, ventriculomegaly, and increased pericerebral cerebrospinal fluid spaces or tumors [13, 63]. Macrocephaly/macrocrania should not be confused with megalencephaly, since a large cranium may be often present with a normal brain size but accompanied just by enlarged pericerebral spaces and ventricles. On the other hand, megalencephaly, when global, is generally associated with macrocrania, since the entire large brain fills the intracranial space and expands it; this may not occur when megalencephaly is unilateral or limited to some lobes [64].

Macrocrania can be easily suspected at prenatal ultrasound, while fetal MRI is performed to confirm and characterize possible malformations of the brain. In the most common form, hemimegalencephaly, cerebral hemisphere asymmetry, cortical anomalies, basal ganglia-ganglionic eminence dysmorphism, and lateral ventricle frontal horn straightening are key to the diagnosis (Fig. 14) [13, 65].

Megalencephaly can be related to PIK3CA-related overgrowth spectrum (PROS). In the

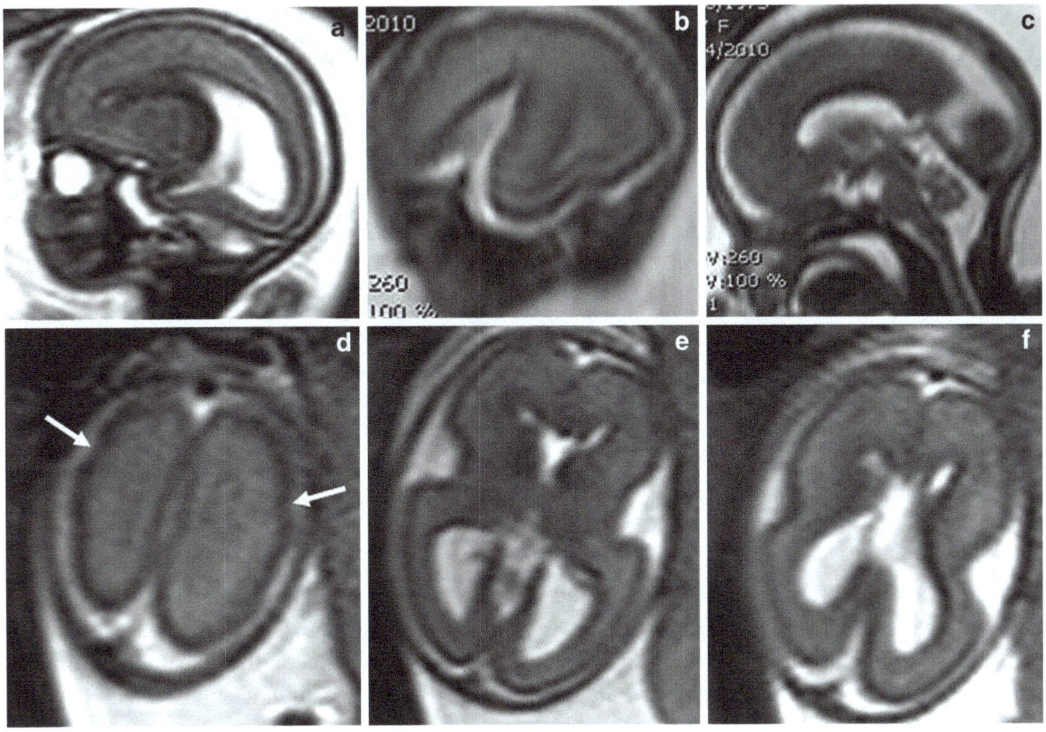

Fig. 14 Megalencephaly with PMG. Fetal MRI at 22 GW (**a–f**) shows a megalencephalic brain with increase in size of the frontal lobes and irregularities of cortical profile (arrows, **d**)

PROS group, megalencephaly is caused by somatic mosaicism of the PIK3CA gene [66]. Megalencephaly associated with macrocrania related to PROS should be differentiated from benign familial macrocrania, an autosomal dominant condition associated with an absolute increase in the head circumference and increased pericerebral CSF spaces and, to a minor extent, with enlarged ventricular size [67].

9 Tuberous Sclerosis Complex

Tuberous sclerosis complex represents a genetic multisystemic neurocutaneous disorder caused by mutations in TSC1 and TSC2 genes. Prenatal diagnosis can detect cortical tubers, subependymal nodules, renal angiomyolipomas, or cardiac rhabdomyoma. Prenatal ultrasound can detect cardiac rhabdomyoma from 20 weeks of gestation onwards [68].

Fetal MRI can detect cortical tubers and subependymal nodules. Subependymal nodules are localized along the margins of the lateral ventricles and appear hypointense on T2-weighted images. Cortical tubers appear hypointense on T2-weighted and hyperintense on T1-weighted images [69]. The exact accuracy of fetal MRI in detecting brain features of TSC is not clear, especially for early gestational ages; therefore, caution should be considered when ruling out possible brain involvement in fetuses with cardiac rhabdomyomas on the sole basis of MRI.

10 Holoprosencephaly

Holoprosencephaly (HPE) is the most common forebrain malformation, presenting as an incomplete midline cleavage of the two hemispheres in variable degrees combined with other midline structures and facial anomalies. The three main

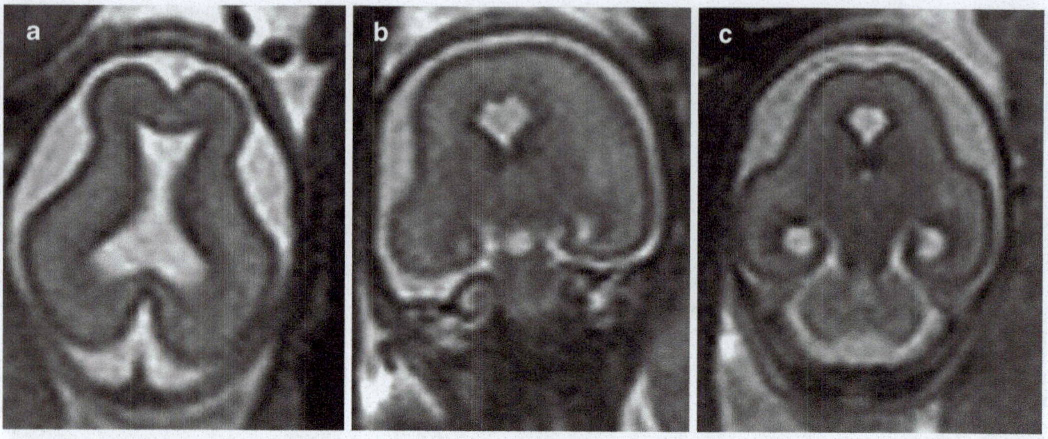

Fig. 15 Semilobar holoprosencephaly at 21 GW. Fusion of the frontal lobes with absence of septum pellucidum; of note, typical keyhole shape of the midline holoventricle in the coronal planes is visualized (**b**, **c**)

forms in decreasing order of severity are the alobar, semilobar, and lobar HPE [70]. The first two have a pathognomonic appearance at US examination, even in the early developmental stages. The mild form of lobar HPE can be suspected by the shape of the frontal horns and corpus callosum, but in some cases, MRI is required for diagnosis confirmation (Fig. 15). Other imaging findings of lobar HPE include wide communication between the lateral third ventricles and the absence of septum pellucidum.

11 Intraventricular Malformations

The most common intraventricular anomaly is represented by choroid plexus cysts. The cysts can be unilateral or bilateral leading to asymmetry with mild to moderate ventriculomegaly (Fig. 16). They can be associated with other malformations (especially in patients with trisomy 18 and 21), but when isolated they are usually considered benign. The differentiation of a choroid plexus cyst from posthemorrhagic changes with synechiae can be challenging at US exam. MRI, and in particular FLAIR sequences, can demonstrate the difference in signal between pure intraventricular CSF and choroid plexus cyst because of the higher protein content of the latter leading to an increased signal intensity. In addition, T1 helps to rule out any hemorrhagic components. The absence of synechiae is used for the differentiation from infective ependymitis or intraventricular hemorrhage [71].

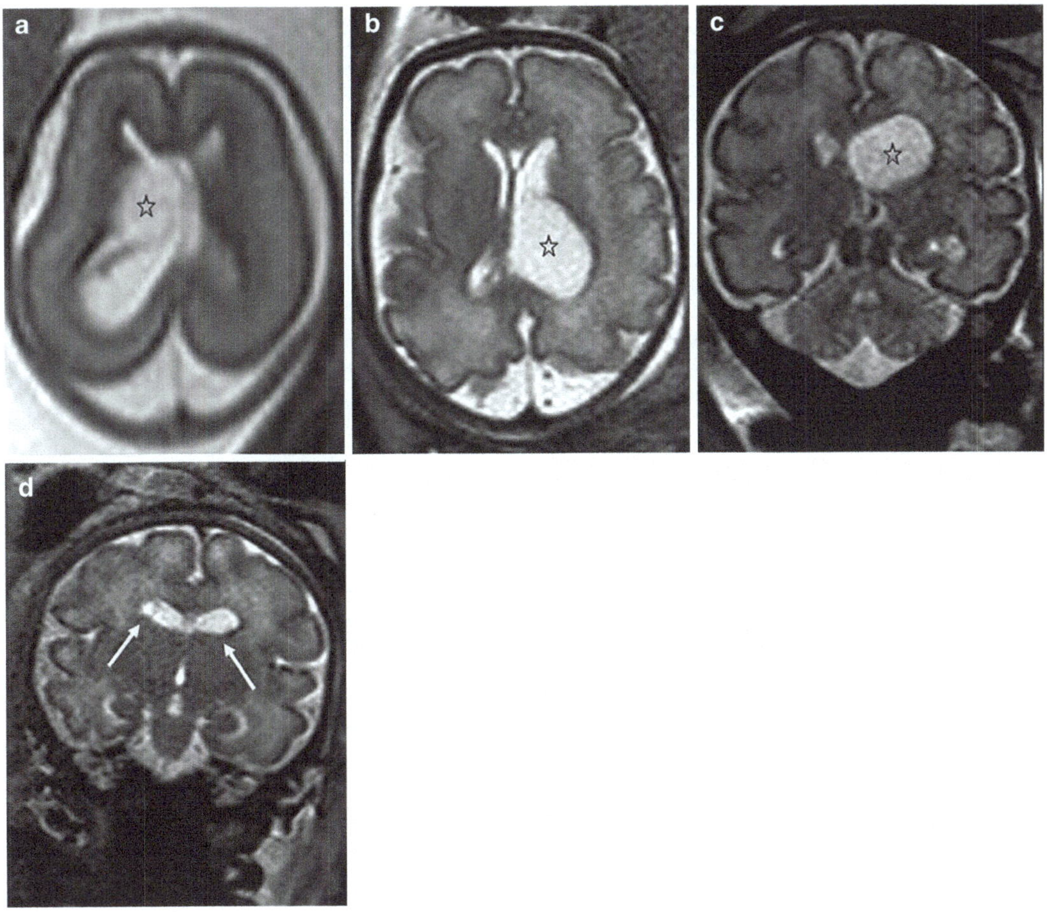

Fig. 16 Intraventricular cysts: right-sided cyst (star) at 21 GW, causing asymmetry and unilateral enlargement of the lateral ventricle (**a**); left-sided intraventricular cyst at 31 GW (**b**, **c**); small bilateral cysts (arrows) at 34 GW (**d**)

12 Vascular Malformations

Dural sinus malformations (DSM) are rare vascular malformations characterized by abnormal development of the posterior sinuses (transverse, sigmoid sinus, and/or confluence of sinuses), usually related to abnormal arterial feeding-shunting. According to their location, they can be divided into posterior and lateral. Posterior DSM is the most frequent variant, usually affecting the torcular or superior sagittal sinus (Fig. 17). The second type is located on the lateral sinuses or jugular bulbs. DSMs can be of large size leading to mass effect on the brain parenchyma; spontaneous thrombosis is often described with regression of the anomaly and halting possible complications. US can identify the lesion, but color Doppler imaging is not always informative enough to describe the flow in the lumen given the low flow velocity. Fetal MRI can confirm the presence of DSM, define possible shunts, and demonstrate any additional brain changes resulting of venous hypertension [72].

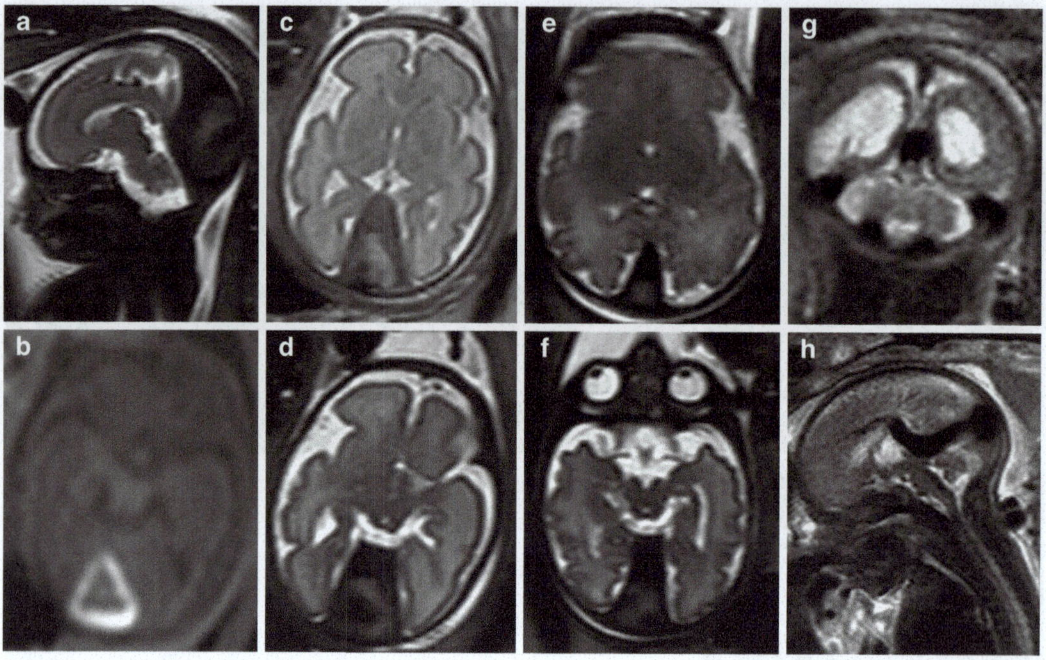

Fig. 17 Vascular malformations. Posterior dural sinus malformation at 30 GW (**a–d**) with spontaneous thrombosis and size reduction during the follow-up exam at 34 GW (**e, f**); Vein of Galen aneurysmal malformation visualized at 26 GW (**g, h**)

The vein of Galen aneurysmal malformation (VGAM) is the most common intracranial arteriovenous shunt malformation in the fetal-neonatal period (Fig. 17). Depending on the development mechanism and the angioarchitecture, VGAMs can be divided into choroidal and mural variants. The choroidal type is a result of the persistence of the primitive choroidal circulation and the median prosencephalic vein (MProsV) of Markowski. The mural type is characterized by a dural arteriovenous fistula in the wall of the vein of Galen, developed around 11th gestational week, and it has a better postnatal outcome. MR can identify predictor signs that can help in the treatment strategy as it can help the recognition of the cases with potential aggressive neonatal presentation and of those which can be safely embolized at a later stage; identification of a stenotic superior sagittal sinus, presence of pseudofeeders (i.e., enlarged middle cerebral artery branches that do not appear to feed the malformation directly), and evidence of prenatal brain injury are negative predictors; also, large size of the venous pouch is associated with worse postnatal outcomes [73].

13 Eye Globe, Optic Nerve, and Inner Ear Anomalies

Common eye globe anomalies include microphthalmia and optic nerve head colobomas. While microphthalmia can be detected during routine US, optic nerve head colobomas may not be easily recognized (Fig. 18). MR can confirm the presence of morning glory malformation and exclude other brain malformations. The most common anomalies of the optic nerve are agenesis or marked hypoplasia. The absence of chiasm is rarely demonstrated in fetal MR studies [74].

Since the labyrinth and the cochlea have fluid content, their size and shape can be depicted with specific MR techniques such as BALANCE and TRUE-fisp. The persistence of any anomaly of the inner ear should raise suspicion for a potential malformation complex. Abnormal findings affecting the modiolus or semicircular canals are rarely visualized in the fetal stage. The reported findings are more often cystic, uni, or bilateral cochlear malformations [74].

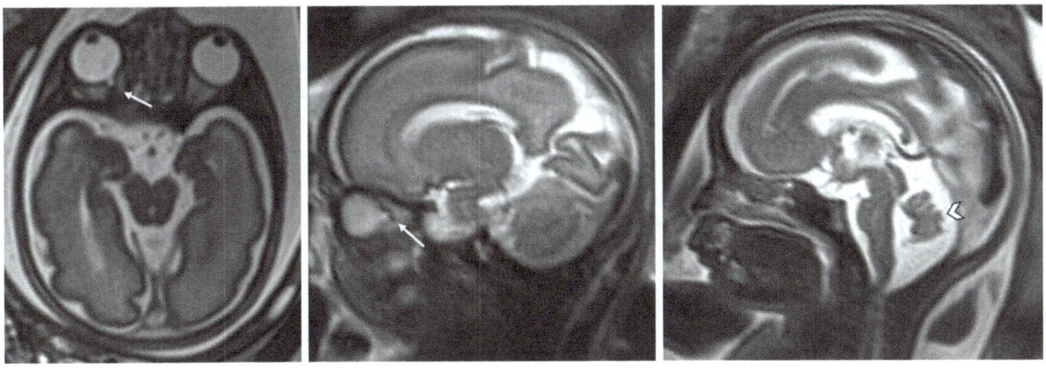

Fig. 18 Fetal MR at 30 GW—right-sided coloboma (arrows) combined with vermian hypoplasia (arrowhead)

14 Pituitary Region Anomalies

The anomalies in the sellar region are rarely seen prenatally. The MR exams aimed at the visualization of the pituitary stalk and its morphology. The absence of a pituitary stalk can be associated with other malformations (such as callosal dysgenesis, agenesis of the septum pellucidum, or cortical malformations) in the context of septo-optic dysplasia. Other characteristic MR features can be suggestive of pituitary dwarfism or an early indicator of potential neonatal severe hypoglycemia. In cases of not conclusive results of the first exam, a follow-up may be performed with a specific focus on that area [74].

References

1. Fric R, Eide PK. Chiari type 1-a malformation or a syndrome? A critical review. Acta Neurochir. 2020;162(7):1513–25.
2. Raybaud C, Jallo GI. Chiari 1 deformity in children: etiopathogenesis and radiologic diagnosis. Handb Clin Neurol. 2018;155:25–48.
3. Righini A, Parazzini C, Doneda C, Arrigoni F, Rustico M, Re TJ, et al. Fetal MRI features related to the Chiari malformations. Neurol Sci. 2011;32(Suppl 3):S279–81.
4. Iruretagoyena JI, Trampe B, Shah D. Prenatal diagnosis of Chiari malformation with syringomyelia in the second trimester. J Matern Fetal Neonatal Med. 2010;23(2):184–6.
5. Palumbo G, Arrigoni F, Peruzzo D, Parazzini C, D'Errico I, Agazzi GM, et al. Onset of Chiari type 1 malformation: insights from a small series of intrauterine MR imaging cases. Neuroradiology. 2023;65(9):1387–94.
6. Masse O, Kraft E, Ahmad E, Rollins CK, Velasco-Annis C, Yang E, et al. Abnormal prenatal brain development in Chiari II malformation. Front Neuroanat. 2023;17:1116948.
7. Albert GW. Chiari malformation in children. Pediatr Clin N Am. 2021;68(4):783–92.
8. Adzick NS, Thom EA, Spong CY, Brock JW 3rd, Burrows PK, Johnson MP, et al. A randomized trial of prenatal versus postnatal repair of myelomeningocele. N Engl J Med. 2011;364(11):993–1004.
9. Nagaraj UD, Bierbrauer KS, Zhang B, Peiro JL, Kline-Fath BM. Hindbrain herniation in Chiari II malformation on fetal and postnatal MRI. AJNR Am J Neuroradiol. 2017;38(5):1031–6.
10. Dovjak GO, Diogo MC, Brugger PC, Gruber GM, Weber M, Glatter S, et al. Quantitative fetal magnetic resonance imaging assessment of cystic posterior fossa malformations. Ultrasound Obstetr Gynecol. 2020;56(1):78–85.
11. Pinto J, Paladini D, Severino M, Morana G, Pais R, Martinetti C, et al. Delayed rotation of the cerebellar vermis: a pitfall in early second-trimester fetal magnetic resonance imaging. Ultrasound Obstetr Gynecol. 2016;48(1):121–4.
12. Conte G, Caschera L, Parazzini C, Cinnante C, Izzo G, Talenti G, et al. Prenatal magnetic resonance imaging within the 26th week of gestation may predict the fate of isolated upward rotation of the cerebellar vermis: insights from a multicentre study. Eur Radiol. 2020;30(4):2161–70.
13. Fileva N, Severino M, Tortora D, Ramaglia A, Paladini D, Rossi A. Second trimester fetal MRI of the brain: through the ground glass. J Clin Ultrasound. 2023;51(2):283–99.
14. Whitehead MT, Vezina G, Schlatterer SD, Mulkey SB, du Plessis AJ. Taenia-tela choroidea complex and choroid plexus location help distinguish Dandy-Walker malformation and Blake pouch cysts. Pediatr Radiol. 2021;51(8):1457–70.

15. Miller E, Orman G, Huisman T. Fetal MRI assessment of posterior fossa anomalies: a review. J Neuroimaging. 2021;31(4):620–40.
16. Robinson AJ. Inferior vermian hypoplasia--preconception, misconception. Ultrasound Obstetr Gynecol. 2014;43(2):123–36.
17. Conte G, Milani S, Palumbo G, Talenti G, Boito S, Rustico M, et al. Prenatal brain MR imaging: reference linear biometric centiles between 20 and 24 gestational weeks. AJNR Am J Neuroradiol. 2018;39(5):963–7.
18. Triulzi F, Parazzini C, Righini A. Magnetic resonance imaging of fetal cerebellar development. Cerebellum. 2006;5(3):199–205.
19. Whitehead MT, Barkovich MJ, Sidpra J, Alves CA, Mirsky DM, Oztekin O, et al. Refining the neuroimaging definition of the Dandy-Walker phenotype. AJNR Am J Neuroradiol. 2022;43:1488.
20. Severino M, Huisman T. Posterior fossa malformations. Neuroimaging Clin N Am. 2019;29(3):367–83.
21. Krajden Haratz K, Oliveira Szejnfeld P, Govindaswamy M, Leibovitz Z, Gindes L, Severino M, et al. Prenatal diagnosis of rhombencephalosynapsis: neuroimaging features and severity of vermian anomaly. Ultrasound Obstetr Gynecol. 2021;58(6):864–74.
22. Ishak GE, Dempsey JC, Shaw DW, Tully H, Adam MP, Sanchez-Lara PA, et al. Rhombencephalosynapsis: a hindbrain malformation associated with incomplete separation of midbrain and forebrain, hydrocephalus and a broad spectrum of severity. Brain. 2012;135(Pt 5):1370–86.
23. Pasquier L, Marcorelles P, Loget P, Pelluard F, Carles D, Perez MJ, et al. Rhombencephalosynapsis and related anomalies: a neuropathological study of 40 fetal cases. Acta Neuropathol. 2009;117(2):185–200.
24. Guduru M, Powers A, Love T, Beavers A. Second trimester fetal MRI features in a fetus with TUBB3 gene mutation. Radiol Case Rep. 2021;16(2):381–3.
25. Amir T, Poretti A, Boltshauser E, Huisman TA. Differential diagnosis of ventriculomegaly and brainstem kinking on fetal MRI. Brain Dev. 2016;38(1):103–8.
26. Stroustrup Smith A, Levine D, Barnes PD, Robertson RL. Magnetic resonance imaging of the kinked fetal brain stem: a sign of severe dysgenesis. J Ultrasound Med. 2005;24(12):1697–709.
27. Beke A, Bartek V, Simonyi A. Fetal craniospinal malformations: aetiology and diagnosis. Ectopic Pregnancy and Prenatal Diagnosis. 2022.
28. Mitchison HM, Valente EM. Motile and non-motile cilia in human pathology: from function to phenotypes. J Pathol. 2017;241(2):294–309.
29. Poretti A, Vitiello G, Hennekam RC, Arrigoni F, Bertini E, Borgatti R, et al. Delineation and diagnostic criteria of oral-facial-digital syndrome type VI. Orphanet J Rare Dis. 2012;7:4.
30. Severino M, Tortora D, Pistorio A, Ramenghi LA, Napoli F, Mancardi MM, et al. Expanding the spectrum of congenital anomalies of the diencephalic-mesencephalic junction. Neuroradiology. 2016;58(1):33–44.
31. Accogli A, Goergen S, Izzo G, Mankad K, Krajden Haratz K, Parazzini C, et al. L1CAM variants cause two distinct imaging phenotypes on fetal MRI. Ann Clin Transl Neurol. 2021;8(10):2004–12.
32. Cabet S, Karl K, Garel C, Delius M, Hartung J, Lesca G, et al. Two different prenatal imaging cerebral patterns of tubulinopathy. Ultrasound Obstetr Gynecol. 2021;57(3):493–7.
33. Hagege R, Krajden Haratz K, Malinger G, Ben-Sira L, Leibovitz Z, Heron D, et al. Spectrum of brain malformations in fetuses with mild tubulinopathy. Ultrasound Obstetr Gynecol. 2023;61(6):740–8.
34. Brar BK, Thompson MG, Vora NL, Gilmore K, Blakemore K, Miller KA, et al. Prenatal phenotyping of fetal tubulinopathies: a multicenter retrospective case series. Prenat Diagn. 2022;42(13):1686–93.
35. Boitor-Borza D, Kovacs T, Stamatian F. Ganglionic eminence within the early developing brain visualized by 3D transvaginal ultrasound. Med Ultrason. 2015;17(3):289–94.
36. Righini A, Cesaretti C, Conte G, Parazzini C, Frassoni C, Bulfamante G, et al. Expanding the spectrum of human ganglionic eminence region anomalies on fetal magnetic resonance imaging. Neuroradiology. 2016;58(3):293–300.
37. Goergen SK, Alibrahim E, Christie J, Dobrotwir A, Fahey M, Fender L, et al. The fetus with ganglionic eminence abnormality: head size and extracranial sonographic findings predict genetic diagnoses and postnatal outcomes. AJNR Am J Neuroradiol. 2021;42(8):1528–34.
38. Scarabello M, Righini A, Severino M, Pinelli L, Parazzini C, Scola E, et al. Ganglionic eminence anomalies and coexisting cerebral developmental anomalies on fetal MR imaging: multicenter-based review of 60 cases. AJNR Am J Neuroradiol. 2021;42(6):1151–6.
39. Sepulveda W, Sepulveda F, Ranzini AC. Role of fetal magnetic resonance imaging in differentiating isolated septal agenesis from septo-optic dysplasia: case study and review. Fetal Diagn Ther. 2023;50(3):165–74.
40. Shinar S, Blaser S, Chitayat D, Selvanathan T, Chau V, Shannon P, et al. Long-term postnatal outcome of fetuses with prenatally suspected septo-optic dysplasia. Ultrasound Obstetr Gynecol. 2020;56(3):371–7.
41. Jarre A, Llorens Salvador R, Montoliu Fornas G, Montoya FA. Value of brain MRI when sonography raises suspicion of agenesis of the corpus callosum in fetuses. Radiologia. 2017;59(3):226–31.
42. Ketonen L.M, Hiwatashi A, Sidhu R., Westesson P-L. Pediatric brain and spine: an atlas of MRI and spectroscopy. 2005;18(2).
43. Romaniello R, Arrigoni F, De Salvo P, Bonaglia MC, Panzeri E, Bassi MT, et al. Long-term follow-up in a cohort of children with isolated corpus callosum agenesis at fetal MRI. Ann Clin Transl Neurol. 2021;8(12):2280–8.

44. Manor C, Rangasami R, Suresh I, Suresh S. Magnetic resonance imaging findings in fetal corpus callosal developmental abnormalities: a pictorial essay. J Pediatr Neurosci. 2020;15(4):352–7.
45. Masnada S, Chiara D, Giana I, Manuela F, Marco S, Andrea A, et al. Aicardi syndrome: key fetal MRI features and prenatal differential diagnosis. Neuropediatrics. 2020;51(4):276–85.
46. Vola EA, Griffiths PD, Parazzini C, Palumbo G, Scola E, Severino M, et al. Complete agenesis of corpus callosum and unilateral cortical formation anomalies detected on fetal MR imaging: a phenotype strongly associated with the male fetuses. Eur Radiol. 2023;33(3):2258–65.
47. Paladini D, Biancotto G, Della Sala F, Severino M, Rossi A. Neurosonographic and MRI diagnosis of fetal cerebral lesions heralding polymicrogyria. Ultrasound Obstet Gynecol. 2023;63(3):293–302.
48. Izzo G, Toto V, Doneda C, Parazzini C, Lanna M, Bulfamante G, et al. Fetal thick corpus callosum: new insights from neuroimaging and neuropathology in two cases and literature review. Neuroradiology. 2021;63(12):2139–48.
49. Arrigoni F, Romaniello R, Peruzzo D, Righini A, Parazzini C, Colombo P, et al. Aberrant supracallosal longitudinal bundle: MR features, pathogenesis and associated clinical phenotype. Eur Radiol. 2016;26(8):2587–96.
50. Lerman-Sagie T, Leibovitz Z. Malformations of cortical development: from postnatal to fetal imaging. Can J Neurol Sci. 2016;43(5):611–8.
51. Moltoni G, Talenti G, Righini A. Brain fetal neuroradiology: a beginner's guide. Transl Pediatr. 2021;10(4):1065–77.
52. Righini A, Zirpoli S, Mrakic F, Parazzini C, Pogliani L, Triulzi F. Early prenatal MR imaging diagnosis of polymicrogyria. AJNR Am J Neuroradiol. 2004;25(2):343–6.
53. Righini A, Parazzini C, Doneda C, Avagliano L, Arrigoni F, Rustico M, et al. Early formative stage of human focal cortical gyration anomalies: fetal MRI. AJR Am J Roentgenol. 2012;198(2): 439–47.
54. Okamura K, Murotsuki J, Sakai T, Matsumoto K, Shirane R, Yajima A. Prenatal diagnosis of lissencephaly by magnetic resonance image. Fetal Diagn Ther. 1993;8(1):56–9.
55. Tonni G, Pattacini P, Bonasoni MP, Araujo E Jr. Prenatal diagnosis of lissencephaly type 2 using three-dimensional ultrasound and fetal MRI: case report and review of the literature. Rev Bras Ginecol Obstet. 2016;38(4):201–6.
56. Williams F, Griffiths PD. In utero MR imaging in fetuses at high risk of lissencephaly. Br J Radiol. 2017;90(1072):20160902.
57. Lerman-Sagie T, Pogledic I, Leibovitz Z, Malinger G. A practical approach to prenatal diagnosis of malformations of cortical development. Eur Jo Paediatr Neurol. 2021;34:50–61.
58. Ghai S, Fong KW, Toi A, Chitayat D, Pantazi S, Blaser S. Prenatal US and MR imaging findings of lissencephaly: review of fetal cerebral sulcal development. Radiographics. 2006;26(2):389–405.
59. Yue-Ru B, Pei-Yin T, Yueh-Chin C, Chiung-Hsin C, Fong-Ming C. Prenatal diagnosis of fetal Schizencephaly by ultrasonography and magnetic resonance imaging. J Med Ultrasound. 2012;20(3):162–8.
60. Nabavizadeh SA, Zarnow D, Bilaniuk LT, Schwartz ES, Zimmerman RA, Vossough A. Correlation of prenatal and postnatal MRI findings in schizencephaly. AJNR Am J Neuroradiol. 2014;35(7):1418–24.
61. Zajac-Mnich M, Kostkiewicz A, Guz W, Dziurzynska-Bialek E, Solinska A, Stopa J, et al. Clinical and morphological aspects of gray matter heterotopia type developmental malformations. Pol J Radiol. 2014;79:502–7.
62. Nagaraj UD, Peiro JL, Bierbrauer KS, Kline-Fath BM. Evaluation of subependymal gray matter heterotopias on fetal MRI. AJNR Am J Neuroradiol. 2016;37(4):720–5.
63. Pavone P, Pratico AD, Rizzo R, Corsello G, Ruggieri M, Parano E, et al. A clinical review on megalencephaly: a large brain as a possible sign of cerebral impairment. Medicine. 2017;96(26):e6814.
64. Severino M, Geraldo AF, Utz N, Tortora D, Pogledic I, Klonowski W, et al. Definitions and classification of malformations of cortical development: practical guidelines. Brain. 2020;143(10):2874–94.
65. Romero XC, Molina FS, Pastor E, Amaya F. Hemimegalencephaly: 2D, 3D ultrasound and MRI correlation. Fetal Diagn Ther. 2011;29(3):257–60.
66. Park HJ, Shin CH, Yoo WJ, Cho TJ, Kim MJ, Seong MW, et al. Detailed analysis of phenotypes and genotypes in megalencephaly-capillary malformation-polymicrogyria syndrome caused by somatic mosaicism of PIK3CA mutations. Orphanet J Rare Dis. 2020;15(1):205.
67. Biran-Gol Y, Malinger G, Cohen H, Davidovitch M, Lev D, Lerman-Sagie T, et al. Developmental outcome of isolated fetal macrocephaly. Ultrasound Obstet Gynecol. 2010;36(2):147–53.
68. Santana EFM, Esteves AMF, Delorenzo DG, Hygino C, Werner H, Araujo JE. Tuberous sclerosis complex: prenatal diagnosis using ultrasound and magnetic resonance imaging-a report of two cases. Indian J Radiol Imaging. 2023;33(1):113–6.
69. Dragoumi P, O'Callaghan F, Zafeiriou DI. Diagnosis of tuberous sclerosis complex in the fetus. Eur J Paediatr Neurol. 2018;22(6):1027–34.
70. Ramakrishnan S, Gupta V. Holoprosencephaly. StatPearls. Treasure Island (FL) with ineligible companies. Disclosure: Vikas Gupta declares no relevant financial relationships with ineligible companies. 2023.
71. Falanga G, Moscatelli M, Izzo G, Parazzini C, Doneda C, Righini A. Single-shot version of FLAIR sequence in the detection of intraventricular anomalies: prelimi-

nary experience in fetal MR imaging. J Comput Assist Tomogr. 2018;42(3):487–91.

72. Rossi A, De Biasio P, Scarso E, Gandolfo C, Pavanello M, Morana G, et al. Prenatal MR imaging of dural sinus malformation: a case report. Prenat Diagn. 2006;26(1):11–6.
73. Arko L, Lambrych M, Montaser A, Zurakowski D, Orbach DB. Fetal and neonatal MRI predictors of aggressive early clinical course in vein of Galen malformation. AJNR Am J Neuroradiol. 2020;41(6):1105–11.
74. Righini A, Tortora M, Izzo G, Doneda C, Arrigoni F, Palumbo G, et al. Cutting-edge applications of fetal MR neuro-imaging in clinical routine: a pictorial essay. Neuroradiology. 2023;65(12):1813–23.